# DOCUMENTS
## OF
# WEST INDIAN
# HISTORY

## FROM THE SPANISH DISCOVERY
## TO
## THE BRITISH CONQUEST OF JAMAICA

By

## DR. ERIC WILLIAMS

B.A., D.Phil. (Oxon.)
*Assistant Professor of Social and Political Science*
*Howard University*

Former Prime Minister of
Trinidad & Tobago

*New Introduction by*

## EDWARD SCOBIE

**Brooklyn New York**
**11201**

# ERRATA

p. 129, Doc. No. 112
source under Title: read *Indis* for *Indias*

p. 208, Doc. No. 192
source under Title: read *1615 Edition* for *1615, Edition*

p. 223, Doc. No. 207
source under Title: read *Philip* for *Phillip*

p. 223, Doc. No. 209
source under Title: read *Reviv'd* for *Revised*

*To the young people of the West Indies*
*as an aid in their struggle against the legacy,*
*the mentality and the fragmentation of colonialism*

*DOCUMENTS OF WEST INDIAN HISTORY.* © by Eric Williams. No part of this book may be reproduced in any form or by any means including electronic, mechanical or photocopying or stored in a retrieval system without permission in writing from the publisher except by a reviewer who may quote brief passage to be included in a review.

First published 1963 by PNM Publishing Co., LTD

Introduction Copyright © 1994 by. Edward Scobie
All rights reserved..

**COVER DESIGN**: *A&B BOOKS PUBLISHERS*
**LETTERING**: *INDUSTRIAL FONTS & GRAFIXS*
**COVER PHOTO**: *DOMINICAN DANCERS:'AGOSTINO BRUNIAS 1770-1796*

ISBN 1-881316-66-1

Reprinted 1994
by

## A&B BOOKS PUBLISHERS
**149 Lawrence Street**
**Brooklyn, New York,11201**
**(718)596-3389**

94 95 96 97     4 3 2 1

# CONTENTS

# INTRODUCTION

In intellectual, as in political, matters the Caribbean is a geographical expression. There is no history of the Caribbean area as a whole. Indeed, histories worthy of the name exist for only a few of the Caribbean territories.

After more than four and a half centuries of metropolitan control, shared among several countries of Europe and America, all that we can boast of is a few monographs, the product of a metropolitan scholarship that has been fragmented, irregular, sporadic, and often pathetically inaccurate and prejudiced. Few "colonials" have to date extended their nationalism to the cultural field and dedicated themselves to the task of writing — or rewriting, where necessary — their own history.

The present publication is designed to fill this gap and to correct this deficiency. Its scope is the entire West Indian area, including the Guianas — whether their connections have been or are British or French, Spanish or American, Dutch or Danish, or whether they have discarded or are about to discard the alien rule of previous centuries.

Its goal is the cultural integration of the entire area, a synthesis of existing knowledge, as the essential foundation of the great need of our time, closer collaboration among the various countries of the Caribbean with their common heritage of subordination to and dictation by outside interests.

The series thus aims at bringing together, in English, the available scholarship and research on the West Indian area, whatever the original language of publication. It thus will embrace the great collections whether public or private—among the Spanish, the works of Las Casas, Navarrete, Herrera, Oviedo and the little-known Saco of Cuba; among the French, the monumental collection of Moreau de Saint Mery and the works of Schoelcher; among the British, the Calendars of State Papers, the Parliamentary Debates and Hansard, reports of Commissions, the works of the Hakluyt Society, and the more modern docmentary selections of Harlow, Bell and Morrell, and Eric Williams; among the Americans, the great collections of the Carnegie Institution by Stock and Donnan.

The series originated in the author's personal reseaches on West Indian history beginning with abolition and emancipation in the British West Indies. The expansion to the larger Caribbean area was facilitated by a Rosenwald Fellowship which permitted research in the Havana archives in 1940 and by a Carnegie grant which permitted travel and research in Europe, from Copenhagen to Seville, in 1953. Some collaboration with the Social Science Research Centre of the University of Puerto Rico, involving mainly translations and typing aid, is also gratefully acknowledged.

The undertaking was begun over ten years ago, but increasing pressures and commitments relegated it to cold storage, until more propitious and leisurely times. The recent reappraisal of the role of the University of the West Indies following on its emancipation from British tutelage, and the decision to make West Indian studies compulsory at the very time when a large accession to its clientele, in decentralised colleges of arts, has been agreed to, make more necessary than ever the provision of appropriate West Indian materials.

So the assignment has once more been brought into the light of day. It was no easy matter to complete it, far from the metropolitan research centres, in the midst of official responsibilities and political commitments. The resurrection took place in Tobago at Easter of 1963 and the work has been done in such odd moments as could be snatched from other chores — a little in Barbados, some in Jamaica, more in Trinidad, a little in Curacao, and the final bits put together in Tobago. If the combination of the national responsibility of the head of a government and the personal hobby of the student has resulted in blemishes, untidiness and obvious evidence of haste, the author can only reply — however arrogant it may sound — that West Indian development in any field today is an urgent and not a leisurely matter, and that it is much better to have tried to play both roles than to have played neither.

A rapid appraisal of the possibility of condensing the voluminous data into a single manageable volume was quickly rejected — too much injustice would have been done thereby to West Indian history. Thus it is that the present work has been planned in five volumes, divided at convenient watersheds, as follows:

Vol. I, 1492 — 1655 : From the Spanish Discovery to the British Conquest of Jamaica

Vol. II, 1656 — 1783 : To the Independence of the United States of America

Vol. III, 1784 — 1897 To the bankruptcy of the British West Indian Sugar Industry

Vol. IV, 1898 — 1941 : From the Spanish-American War to the United States/United Kingdom Leased Bases Agreement

Vol. V. 1942 — 1962 : From the emergence of Puerto Rican democracy to the Independence of Jamaica and Trinidad and Tobago.

The book is based on the collation of documentary material in almost every case contemporary with the period under discussion. Unlike those anthologies in which heterogeneous documents are collected, with no pattern and according to no plan, the documents are divided up according to subject matter into distinct chapters. Each document, in addition, has been given a title which, it is hoped, will assist in the telling of the West Indian story — in pointing a moral as well as adorning the tale.

The first volume of the series is now presented to the West Indian citizen and student and to the interested metropolitan public, as the intellectual cement of the edifice of Caribbean collaboration which has no future whatsoever unless it is the work of West Indian architects, and these are like blind men if their past continues to remain inaccessible to them.

It is the answer to those philistines who, inside and outside the West Indies, deny that the West Indies have a history or, where they do concede that we have, bleat that the West Indies must not divorce themselves from the metropolitan intellectual comments. In so far as there is any substance in either this metropolitan contempt or this colonial servility, then the answer is to be found in a series which deals with metropolitan history in so far as it affects and has relevance for the West Indies. For example, the defeat of the Spanish Armada by England is presented in its West Indian context, as dealing a mortal blow to the Spanish monopoly in the Caribbean. Or, again, the rise of Cromwell and the struggle with the royal autocracy in England emerges, in West Indian history, as Cromwell's Western Design or the protests of Barbadian democracy against British efforts to control its trade. Similarly, Spanish history, so neglected in British colonies, is seen in its best light in the contributions of Las Casas to West Indian society.

For over four and a half centuries the West Indies have been the pawns of Europe and America. Across the West Indian stage the great characters, political and intellectual, of the Western World strut and fret their hour — Louis XIV and Bonaparte, Chatham and Pitt, Castlereagh and Canning, John Stuart Mill and Carlyle, Clarkson and the Abbe Raynal, Victor Schoelcher and Jose Marti, Jefferson and Adams, Joseph Chamberlain and Theodore Roosevelt, the ancien regime and the Revolution of 1789, Gladstone and Disraeli, Cobden and Bright, Russell and Palmerston, the mercantilists and the Manchester School. The beet sugar industry of Prussia, slave labour from Africa, contract labour from India and China, Christianity, Hinduism and Islam — all have left their mark on our West Indian society. Of the West Indies more than of most geographical areas is it possible to say that we are one world.

Far, therefore, from this effort to cultivate West Indian historical materials and rescue them from scorn and oblivion being dismissed as cultural autarchy, the presentation of Europe and America in the West Indian context can confidently be expected to throw new light on many European and American situations and personalities, and open up new avenues of research where these are concerned.

It may not, after all, amount to very much in a world in which independent West Indian pigmies strive to maintain their existence against giant international corporations and in which tiny West Indian communities separated by miles of sea try to live side by side with nations migrating to outer space. But let us in the West Indies not be dismayed. Small though we may be, let us take heart, as the late Pope John XXIII sought to encourage the author, in the reminder that the Lord will hasten in his time that a little one shall become a thousand, and a small one a strong nation.

ERIC WILLIAMS

Port-of-Spain,
Trinidad and Tobago,
August 31, 1966.

# FOREWORD TO VOLUME I

This, the first volume of the series of Documents of West Indian History, covers the period from the discovery of the West Indies by Columbus in 1492 down to the British conquest of Jamaica in 1655. Britain's conquest represented the first successful breach in the Spanish claim to monopoly, the first permanent conquest of a territory occupied by the Spaniards as distinct from settlement of islands like Barbados or St. Kitts which were not physically occupied by the Spaniards. It constituted therefore the first practical repudiation of the Papal Donation of the New World to Spain.

The period covered by this volume is therefore the period of the Spanish monopoly and the international competition thereby engendered. In this period the foundations were laid of West Indian political development, of the West Indian social structure, and of the West Indian character and psychology.

These foundations, in general outline, were as follows :

**(1)    The relations of the metropolitan countries with weaker races.** Spain's relations with the Aboriginal Indians, the **encomienda**, slavery, the slave trade within the Caribbean and even to Spain itself, were the foundations on which the slavery of Africans and the indenture of natives of India were subsequently erected. The Spanish controversy over the character of the Aboriginal Indians anticipated the later controversies over the character of the Negroes and the Hindus. Indian **encomienda** and Negro slavery betrayed the same legislative weaknesses, the same impotence of pious appeals to individual conscience.

It must be conceded, however, that no other metropolitan record can achieve the absurdity of the Requisition or the fatuousness of the Spanish determination to make the Aboriginal Indians walk and dress like "rational men."

**(2)    The metropolitan monopoly of West Indian trade and production.** The extreme centralisation and the almost incredible bureaucracy established by the Spaniards were not indistinguishable from the mercantilist philosophy and the crown colony system of later centuries. The bankruptcy, moral and material, of the Spanish monopoly differed in degree only and not in kind from the subsequent experience of Spain's rivals.

**(3)    The organisation and structure of the sugar industry.** The experience of Hispaniola was later carried over to other West Indian areas, Barbados, Martinique and Jamaica. The social character of sugar production was clearly established in early Hispaniola — large capital investment, the latifundia and the plantocracy, production for export, and slavery.

**(4)    The establishment of the West Indian class and race structure, white capital exploiting coloured labour.** The value of the West Indies as outlets for metropolitan undesirables was recognised as much by Spain in Hispaniola as by England in Barbados and France in Martinique, and all over the West Indies the high market value of the white skin and the metropolitan antecedents, however lowly and humble, set a pattern which is still one of the principal obstacles to rational social development in contemporary Tobago. Their lordly airs, their arrogance, their conspicuous consumption, their extravagant living — these, transmitted to those at whose expense they lived so well, have become the social climbing and the insatiable individual ambition which are today the worst legacy of metropolitan misrule.

The West Indian story is presented through the eyes and mouths of the actors themselves. It corrects various inaccuracies and distortions. The easy and conventional charge of barbarity against the Spaniards is seen against the background of the humanity of Las Casas, the most important metropolitan figure who has ever crossed the West Indian stage, and whose single handed advocacy of the cause and rights of the Aboriginal Indians, relentless opposition to metropolitan imperialism, and tireless dedication to the cause of human rights both by voice and by pen constitute the finest chapter in metropolitan relations with the West Indies. The typically British arrogation of primacy in the battle for the abolition of slavery can be seen in the context of the condemnation of the slave trade and slavery by the seventeenth century Spanish prelates as inhuman, unjust and impolitic. The general assumption of metropolitan military superiority over the weaker races, and the colonial acceptance of the resultant inferiority, will be disturbed by the picture of Spanish knights in armour and on horseback, armed with lance and assisted by bloodhounds, winning great victories over Indians with painted faces (as in a Trinidad carnival) and armed with bows and arrows (a disparity immortally ridiculed by Diego Rivera's canvases); and by the British conquest of Jamaica by an army running from crabs and shooting at fireflies.

The two dominant themes of this first volume are race relations and monopoly. The dominant figure is Las Casas, who, as Protector of the Aboriginal Indians, anticipates the later crusades of the Englishman Clarkson and the Frenchman Schoelcher in defence of the African slaves.

One other aspect of the story presented herein warrants some mention in the light of contemporary conditions in the West Indies. It is Columbus' lyrical descriptions of the West Indian islands and especially of Hispaniola, the land he loved. He is really the first of the "tourists". To anyone with experience of the European winters or the incredible summer heat of Spain, the West Indies must have appeared as an earthly paradise.

The first volume sets the stage for all subsequent West Indian history. A century and a half of European power politics over possession of West Indian territory ends with the emergence of a "West Indian" movement for self-government and independence. In these days of West Indian self-determination in the face of continued outside interference in West Indian affairs, it is timely and valuable to be reminded of this first and modest claim of the West Indians themselves as the beneficiaries of Adam's Will.

# PROLOGUE

## The European Background

Columbus was no visionary, seeking a New World in whose existence no one but himself believed.

Europe was ready, in every sense of the word, for the great adventure.

(1) Europe had developed, in embryo, the economic foundations which stimulated overseas expansion. The dawn of the capitalist era with its large scale production had begun in England, some forty years before Columbus' first voyage.

**The History of Jack of Newbury, called The Clothier of England, ca. 1450.**

"Jack had,
In one room two hundred looms all going.
Two hundred boys winding quills.
An hundred women carding.
In another room, two hundred maids spinning.
One hundred and fifty boys picking wool.
Fifty shearmen.
Eight toers.
Forty dyers in the dye house.
Twenty men in a fulling-mill.
In his own house he kept a butcher, a baker, a brewer, five cooks, and six scullion boys. He spent every week ten fat oxen in his house, besides butter, cheese, fish, etc...."

(2) Europe had developed the germ of the economic theory which was to dominate the national state in the age of overseas expansion. Eight years before Columbus' first voyage the national concern with gold and over the drain of bullion was thus enunciated:

**The Estates General of France, 1484.**

"Money is in the body politic what blood is in the human body; it is then necessary to examine what purgings the monarchy has undergone in the last century. The first was in the time of the popes Alexander and Martin, who in the space of four years took out of this kingdom sums so considerable that they were reckoned at more than two millions of gold."

(3) Europe also had the economic organisation for any potential colonies. The sugar industry was well established in the Mediterranean in the fifteenth century. Forty-four years before Columbus' first voyage, the industry in Cyprus was thus described by an Italian traveller :

**Casola, Viagio a Gerusalamme, 1449**

"The abundance of sugar cane and its magnificence in Cyprus are beyond description. The patrician, Francisco Cornaro of Venice, has at Limasso a great estate, Episcopia, where so much sugar is made that I believe there must be enough for the whole world. The best goes to Venice and every year more is sold. In this area it is impossible to believe that anyone can starve. It is charming to see how the best qualities and the inferior grades are made, and how the people, nearly 400, are employed, some here, some there. There are so many sorts of apparatus that I thought I was in another world, and the boilers are so large that if I described them nobody would believe me. Moreover, all the people are paid every Saturday."

(4) Gold mining and sugar production obviously required labour. Long before Columbus' first voyage, Europe had established contact with Africa where it encountered a high level of civilisation that it was later to destroy. African civilisation before European slavery and the European slave trade was described a century and a half before Columbus' first voyage by the Moorish traveller, Ibn Battuta. One example is his description of the Mandingan Empire of Mali.

Ibn Battuta, **Travels in Asia and Africa,** 1325-1354

"My stay at Iwalatan lasted about fifty days; and I was shown honour and entertained by its inhabitants. It is an excessively hot place, and boasts a few small date-palms, in the shade of which they sow watermelons. Its water comes from underground water beds at that point, and there is plenty of mutton to be had. The garments of its inhabitants, most of whom belong to the Massufa tribe, are of fine Egyptian fabrics. Their women are of surpassing beauty, and are shown more respect than the men. The state of affairs amongst these people is indeed extraordinary. Their men show no signs of jealousy whatever; no one claims descent from his father, but on the contrary from his mother's brother. A person's heirs are his sister's sons, not his own sons. This is a thing which I have seen nowhere in the world except among the Indians of Malabar. But those are heathens; these people are Muslims, punctilious in observing the hours of prayer, studying books of law, and memorizing the Koran.... one has the impression that Mandingo was a real state whose organisation and civilisation could be compared with those of the Musselman kingdoms or indeed the Christian kingdoms of the same epoch."

(5) Europe thus had, in Africa, the manpower for colonial expansion and development. It needed only to rationalise its use of this manpower. Forty years before Columbus' first voyage, the Portuguese provided the rationalisation of what became, in the four subsequent centuries, the Negro slave trade.

Gomes Eannes de Azurara, **The Chronicle of the Discovery and Conquest of Guinea,** Lisbon, 1453

*"Wherein the author reasoneth somewhat concerning the pity inspired by the captives, and of how the division was made.*

"O, Thou heavenly Father — who with Thy powerful hand, without alteration of Thy divine essence, governest all the infinite company of Thy Holy City, and controllest all the revolutions of higher worlds, divided into nine spheres, making the duration of ages long or short according as it pleaseth Thee — I pray Thee that my tears may not wrong my conscience, for it is not their religion but their humanity that maketh mine to weep in pity for their sufferings. And if the brute animals, with their bestial feelings, by a natural instinct understand the sufferings of their own kind, what wouldst Thou have my human nature to do on seeing before my eyes that miserable company, and remembering that they too are of the generation of the sons of Adam?

"On the next day, which was the 8th of the month of August, very early in the morning, by reason of the heat, the seamen began to make ready their boats, and to take out captives, and carry them on shore, as they were commanded. And these, placed altogether in that field, were a marvellous sight, for amongst them were some white enough, fair to look upon, and well proportioned; others were less white like mulattoes; others again were as black as Ethiops, and so ugly, both in features and in body, as almost to appear (to those who saw them) the images of a lower hemisphere. But what heart could be so hard as not to be pierced with piteous feeling to see that company? For some kept their heads low and their faces bathed in tears, looking one upon another; others stood groaning very dolorously, looking up to the height of heaven, fixing their eyes upon it, crying out loudly, as if asking help of the Father of Nature; others struck their faces with the palms of their hands, throwing themselves at full length upon the ground; others made their lamentations in the manner of a dirge, after the custom of their country. And though we could not understand the words of their language, the sound of it right well accorded with the measure of their sadness. But to increase their sufferings still more, there now arrived those who had charge of the division of the captives, and who began to separate one from another, in order to make an equal partition of the fifths and then was it needful to part fathers from sons, husbands from wives, brothers from brothers. No respect was shewn either to friends or relations, but each fell where his lot took him.

"O powerful Fortune, that with thy wheels doest and undoest, compassing the matters of this world as pleaseth thee, do thou at least put before the eyes of that miserable race some understanding of matters to come, that they may receive some consolation in the midst of their great sorrow. And you who are so busy in making that division of the captives, look with pity upon so much misery; and see how they cling one to the other, so that you can hardly separate them.

"And who could finish that partition without very great toil? for as often as they had placed them in one part the sons, seeing their fathers in another, rose with great energy and rushed over to them; the mothers clasped their other children in their arms, and threw themselves flat on the ground with them, receiving blows with little pity from their own flesh, if only they might not be torn from them.

"And so troublously they finished the partition, for besides the toil they had with the captives, the field was quite full of people, both from the town and from the surrounding villages and districts, who for that day gave rest to their hands (in which lay their power to get their living) for the sole purpose of beholding this novelty. And with what they saw, while some were weeping and others separating the captives, they caused such a tumult as greatly to confuse those who directed the partition.

"The Infant was there, mounted upon a powerful steed, and accompanied by his retinue, making distribution of his favours, as a man who sought to gain but small treasure from his share; for of the forty-six souls that fell to him as his fifth, he made a very speedy partition of these (among others), for his chief riches lay in (the accomplishment of) his purpose; for he reflected with great pleasure upon the salvation of those souls that before were lost.

"And certainly his expectation was not in vain; for....as soon as they understood our language they turned Christians with very little ado; and I who put together this history into this volume, saw in the town of Lagos boys and girls (the children and grandchildren of those first captives, born in this land) as good and true Christians as if they had directly descended, from the beginning of the dispensation of Christ, from those who were first baptised."

(6) Europe, equipped intellectually, economically and with manpower for overseas expansion, had also the scientific certainty that the New World existed, awaiting only its discoverer. Columbus was certain of this nearly twenty years before his first voyage.

Pablo Toscanelli to Christopher Columbus, June 25, 1474

"I received your letter with everything you sent me, for which I am very much obliged. I praise your intention to travel West; and I am sure that you have seen from my letter that the voyage you wish to undertake is not as difficult as people think; on the contrary, the ship's course is certain, due to the conditions which I have pointed out. You would be entirely convinced if you had, as I have, talked to many persons who have been in these countries. You may be sure you will find powerful kingdoms, a great many populated and rich cities, and provinces with an abundance of precious stones. And it will be cause of great pleasure for the King and the Princes who rule these far away lands, to open the way for them to communicate with the Christians, in order to have themselves instructed in the Catholic Religion and in all the sciences which we possess. For this reason, and for many others which I could mention, I am not surprised to see that you have as great a heart as the whole Portuguese Nation, where there have always been outstanding men in all enterprises."

(7) Europe had, not only the scientific certainty, but also the scientific equipment to undertake, exploit and consolidate its discoveries. The great scientific achievements of the fifteenth century ensured this.

Francis Bacon, Novum Organum, 1620

"It is well to observe the force and virtue and consequence of discoveries, and these are to be seen nowhere more conspicuously than in those three which were unknown to the ancients....namely, printing, gunpowder, and the magnet. For these three have changed the whole face and state of things throughout the world, the first in literature, the second in warfare, and the third in navigation. Whence have followed innumerable changes, in so much that no empire, no sect, no star seems to have exerted greater power and influence in human affairs than these mechanical discoveries."

(8) The question remained, who was to win the prize? England was well in line, but lost her opportunity.

Richard Hakluyt, **The Principal Navigations, Voyages, Traffiques and Discoveries of the English Nation**, London, 1599

"The offer of the discovery of the West Indies by Christopher Columbus to King Henry the seventh in the year 1488 the 13 of February: with the King's acceptation of the offer, & the cause whereupon he was deprived of the same: recorded in the thirteenth chapter of the history of Don Fernand Columbus of the life and deeds of his father Christopher Columbus.

"Christopher Columbus fearing lest if the King of Castile in like manner (as the King of Portugal had done) should not condescend unto his enterprise, he should be enforced to offer the same again to some other prince, & so much time should be spent therein, sent into England a certain brother of his which he had with him, whose name was Bartholomew Columbus, who, albeit he had not the Latin tongue, yet nevertheless was a man of experience and skilful in sea causes, and could very well make sea cards & globes, and other instruments belonging to that profession, as he was instructed by his brother. Wherefore after that Bartholomew Columbus was departed for England, his luck was to fall into the hands of pirates, which spoiled him with the rest of them which were in the ship which he went in. Upon which occasion, and by reason of his poverty and sickness which cruelly assaulted him in a country so far distant from his friends, he deferred his ambassage for a long while, until such time as he had gotten somewhat handsome about him with making of sea cards. At length he began to deal with King Henry the seventh the father of Henry the eighth, which reigneth at this present: unto whom he presented a map of the world....after he had seen the map, and that which my father Christopher Columbus offered unto him, he accepted the offer with joyful countenance, and sent to call him unto England. But because God had reserved the said offer for Castile, Columbus was gone in the mean space, and also returned with the performance of his enterprise...."

(9) England's loss was Spain's gain. Spain in 1492 was exactly ready for the overseas adventure—a centralised monarchy, a national state, a militant Church, all basking in the sunshine of a successful war against the intruder and the infidel, the Moors.

**King Abu Abdallah to King Ferdinand of Spain, 1492**

"We are now thy subjects, O powerful and exalted King. The city and kingdom we resign to thee, for such is the will of Allah. We trust that thou wilt use thy triumph with clemency and generosity."

# INTRODUCTION

C.L.R. James who once shared a closeness with Dr. Eric Williamps based on mutual respect for each other, in 1960 gave this appraisal of Williams in the light of historical research:

*Williams has been tireless in his pursuit of original material and information about West Indian history.*

When one looks back at Dr. Williams' prodgious output of historical studies on the Caribbean there can be no doubt about C.L.R's truth concerning Williams. But it is not his output that is so important, it is the quality of his works; and, of the utmost consequence that he exposed the big lie of western academia, in all its shameful wickedness:that civilization was not, as those plunderers of empire lands had shouted, repeat not, "the product of the white races, and, that the non-white world came into its orbit only with the intervention of the Europeans."

Williams began his history way back in the late years of the 1930s when he started to shake the pundits of Oxford with his Ph.D. dissertation. Its material was to form the substance of his classic study "Capitalism and Slavery." At that time Williams had already been very familiar with the knowledge of earlier civilizations in Ghana and Songhay, even though as he himself observed, "for the most part [it was] less accessible than it is today, with the work of Davidson and others." By then, however, he had researched, and was acquainted with, the works of Frobenius, Delafosse and Torday, Leo Africanus and Ian Batuta, Mungo Park and Marco Polo; scholars who had written about the golden ages of African civilization well before the Columbus encounter in the fifteenth century which triggered off the beginning of the Atlantic Slave Trade and Slavery.

It was this unhappy encounter that brought about the relentless destruction of the people of Africa, their traditions, their lands, and their resources, leaving Africa sucked dry and underdeveloped. The late President Kwame Nkrumah of Ghana once predicted that in the same way that imperialism saw the light of birth in Africa it would suffer the twilight of death on that very same continent. This prediction must not be taken too lightly. Today, with a new millennium almost on the doorstep of the old one, we have seen the collapse of empires. European nations that had grown obese and vulgar on the fat of African lands when they partitioned off, at the Berlin Conference in 1884, large chunks of Africa to satiate their greed for gold and other minerals, are now closing their doors and busily trying to build a European economic and constitutional bastion of whiteness in order to survive. A totally lily-white Europe will not, and cannot save them. Their historical behavior to each other shows otherwise. The crumbling of walls will not change the path of history. One only has to read their own histories, written by themselves, to understand their situation at this present time.

No scholar was more aware of that fact than Dr. Eric Williams. In his researches and his writings of the history of the West Indies Williams, - even though he had to seek material from the documents and papers of European and British imperialists and colonizers - made the West Indian man "the master and not the slave of the relations in which he is involved." Using material from documents that had been given royal, ecclesiastical and legal power and might by imperial and colonial so-called conquerors, Dr. Eric Williams exposed the humbug, hypocrisy, arrogance and racism of men who had already been fired with the flames of empire in tropical lands across the many many thousands of nautical miles from the North Sea and the English Channel. Out of Williams' pen grew a new Caribbean man, a new Caribbean woman, a new Caribbean land.

Naturally, there were those, - still relics of empire, - who tried to deride him; to seek to minimize and reject his scholarship. There are still minor portions of those around in this very late day and ultra late age who seek to perpetuate that pettiness and jealousy. What they could not see, and still cannot see, was that Dr. Eric Williams was no historical researcher who dwelt in an ivory tower of scholarship. He was well aware that this research had to be employed in public policy. He remained convinced that it was only in this way, the Caribbean could be truly free from the strictures of colonialism, and too, neo-colonialism.

The attitude of his detractors, primarily political fellow travelers, almost totally devoid of the knowledge of the ravages which were enumerated in the chronicles of colonial history, reached a point of hysteria. This came about when Williams brought out, what was described as "a masterpiece of political and sociological analysis" entitled Massa Day Done in 1961. Some members of the Democratic Labour Party (DLP) in paroxysms of indignation wrote a letter to the Trinidad Guardian newspaper on March 5, 1961, calling on Dr. Eric Williams to withdraw what it called the wicked statement Massa Day Done, and to make an unqualified apology to introducing it."

They claimed that Williams was stirring up racial antagonism. Williams replied to them that Massa Day Done was not a racial term but a symbol of a bygone age. He went on to say that "Massa Day Done is a social phenomenon: Massa Day Done connotes a political awakening and a social revolution." This "band of obscurantist politicians," as Williams termed the DLP politicians, could not see and understand the connection between the history of colonialism and the politics of colonialism. That both are intertwined in the social and economic fabric of the Caribbean and are the prime causes of the backwardness and underdevelopment that still plague the islands of the Antilles. Lands that were once cherished as the jewels and gems of empire during the bygone centuries when sugar was king; and the islands a rich haven for mercantilist rogues, brigands and brethrens of the coast.

Naturally, Williams refused categorically to accede to the spineless request of the Democratic Labour Party members whom he styled "this pack of benighted idiots." His terse reply was given with the biting acidity and sarcasm for which the Doctor was well-known:

> *I categorically refuse to withdraw my statement or to make any apology for it, qualified or unqualified. I repeat more emphatically than when I said it the first time Massa Day Done. I accuse the DLP of being the stooge of the Massas who still exist in our society.*

As recently as October 24, 1993, the Trinidad Guardian had to ask on its front page "why treat Williams so?" The paper was referring to a statement made by a Trinidadian, Professor Dr. Selwyn Cudjoe, who "complained of being kicked from the pillar to post in a effort to launch a book, *Eric E. Williams Speaks*, on the legacy of former Prime Minister Dr. Eric Williams." Among those present at that launching at the Holiday Inn's Teak Room in Trinidad was Williams' daughter Erica Connell who flew there especially for the occasion.

Dr. Cudjoe made it quite obvious that this political pettiness, born out a crucible of colonial brew, still existed, eating at the marrow and minds of men who are still the victims of an empire, now long time dead and gone, but not yet entirely laid to rest. Dr. Cudjoe had to remind the packed Teak Room that the publication of a scholar's or politician's or an economist's speeches was merely a way of "immemorialising them, and was an example of the eternal gratitude and respect that a nation always showed its citizens who have performed outstandingly and well." Dr. Cudjoe went on to lament the sad fact that his attempt to launch this project was being "laden with political symbolism and paranoid distrust."

Dr. Cudjoe's final observation on the reasons for the honoring of a great mind of the Caribbean soil brought back to mind many significant factors in the make-up of Dr. Williams: the tireless researcher in digging out primary source material on the West Indies in whatever country it may be deposited; the brilliant scholar-historian who could use the historical data to write major studies on the Caribbean that removed its people from the fringes of colonialism and placed them at center-stage in their own affairs;the iron-willed politician who took Trinidad and Tobago from the clutches of colonial rule to sovereign independence;and the committed Caribbean nationalist who could stand strong against the economic choke-hold of the superpowers. These were the outstanding attributes that Dr. Eric Williams exhibited during his fruitful life on this planet. Dr. Cudjoe repeated that , far from being a morsel of political propaganda, his book *Eric E. Williams Speaks, was* about "the genesis of an academic event and some of the considerations that led to its growth and development of national consciousness." As Dr. Cudjoe summed up, Dr. Eric Williams' words speeches and writings did just that.

One is forced to ask how many of those present at that function remembered that it was Dr. Eric Williams who first took and researched the documents of West Indian history. A history written by imperialists, colonialists and other white supremacists who had no love, and only contempt for the West Indies, its indigenous population, and the Africans transported there in the packed bellies of wood-wormed slave vessels. It was this same Dr. Eric Williams who used their own words to beat the arrogance out of them with his scholarship and brilliance. For, all these documents reveal an imperial tone that you can cut with a carving knife. It is cold-blooded, authoritative, officious, patronizing, like the voice of the lord and master thundering and pontificating from above to "creatures with the minds of children and the habits of brutes."

Dr. Eric Williams' first volume on *Documents of West Indian History* is dated from 1492 to 1655; in other words from the arrival of the man Columbus to the removal of the Spanish from the island of Jamaica by the British. The book is structured in eight chapters, beginning with chapter One - The Discovery of the West Indies, and going through the entire gamut of conquest and colonization to The Early Organization of the Non-Spanish Colonies. The finding and selecting of the documents was a long and arduous undertaking. But that is not all. It is how these documents were shaped later by Dr. Williams himself and other conscious Caribbean writers to present a new Caribbean; the real Caribbean people, not as stunned victims of slavery and colonialism, but men and women in their own right who can - not only write their own history - but are masters and mistresses of their own destiny. As men and women, –in the words of one of our powerful writers, George Lamming, –who were going to stop being tenants on our own Caribbean lands, and take over the ownership; where, as Jean Jacques Dessalines once said to the Haitian people there will be no masters, no servants, no slaves.

Finally, in ending this introduction let us go back to the beginning with the appraisal of Dr. Eric Williams' research and scholarship by his one-time friend, C.L.R. James. In doing that I want to impress on the minds of our young and future leaders that genius is ninety-nine percent perspiration and one percent brains. C.L.R's observation of the early

Williams, the young Williams, when he was carrying out his searches for historical data brings out clearly the claim that I just made about genius. James noted that:

> *Williams spent vacations traveling over Europe in Holland, in Copenhagen, in Spain, digging out original material on the West Indies that has been buried for centuries. When I was preparing the Black Jacobins I had to leave Paris and spend some days in Bordeaux and in Nantes. I was interested to hear from Williams that he also, in pursuit of material on the slave trade and the West Indies, had to visit those two cities. He has written and I also have a copy to which I regularly refer, an absolutely magnificent manuscript which deals with the history of all the West Indian islands from Cuba to Trinidad. I am certain that no such history of the West exists anywhere else.*

Such an assessment of the scholarship and stature of Eric Williams, coming from someone like C.L.R. James, a scholar moving in that same rarefied air of brilliance as Williams, must be taken very seriously indeed; in spite of the falling apart of these two giants in their later years.

Again, James like others who knew Williams and his historical writings from his beginning years speak of his utter loathing of colonialism in any of its objectionable forms. James phrased it in this way:

> *To have arrived at so completely a nationalist outlook carries with it certain dangers, certain not merely inevitable and necessary dangers, necessary because you have to arm yourself at all points to resist the encroachments of powerful enemies of the as yet immature national personality. Williams' education and general knowledge and understanding of western culture stand him in good stead.*

Among the powerful enemies joining forces against the nationalism of Dr. Eric Williams were the colonial office of London, England, and the U.S. State Department, of Washington, D.C. James saw their partnership as a "frantic desire to bend to their purposes, to humiliate and to exploit a small people in their long overdue effort to stand on their own feet and express themselves as an independent nationalist community." James carried on his condemnation of the colonial office and the State Department by finding them "guilty of one of the most willful, unnecessary, cruel and sordid pieces of bullying in all the wretched history of imperialism."

C.L.R. James was talking about the colonial years before independence. He ended his indictment of these bodies by observing:

*Instead of recognizing what Dr. Williams represents, and he represents the future of the West Indies, they descend on to the meanest and most contemptible tricks and dodges, ready to ally themselves with self-seeking, discredited and even grossly dishonoured and dishonourable elements in the population.*

But Dr. Eric Williams' contribution to the history of the Caribbean cannot be dismissed. It was the Doctor who took the documents of the false conquerors of lands and people and formed them into weapons against the conquest and greed of those who wrote them. Today, among the millions of liberated thinkers, their histories are not taken seriously and are viewed as archaic museum pieces, not even worth the papers on which their arrogance was inscribed. It was with this thought in mind and that mood that I read Dr. Eric Williams *Documents of West Indian History*. Their value today lies merely as historical data to be used by those who wish to find out how these men from European nations carved out a life of prosperity on the backs of those they once held in colonial bondage.

For that information we must remain eternally grateful to Dr. Eric Williams who showed us how to collect the evidence of history and how to use it for our own liberation.

Edward Scobie
November 20, 1993

# CHAPTER I
# The Discovery of the West Indies

## No. 1 — THE DISCOVERY CONTRACT

*(Articles of Agreement between the Sovereigns of Spain and Christopher Columbus, April 17, 1492)\**

The things prayed for, and which Your Highnesses give and grant to Don Cristobal Colon as some recompense for what he is to discover in the Oceans, and for the voyage which now, with the help of God, he has engaged to make therein in the service of Your Highnesses, are the following :

Firstly, that Your Highnesses, as actual Lords of the said Oceans, appoint from this date the said Don Cristobal Colon to be your Admiral in all those islands and mainlands which by his activity and industry shall be discovered or acquired in the said oceans, during his lifetime, and likewise, after his death, his heirs and successors one after another in perpetuity, with all the preeminences and prerogatives appertaining to the said office. . . .

Likewise, that Your Highnesses appoint the said Don Cristobal Colon to be your Viceroy and Governor General in all the said islands and mainlands. . . . which, as aforesaid, he may discover and acquire in the said seas; and that for the government of each and any of them he may make choice of three persons for each office, and that Your Highnesses may select and choose the one who shall be most serviceable to you; and thus the lands which our Lord shall permit him to discover and acquire for the service of Your Highnesses, will be the better governed.

Item, that of all and every kind of merchandise, whether pearls, precious stones, gold, silver, spices, and other objects of merchandise whatsoever, of whatever kind, name and sort, which may be bought, bartered, discovered, acquired and obtained within the limits of the said Admiralty, Your Highnesses grant from now henceforth to the said Don Cristobal, and will that he may have and take for himself, the tenth part of the whole, after deducting all the expenses which may be incurred therein, so that of what shall remain clear and free he may have and take the tenth part for himself, and may do therewith as he pleases, the other nine parts being reserved for Your Highnesses. . . .

\*Cited in E. G. Bourne (ed.), *The Northmen, Columbus and Cabot, 985-1503*, New York, 1906, pp. 77-80.

Item, that in all the vessels which may be equipped for the said traffic and business, each time and whenever and as often as they may be equipped, the said Don Cristobal Colon may, if he chooses, contribute and pay the eighth part of all that may be spent in the equipment, and that likewise he may have and take the eighth part of the profits that may result from such equipment....

## No. 2 — PROVIDING A CREW FOR THE VOYAGE
### (Ferdinand and Isabella, King and Queen of Spain, to the Royal Officials, April 30, 1492)*

Be it known that we have sent Christopher Columbus across the Ocean, to undertake useful enterprises in our service; and in order to obtain the crew he needs in the three vessels for the voyage, it is necessary to promise safety to those persons, for otherwise they would not want to go with him on the said voyage.... And we hereby promise safety to each and every person who will go on the said vessels with the said Christopher Columbus....so that no harm or evil, and no injury will befall their persons or their property, nor any of their possessions because of any crime they might have done or committed up to the date of this letter, during the time of their voyage and the time spent there including their return voyage home and for two months afterwards. We, therefore, command each and every one of you in your place, and jurisdictions, not to take account of any criminal cause, regarding the persons who may go with the said Christopher Columbus on the said three vessels, during the aforesaid time.

## No. 3 — THE DISCOVERY OF THE WEST INDIES
### ("Journal of the First Voyage of Christopher Columbus", 1492-1493)**

I left the city of Granada on the 12th day of May, in the same year of 1492, being Saturday, and came to the town of Palos, which is a seaport, where I equipped three vessels well suited for such service; and departed from that port, well supplied with provisions and with many sailors, on the 3rd of August of the same year, being Friday, half an hour before sunrise, taking the route to the islands of Canaria....

*Cited in Martin Fernandez de Navarrete, Coleccion de los Viages y Descubrimientos que hicieron por Mar los Espanoles desde Fines del Siglo XV, (Madrid, 1825-1837), 1945 Edition, Editorial Guarania, Buenos Aires, Tomo II, Num. IX, pp. 25—26.
**Cited in Bourne op. cit., pp. 90-91, 108-110, 118, 173, 215, 218 226-227, 238-239, 241, 244, 257-258.

### Wednesday, 10th of October

....Here the people could endure no longer. They complained of the length of the voyage. But the Admiral cheered them up in the best way he could, giving them hopes of the advantages they might gain from it. He added that, however much they might complain, he had to go to the Indies, and that he would not go until he found them, with the help of our Lord.

### Thursday, 11th of October

....The land was first seen by a sailor named Rodrigo de Triana.... the Admiral asked and admonished the men to keep a good look-out on the forecastle, and to watch well for land; and to him who should first cry out that he saw land, he would give a silk doublet, besides the other rewards promised by the Sovereigns, which were 10,000 maravedis to him who should first see it. At two hours after midnight the land was sighted at a distance of two leagues. They shortened sail, and lay by under the mainsail without the bonnets.

### Friday, 12th of October

The vessels were hove to, waiting for daylight; and on Friday they arrived at a small island of the Lucayos, called, in the language of the Indians, Guanahani*....The Admiral went on shore in the armed boat.... The Admiral took the royal standard, and the captains went with two banners of the green cross, which the Admiral took in all the ships as a sign, with an F and a Y** and a crown over each letter.... The Admiral....said that they should bear faithful testimony that he, in presence of all, had taken, as he now took, possession of the said island for the King and for the Queen, his Lords....

### Tuesday, 16th of October

I sailed from the island of Santa Maria de la Concepcion at about noon, to go to Fernandina Island,*** which appeared very large to the westward....

### Sunday, 9th of December

....At the upper end there are the mouths of two rivers, with the most beautiful champaign country, almost like the lands of Spain: these even have the advantage; for which reasons the Admiral gave the name of the said island Isla Espanola.

* Generally identified as Watling Island.
** For Ferdinand and Isabella, the King and Queen of Spain.
*** Cuba.

### Sunday, 6th of January

....The Admiral also heard of an island further east, in which there were only women, having been told this by many people. He was also informed that Yamaye* and the island of Espanola were ten days' journey in a canoe from the mainland, which would be about 70 or 80 leagues, and that there the people wore clothes.

### Wednesday, 9th of January

....On the previous day, when the Admiral went to the Rio del Oro, he saw three mermaids,** which rose well out of the sea; but they are not so beautiful as they are painted, though to some extent they have the form of a human face..

### Tuesday, 15th of January

....The intercourse at Carib*** would, however, be difficult, because the natives are said to eat human flesh.... the Admiral determined to go there, as it was on the route, and thence to Matinino,**** which was said to be entirely peopled by women, without men. He would thus see both islands, and might take some of the natives....

### Thursday, 14th of February

This night the wind increased, and the waves were terrible.... At sunrise the wind blew still harder, and the cross sea was terrific.... the Admiral and all the crew made a vow that, on arriving at the first land, they would all go in procession, in their shirts, to say their prayers in a church dedicated to Our Lady.

Besides these general vows made in common, each sailor made a special vow; for no one expected to escape, holding themselves for lost, owing to the fearful weather from which they were suffering.... that the Sovereigns might still have information, even if he perished in the storm, he took a parchment and wrote on it as good an account as he could of all he had discovered, entreating anyone who might pick it up to deliver it to the Sovereigns. He rolled this parchment up in waxed cloth, ordered a large wooden barrel to be brought, and put it inside, so that no one else knew what it was. They thought that it was some act of devotion, and so he ordered the barrel to be thrown into the sea....

### Monday, 18th of February

....He pretended to have gone over more ground, to mislead the pilots and mariners who pricked off the charts, in order that he might remain master of that route to the Indies, as, in fact, he did. For none of the others kept an accurate reckoning, so that no one but himself could be sure of the route to the Indies.

*Jamaica.       **Manatís, or sea-cows.
*** Puerto Rico.        **** Martinique.

### Friday, 15th of March

....At noon, with the tide rising, they crossed the bar of Saltes, and reached the port which they had left on the 3rd of August of the year before.... "I know respecting this voyage", says the Admiral, "that he has miraculously shown his will, as may be seen from this journal, setting forth the numerous miracles that have been displayed in the voyage, and in me who was so long at the court of Your Highnesses, working in opposition to and against the opinions of so many chief persons of your household, who were all against me, looking upon this enterprise as folly. But I hope, in our Lord, that it will be a great benefit to Christianity, for so it has ever appeared". These are the final words of the Admiral Don Cristoval Colon respecting his first voyage to the Indies and their discovery.

---

### No. 4—COLUMBUS' DESCRIPTION OF THE WEST INDIES ("Journal of the First Voyage of Christopher Columbus", 1492-1493)*

### Tuesday, 16th of October

....I saw many trees very unlike those of our country. Many of them have their branches growing in different ways and all from one trunk, and one twig is one form, and another in a different shape, and so unlike that it is the greatest wonder in the world to see the great diversity; thus one branch has leaves like those of a cane, and others like those of a mastick tree....

### Friday, 19th of October

....I can never tire my eyes in looking at such lovely vegetation, so different from ours. I believe that there are many herbs and many trees that are worth much in Europe for dyes and for medicines; but I do not know them, and this causes me great sorrow.... I found the smell of the trees and flowers so delicious that it seemed the pleasantest thing in the world....

### Wednesday, 14th of November

....he saw so many islands that he could not count them all, with very high land covered with trees of many kinds, and an infinite number of palms. He was much astonished to see so many lofty islands; and assured the Sovereigns that the mountains and isles he had seen since yesterday seemed to him to be second to none in the world; so high and clear of clouds and snow, with the sea at their bases so deep....

*Cited in Bourne, op. cit., pp. 119, 123, 147-148, 181-182, 189-190, 193.

### Sunday, 16th of December

.... This land is cool, and the best that words can describe. It is very high, yet the top of the highest mountain could be ploughed with bullocks; and all is diversified with plains and valleys. In all Castile there is no land that can be compared with this for beauty and fertility.... Your Highnesses may believe that these lands are so good and fertile, especially those of the island of Espanola, that there is no one who would know how to describe them, and no one who could believe if he had not seen them....

### Friday, 21st of December

.... I have traversed the sea for 23 years, without leaving it for any time worth counting, and I saw all the east and the west, going on the route of the north, which is England, and I have been to Guinea, but in all those parts there will not be found the perfection of harbours.... this one is better than all others, and will hold all the ships of the world, secured with the oldest cables.... This port is very good for all the winds that can blow, being enclosed and deep.... Any ship may lie within it without fear that other ships will enter at night to attack her, because although the entrance is over two leagues wide, it is protected by reefs of rocks which are barely awash.... It is the best harbour in the world, and the Admiral gave it the name of Puerto de la Mar de Santo Tomas, because to-day it was that Saint's day. The Admiral called it a sea, owing to its size.

---

## No. 5 — THE MISCONCEPTION OF COLUMBUS

*("Journal of the First Voyage of Christopher Columbus", 1492-1493)\**

### Saturday, 13th of October

.... But, in order not to lose time, I intend to go and see if I can find the island of Cipango\*\*....

### Tuesday, 16th of October

.... This island \*\*\* is very large, and I have determined to sail round it, because, so far as I can understand, there is a mine in or near it.... and to navigate until I find Samaot, which is the island or city where there is gold, as all the natives say who are on board....

### Sunday, 21st of October

.... I shall then shape a course for another much larger island, which I believe to be Cipango, judging from the signs made by the Indians I bring with me. They call it Cuba....

\*Cited in Bourne, *op. cit.*, pp. 113, 118-119, 126-128, 131, 148, 197-198.
\*\* Japan.        \*\*\* Cuba.

I am still resolved to go to the mainland and the city of Guisay, and to deliver the letters of your Highnesses to the Gran Can, requesting a reply and returning with it....

*Tuesday, 23rd of October*

I desired to set out to-day for the island of Cuba, which I think must be Cipango, according to the signs these people make, indicative of its size and riches, and I did not delay any more here....

*Wednesday, 24th of October*

....I cannot understand their language, but I believe that it is of the island of Cipango that they recount these wonders. On the spheres I saw, and on the delineation of the map of the world, Cipango is in this region....

*Sunday, 28th of October*

....He understood that large ships of the Gran Can came here, and that from here to the mainland was a voyage of ten days....

*Monday, 12th of November*

....There are also precious stones, pearls, and an infinity of spices.... Here also there is a great quantity of cotton, and I believe it would have a good sale here without sending it to Spain, but to the great cities of the Gran Can, which will be discovered without doubt, and many others ruled over by other lords, who will be pleased to serve your Highnesses, and whither will be brought other commodities of Spain and of the Eastern lands....

*Wednesday, 14th of November*

....He believes that these islands are those innumerable ones that are depicted on the maps of the world in the Far East. He believed that they yielded very great riches in precious stones and spices....

*Monday, 24th of December*

....among other places they mentioned where gold was found, they named Cipango, which they called Civao. Here they said that there was a great quantity of gold, and the cacique carried banners of beaten gold....

---

## No. 6 — THE VISION OF COLUMBUS
*("Journal of the First Voyage of Christopher Columbus", 1492-1493)\**

*Wednesday, 26th of December*

....I protested to your Highnesses that all the profits of this my enterprise should be spent in the conquest of Jerusalem, and your Highnesses laughed and said that it pleased them, and that, without this, they entertained that desire.

*Cited in Bourne, *op. cit.*, p. 205.

## No. 7 — THE VISION RECEDES

*(Christopher Columbus to Pope Alexander VI, February 1502)**

This undertaking ** is made with a view to expend what is derived from it in guarding the Holy Sepulchre for Holy Church. After I was there and had seen the land I wrote the king and queen my lords that in seven years I would pay for fifty thousand foot and five thousand horse for the conquest of it, and in five more years fifty thousand more foot and five thousand horse, making ten thousand horse and one hundred thousand foot—Satan has disturbed all this.

---

## No. 8 — COLUMBUS IN ROYAL FAVOUR

*(Ferdinand and Isabella, King and Queen of Spain, to Christopher Columbus, August 16, 1494)***

Don Christopher Columbus, our High Admiral of the Islands of the Indies: We have seen your letters and memorials....; and have felt great pleasure in being made acquainted with all that you have written to us in them; and we return many thanks to the Lord for all, hoping that, with his assistance, your undertaking will be the cause of our holy Catholic faith being still more widely spread; and one of the principal things which pleased us so much in this affair is, its having been invented, commenced, and obtained through your means, labour, and industry. It appears to us, that of all that you told us from the beginning would happen almost the whole has been verified; as if you had seen it before mentioning it to us; and we trust in God, that what yet remains to be known will be verified in like manner; for all which things we are bound in duty to confer favours upon you, such as you shall be perfectly satisfied with. And having reflected upon all that you have written to us, although you express yourself minutely upon everything, which upon reading gives us great pleasure and joy, nevertheless, we should feel greater satisfaction by your writing to inform us how many islands have been discovered up to the present time, and what is the name you have given to each of them; for although you name some of them in your letters, they are not all named; and also the name given to the others by the Indians; and the distance between them; and whatever you have found in each of them; and what is said to be produced in them; and what has been sown since you were there;

*Cited in Navarrete, *op. cit.*, Tomo II, Num. CXLV, p. 328.

** His fourth and final voyage.

***Cited in Navarrete, *op. cit.*, Tomo II, Num. LXXIX, pp. 184-185.

and what has been obtained, the time being already elapsed in which whatever has been sown should be reaped.  And, more especially, we wish to know all the seasons of the year, such as they take place there in each month separately; it appearing to us, from what you say, that there is a great difference in the seasons from what we have here: some wish to know if there are two winters and two summers in the same year. Inform us of every thing for our service; and send us the greatest number possible of falcons, and of all the other birds that are produced there, and that can be had; because we are desirous of seeing them all....

## No. 9 — ROYAL COMMISSION OF ENQUIRY

*(Royal Commission of Ferdinand and Isabella, King and Queen of Spain, to Francisco de Bobadilla, March 21, 1499)\**

Be it known that Christopher, Columbus, our Admiral of the Ocean, of the islands and terra-firma of the Indies, has informed us that while he was away from the said islands in our Court, some persons and a mayor with them rose against the said Admiral and the authorities whom he has appointed there in our name.  When those persons and the said mayor were told not to continue with the said revolt and scandal, they refused to desist, but, on the contrary, kept and keep up the said rebellion, and are stealing and causing other evil, damages and violences against the service of God our Lord and ours, in the said Island.  Wherefore, because it was and is a bad example which deserves to be punished, and it is up to Us, as King and Queen and Lords, to provide for it and remedy it we command this Decree to be given to you....  through it we order you to go now to the said islands and terra-firma of the Indies and inquire into the situation and, as best and as diligently as you can, ascertain and learn the truth of all that has been said, who and what persons rose in rebellion against the said Admiral and our authorities, and for what cause and reason, and what robbery and evil and damages they have done, and everything else which in relation to this needs to be known to be better informed: and when the information has been obtained and the truth known, whomever you may find guilty, *have them arrested* and confiscate their possessions; and.... proceed against them and against those absent with the greatest civil and criminal penalties which you may deem lawful....

*Cited in Navarrete, *op. cit.*, Tomo II, Num. CXXVII, pp. 275-276.

*No. 10—COLUMBUS IN ROYAL DISFAVOUR*
*("Narrative of the Voyage which the Admiral, Don Christo-*
*pher Columbus, made the third time that he came to the*
*Indies, when he discovered Tierra Firme, as he sent it to the*
*Sovereigns from the island of Espanola," October 18, 1498)\**

I have been very much aggrieved in that there has been
sent to inquire into my conduct a man who knew that, if the
report which he sent back were very damaging, he would
remain in charge of the government. Would that it had
pleased Our Lord that Their Highnesses had sent him or
another two years ago, for I know that then I should have
been free from scandalous abuse and infamy, and I should
not have been deprived of my honour or have lost it. God
is just, and He will cause it to be known by whom and how
it was done.

At home they judge me as a governor sent to Sicily or
to a city or two under settled government, and where the
laws can be fully maintained, without fear of all being lost;
and at this I am greatly aggrieved. I ought to be judged as
a captain who went from Spain to the Indies to conquer a
people, warlike and numerous, and with customs and beliefs
very different from ours, a people, living in highlands and
mountains, having no settled dwellings, and apart from us;
and where, by the will of God, I have brought under the
dominion of the king and queen, our sovereigns, another
world, whereby Spain, which was called poor, is now most
rich. I ought to be judged as a captain, who, for so long a
time, down to this day, has borne arms, never laying them
down for an hour, and by knights of the sword and by men
of action, and not by men of letters, unless they had been
as the Greeks or Romans, or as others of the present day of
whom there are so many and so noble in Spain, for in any
other way I am greatly aggrieved, because in the Indies there
is neither a town nor any settled dwelling.

*No. 11—THE DISCOVERER PLEADS FOR JUSTICE*
*(Christopher Columbus to Ferdinand, King of Spain, Jamaica,*
*1503)\*\**

Diego Mendez, and the papers I send by him, will shew
your highness what rich mines of gold I have discovered at
Veragua, and how I intended to have left my brother at River
Belen, if the judgements of heaven and the greatest misfortunes in the world had not prevented it. However, it is

---

\* Cited in C. Jane (ed.), *Select Documents Illustrating the Four Voyages of
Columbus,* Works of the Hakluyt Society, Second Series, No. LXV, London,
1930, Vol. I, pp. 66, 68.

\*\* Cited in *Interesting Tracts relating to the Island of Jamaica,* St. Jago de la
Vega, Jamaica, 1800, pp. 3—5.

sufficient your highness and successors will have the glory
and advantage of all, and that the full discovery and settlement are reserved for happier persons than the unfortunate
Columbus. If God be so merciful to me as to conduct Mendez
to Spain, I doubt not but he will make your highness and
my great mistress understand that this will not only be a
Castile and Leon, but a discovery of a world of subjects,
lands, and wealth, greater than man's unbounded fancy could
ever comprehend, or avarice itselt covet. But neither he, this
paper, nor the tongue of mortal man, can express the an-
guish and afflictions of my mind and body, nor the misery
of my son, brother, and friends; for here already we have
been above ten months lodged upon the open decks of our
ships, that are run ashore and lashed together; those of my
men that were well have mutinied under the Porras of
Sevilla; my friends that were faithful are mostly sick and
dying; we have consumed the Indian's provisions, so they
do abandon us; all therefore are likely to perish by hunger, and
these miseries are accompanied with so many aggravating
circumstances that render me the most wretched object of
misfortune this  world shall ever see, as if the displeasure
of heaven seconded the envy of Spain, and would punish as
criminal those undertakings and discoveries, that former ages
would have acknowledged as great and meritorious.   Good
heaven! and you holy saints that dwell in it, let the king
Don Fernando, and my illustrious mistress Donna Isabella,
know that I am the most miserable man living, and that my
zeal for their service and interest hath brought me to it;
for it is impossible to live and have afflictions equal to mine.
I see, and with horror apprehend, (and for my sake,) those
unfortunate and deserving people's destruction.   Alas! piety
and justice have retired to their habitations above, and it is
a crime to have done or performed too much, as my misery
makes my life a burthen to myself, so I fear the empty
titles of perpetual viceroy and admiral render me obnoxious
to the Spanish nation.   It is visible enough how all methods
are made use of to cut the thread which is breaking, for I
am in my old age, and loaded with unsupportable pains of
the gout, and am now languishing and expiring with that
and other infirmities among savages, where I have neither
medicines nor provisions for the body, priests nor sacraments
for the soul.   My men mutinying, my brother, my son, and
those that are faithful, sick, starving, and dying.   The Indians
have abandoned us; and the governor of St. Domingo,
Obando, has sent rather to see if I am dead, than to succour
us, or carry me alive hence, for his boat neither delivered a
letter nor spoke, or would receive any from us, so I conclude
your highness officers intend here my voyage and life shall

end.  O blessed mother of God, that compassionateth the
miserable and oppressed, why did not cruel Bobadilla kill
me, when he robbed me, and my brother of our dear purchased gold, and sent us for Spain in chains, without hearing,
trial, crime, or shadow of one!  These chains are all the
treasures I have, and shall be buried with me, if I chance to
have a coffin or a grave; for I would have the remembrance
of so unjust and tragic an act die with me, and, for the glory
of the Spanish name, be eternally forgot.  Had it been so
(O blessed virgin!) Obando had not then forced us to be
dying ten or twelve months, and to perish *per* malice as
great as our misfortunes.  O let it not bring a further infamy
on the Castilian name, nor let ages to come know, there
were wretches so vile in this, that thought to recommend
themselves to Don Fernando, by destroying the unfortunate
and miserable Christopher Columbus, not for his crimes, but
for his services in discovering and giving Spain a new world.
It was you, O heaven! that inspired and conducted me to it,
do you therefore weep for me, and shew pity; let the earth,
and every soul in it that loves justice or mercy, weep for me.
And you, O glorified saints of God, that know my innocency
and see my sufferings, have mercy.  If this present age is
too envious or obdurate to weep for me, surely those that
are to be born will do it, when they are told Christopher
Columbus, with his own fortune, at the hazard of his own
and brother's lives, with little or no expense to the crown
of Spain, in twelve years, and four voyages, rendered greater
services than ever mortal man did to prince or kingdom,
yet was made to perish (without being charged with the least
crime) poor and miserable, all but his chains being taken
from him, so that he who gave Spain another world, had
neither in it a cottage for himself nor wretched family.  But
should heaven still persecute me, and seem displeased with
what I have done, as if the discovery of this world may be
fatal to the old, and as a punishment bring my life in this
miserable place to its fatal period; yet do you, O good angels!
(you that succour the oppressed and innocent,) bring this
paper to my great mistress.  She knows how much I have
done, and will believe what I suffer for her glory and service,
and will be so just and pious as not to let the sons and
brothers of him, that has brought to Spain such immense
riches, and added to it vast and unknown kingdoms and
empires, want bread or subsist on alms. She (if she lives)
will consider cruelty and ingratitude will provoke heaven,
and the wealth I have discovered will stir up all mankind
to revenge and rapine, so that the nation may chance to
suffer hereafter, for what envious, malicious, and ungrateful people do now.

*No. 12 — THE LAND COLUMBUS LOVED*
*(Extract from the Last Will and Testament of Christopher*
*Columbus, May 19, 1506)\**
I say to D. Diego, my son, and I command him so long
as he has an income as first-born son and also his inheritance,
to maintain in a Chapel, which is to be built, three Chaplains
who will say three Masses a day: one in honour of the Holy
Trinity, another for the Conception of Our Lady, and the
third for all the faithful departed, *for my soul and for those
of my father, my mother and my wife....* And that, if his
income suffices, he make it an honourable Chapel, and increase the prayers and devotions in honour of the Holy
Trinity, and that if this can be done in Hispaniola which God
gave me miraculously, I would rejoice if it were done where
I invoked the Trinity, that is, in the meadow known as La
Concepcion de la Vega.

*No. 13—INJUSTICE TO THE DISCOVERER*
*(Martin Waldseemuller, Cosmographae Introductio, St. Die,*
*1507)\*\**
In the sixth climate towards the south pole are situated
both the farthest part of Africa recently discovered, and
Zanzibar, the islands of lesser Java and Ceylon, and the
fourth part of the globe which since Americus\*\*\* discovered
it may be called Amerige — i.e., Americ's land or America.

*No. 14 — SPAIN'S DEBT TO COLUMBUS*
*(Gonzalo Fernandes de Oviedo y Valdes, Historia General y*
*Natural de las Indias, Islas y Tierra–Firme del Mar Oceano*
*(1535–1557), Madrid, 1851–1855)\*\*\**
Besides his services to the sovereigns of Castile, all
Spaniards owe him much, for although many of them suffered
and died in the conquest of these Indies, many others became
rich and otherwise advantaged. Yet what is greater is that
in lands so remote from Europe, and where the devil was
served and worshipped, he has been driven out by the
Christians, and our holy Catholic faith and the church of
God established and carried on in this far country, where
there are such great kingdoms and dominions, by the means
and efforts of Cristoval Colon. And more than this, such
great treasures of gold, silver, and pearls, and many other
riches and merchandise, have been brought and will be
brought hence to Spain that no virtuous Spaniard will forget
the benefits bestowed upon his country with God's help by
this first admiral of the Indies.

\*Cited in Navarrete, *op., cit.,* Tomo II, Num. CLVIII, pp. 364-365.
\*\* Cited in E. G. Bourne, *Spain in America,* New York, 1904, pp. 98-99.
\*\*\* Amerigo Vespucci.
\*\*\*\* *Op, cit.,* Primera Parte, Libro Tercero, Cap. IX, 1944 Edition, Editorial
    Guarania, Asuncion del Paraguay, Tomo I, p. 158.

# CHAPTER II

# The Economic Organisation of the Spanish Caribbean

## (i) THE MINING ECONOMY

---

### No. 15—THE LUST FOR GOLD

*("Journal of the First Voyage of Christopher Columbus",
1492-1493)* *

#### Saturday, 13th of October

....I was attentive, and took trouble to ascertain if there was gold. I saw that some of them had a small piece fastened in a hole they have in the nose, and by signs I was able to make out that to the south, or going from the island to the south, there was a king who had great cups full, and who possessed a great quantity....

#### Monday, 15th of October

At 10 we departed with the wind S.W., and made for the south, to reach that other island, which is very large, and respecting which all the men that I bring from San Salvador make signs that there is much gold, and that they wear it as bracelets on the arms, on the legs, in the ears and nose, and around the neck.... I do not wish to stop, in discovering and visiting many islands, to find gold. These people make signs that it is worn on the arms and legs; and it must be gold, for they point to some pieces that I have. I cannot err, with the help of our Lord, in finding out where this gold has its origin....

#### Friday, 19th of October

....my desire is to see and discover as much as I can before returning to your Highnesses, our Lord willing, in April. It is true that in the event of finding places where there is gold or spices in quantity I should stop until I had collected as much as I could. I, therefore, proceed in the hope of coming across such places....

#### Sunday, 21st of October

....Beyond this island (Cuba) there is another called Bosio**, which they also say is very large, and others we shall see as we pass. According as I obtain tidings of gold or spices I shall settle what should be done....

* Cited in Bourne, *The Northmen, Columbus and Cabot*, pp. 112, 116—117, 124, 126—127, 130, 144, 154—155, 184, 186—187, 193, 196, 205, 210, 215, 226.
**Hispaniola. Columbus confused the word with *bohio*, the Indian hut.

### Tuesday, 23rd of October

....I see that there is no gold mine here.... It is better to go where there is great entertainment, so I say that it is not reasonable to wait, but rather to continue the voyage and inspect much land, until some very profitable country is reached, my belief being that it will be rich in spices....

### Sunday, 28th of October

....I went thence in seach of the island of Cuba on a S.S.W. course, making for the nearest point of it.... The Indians say that in this island there are gold mines and pearls, and the Admiral saw a likely place for them and mussel-shells, which are signs of them....

### Monday, 12th of November

....Without doubt, there is in these lands a vast quantity of gold, and the Indians I have on board do not speak without reason when they say that in these islands there are places where they dig out gold, and wear it on their necks, ears, arms, legs, the rings being very large....

### Sunday, 25th of November

....He.... saw some stones shining in its bed like gold. He remembered that in the river Tagus, near its junction with the sea, there was gold; so it seemed to him that this should contain gold, and he ordered some of these stones to be collected to be brought to the Sovereigns....

### Monday, 17th of December

....they said to the Admiral that there was more gold in Tortuga than in Espanola, because it is nearer to Baneque. The Admiral did not think that there were gold mines either in Espanola or Tortuga, but that the gold was brought from Baneque in small quantities, there being nothing to give in return. That land is so rich that there is no necessity to work much to sustain life....He believed that they were very near the source, and that our Lord would point out where the gold has its origin....

### Tuesday, 18th of December

....This day little gold was got by barter, but the Admiral heard from an old man that there were many neighbouring islands, at a distance of one hundred leagues or more, as he understood, in which much gold is found; and there is even one island that is all gold. In the others there was so much that it was said they gather it with sieves, and they fuse it and make bars, and work it a thousand ways. They explained the work by signs....

*Saturday, 22nd of December*

At dawn the Admiral made sail to shape a course in search of the islands which the Indians had told him contained much gold, some of them having more gold than earth....

*Sunday, 23rd of December*

....May our Lord favour me by his clemency, that I may find this gold, I mean the mine of gold, which I hold to be here, many saying that they know it....

*Wednesday, 26th of December*

....He trusted in God that, when he returned from Spain, according to his intention, he would find a tun of gold collected by barter by those he was to leave behind, and that they would have found the mine, and spices in such quantities that the Sovereigns would, in three years, be able to undertake and fit out an expedition to go and conquer the Holy Sepulchre....

*Wednesday, 2nd of January*

He left on that island of Espanola.... 39 men with the fortress.... all the merchandise which had been provided for bartering, which was much, that they might trade for gold. He also left the ship's boat, that they, most of them being sailors, might go, when the time seemed convenient, to discover the gold mine, in order that the Admiral, on his return, might find much gold. They were also to find a good site for a town, for this was not altogether a desirable port; especially as the gold the natives brought came from the east....

*Sunday, 6th of January*

....The Admiral then says: "Thus I am convinced that our Lord miraculously caused that vessel to remain here, this being the best place in the whole island to form a settlement, and the nearest to the gold mines". He also says that he knew of another great island, to the south of the island of Juana,* in which there is more gold than in this island, so that they collect it in bits the size of beans, while in Espanola they find the pieces the size of grains of wheat. They call that island Yamaye.**

*Tuesday, 15th of January*

....To-day he had heard that all the gold was in the district of the town of Navidad, belonging to Their Highnesses....

* Cuba.          * * Jamaica.

## No. 16 — THE GOD OF THE SPANIARDS
*(Bartolome de las Casas, Historia de las Indias (1559).*
*Madrid, 1875)\**

A lord and cacique of the province of Guahaba, named Hatuey, escaped (to Cuba) with as many followers as he could take with him....Knowing the customs of the Spaniards.... he always had his spies who brought him news of conditions in Hispaniola because he was afraid that some day the Spaniards would come to Cuba. And finally, it seems that he learned of the decision of the Spaniards to move to it. Knowing this, one day he gathered all his people .... and he began to talk to them and to remind them of the persecutions which the Spaniards had inflicted on the people of Hispaniola. He said to them.... "Do you know why they persecute us and for what purpose they do it ?" They replied : "They do it because they are cruel and bad." The lord replied : "I will tell you why they do it, and it is this — because they have a lord whom they love very much, and I will show him to you." He had a small basket made of palm, full or partly full of gold, and he said: "Here is their lord, whom they serve and adore.... to have this lord they make us suffer, for him they persecute us, for him they have killed our parents, brothers, all our people and our neighbours and deprived us of all our possessions; for him they seek and illtreat us; and because, as you have already heard, they want to come here and seek only this lord and in order to find him and extract him they will persecute us and annoy us, as they have done before in our own land, therefore, let us dance and entertain him, so that when they come, he shall order them not to do us any harm." They agreed that it was a good idea to entertain him and dance for him; then they began to dance and sing until they were tired, for this was their custom.... Then Hatuey addressed them again saying: "Look, notwithstanding what I have said, let us not hide this lord from the Christians in any place, for, even if we should hide it in our intestines, they would get it out of us; therefore, let us throw it in this river, under the water, and they will not know where it is." Whereupon they threw it in the river. The story was later related by the Indians and published among us.

---

## No. 17 — THE GOLD RUSH
*("Narrative of the Voyage which the Admiral, Don Christo-pher Columbus, made the third time that he came to the Indies, when he discovered Tierra Firme, as he sent it to the Sovereigns from the island of Espanola,"* October 18, 1498)\*\*

\* *Op. cit.*, Libro Tercero, Cap. XXI, edition of Fondo de Cultura Economica, Mexico, 1951, Tomo II, pp. 507-508.
\*\* Cited in Jane, *op. cit.*, Vol. I, p. 68.

To the gold and pearls the gate is already opened, and
they may surely expect a quantity of all, precious stones and
spices and a thousand other things....

The news of the gold which I said that I would give is
that, on the day of the Nativity, being greatly afflicted owing
to my struggles with evil Christians and with the Indians,
and being on the verge of leaving all and escaping with
my life, if possible, Our Lord miraculously consoled me and
said : "Take courage, be not dismayed nor fear; I will provide for all; the seven years, the term of the gold, are not
passed, and in this and in the rest I will give thee redress."
On that day I learned that there were eighty leagues of land
and in every part of them mines; it now appears that they
are all one. Some have collected a hundred and twenty castellanos in a day, others ninety, and it has risen to two hundred and fifty. To collect from fifty to seventy, and many
others from fifteen to fifty, is held to be a good day's work,
and many continue to collect it; the average is from six to
twelve, and any who falls below this is not content. The
opinion of all is that, were all Castile to go there, however in-
expert a man might be, he would not get less than a
castellano or two a day, and so it is up to the present time.
It is true that he who has an Indian collects this amount, but
the matter depends on the Christian.

---

## No. 18 — THE BANKRUPTCY OF THE MINING ECONOMY

*(The City of Puerto Rico, San Juan, to the Empress of Spain,
April, 18, 1533)\**

....All the settlers and residents of this island are heavily
in debt, due to the large number of Negroes they bought on
credit in the hope of mining much gold. Since they have not
found any gold, many are in prison, others have taken to the
woods, and others have been ruined by being forced to sell
everything they own. Much of the blame falls on the storms
of the past years, for these destroyed the farms and they
had to buy their supplies at very high prices. Therefore, their
debts increased. We beseech you to take away the tempta-
tion to fall more heavily in debt to the merchants by forbidding the latter to import any Negroes for a year and a half,
and allowing the settlers to bring them over free of duty for
ten years. Also there should be a moratorium on debts for
five years, as long as they give sufficient security.

* Cited in Alejandro Tapia y Rivera, *Biblioteca Historica de Puerto Rico*,
San Juan, 1945 edition, pp. 309—310.

## (ii) THE AGRICULTURAL ECONOMY

### No. 19 — THE SUBSISTENCE ECONOMY OF THE ABORIGINAL INDIANS

*("Journal of the First Voyage of Christopher Columbus,"*
*1492—1493)\**

#### Tuesday, 16th of October

....I have no doubt that they sow and gather corn all the year round, as well as other things.... Here the fish are so unlike ours that it is wonderful.... I saw neither sheep, nor goats, nor any other quadruped....

#### Tuesday, 6th of November

.... The two Christians met with many people on the road going home, men and women with a half-burnt reed in their hands, being the herbs they are accustomed to smoke.. They saw no quadrupeds except the dogs that do not bark. The land is very fertile, and is cultivated with yams and several kinds of bean different from ours, as well as corn. There were great quantities of cotton gathered, spun, and worked up. In a single house they saw more than 500 *arrobas,\*\** and as much as 4000 *quintals\*\** could be yielded every year. The Admiral said that it did not appear to be cultivated, and that it bore all the year round. It is very fine, and has a large boll. All that was possessed by these people they gave at a very low price, and a great bundle of cotton was exchanged for the point of a needle or other trifle....

#### Sunday, 16th of December

....All this island,\*\*\* as well as the island of Tortuga, is cultivated like the plain of Cordova. They raise on these lands crops of yams, which are small branches, at the foot of which grow roots like carrots, which serve as bread. They powder and knead them, and make them into bread; then they plant the same branch in another part, which again sends out four or five of the same roots, which are very nutritious, with the taste of chestnuts. Here they have the largest the Admiral had seen in any part of the world, for he says that they have the same plant in Guinea. At this place they were as thick as a man's leg. All the people were stout and lusty, not thin, like the natives that had been seen before, and of a very pleasant manner, without religious belief. The trees were so luxuriant that the leaves left off being green, and were dark coloured with verdure. It was a won-

* Cited in Bourne, *The Northmen, Columbus and Cabot*, pp. 119—120, 141—142, 181—182.
** The *arroba* was 25 pounds, and the *quintal* one hundredweight.
***Hispaniola.

derful thing to see those valleys, and rivers of sweet water,
and the cultivated fields, and land fit for cattle, though they
have none, for orchards, and for anything in the world that
a man could seek for.

_____

## No. 20 — TOBACCO CULTIVATION AMONG THE ABORIGINAL INDIANS

*(Gonzalo Fernandes de Oviedo y Valdes, Historia General y
Natural de las Indias, Islas y Tierra-Firme del Mar Oceano
(1535—1557), Madrid 1851—1855)\**

Among the vices practised by the Indians of this
island\*\* there was one that was very bad, which was the use
of certain dried leaves that they call *tabaco* to make them
lose their senses. They do this with the smoke of a certain
plant that, as far as I have been able to gather, is of the
nature of henbane, but not in appearance or form, to judge
by its looks, because this plant is a stalk or shoot four or
five spans or a little less in height and with broad and thick
and soft and furry leaves, and of a green resembling the
colour of the leaves of ox-tongue or bugloss (as it is called
by herbalists and doctors). This plant I am speaking of in
some sort or fashion resembles henbane, and they take it in
this way: the caciques and leading men have certain little
hollow sticks about a handbreadth in length or less and the
thickness of the little finger of the hand, and these tubes
have two round pipes that come together,.... and all in one
piece. And they put the two pipes into the openings of their
nostrils and the other into the smoke of the plant that is
burning or smouldering; and these tubes are very smooth
and well made, and they burn the leaves of that plant
wrapped up and enveloped in the same way the pages of the
court take their smokes: and they take in the breath and
smoke once or twice or more times, as many as they can
stand, until they lose their senses for a long time and lay
stretched out on the ground or in a deep and very heavy
sleep. The Indians who do not have these tubes take this
smoke through hollow stems or reeds, and that instrument
through which they take the smoke, or the aforesaid reeds,
are called by the Indian *tabaco,* and not the plant or the
sleep that overtakes them (as some have thought). This
plant is very highly prized by the Indians, and they grow it
in their gardens and farms for the aforesaid use; they believe that the use of this plant and its smoke is not only a

\* *Op. cit.,* Primera Parte, Libro Quinto, Cap. II, Tomo II, pp. 237—239.
Translation from F. Ortiz, *Cuban Counterpoint, Tobacco and Sugar,* New
York, 1947 (Translation by Harriet de Ones), pp. 120—122.
\*\* Hispaniola.

healthy thing for them, but a very holy thing. And when the cacique or leading man dropped to the ground, his wives (of whom he had many) would pick him up and put him in his bed or hammock, if he had so ordered before he lost his senses; but if he had not so said or ordered, he did not want them to do anything but leave him there on the ground until that drunkenness or sleep passed from him. I cannot understand what pleasure they get from this act, unless it is the desire to drink, which they do before they take the smoke or tobacco, and some drink so much of a kind of wine they make that they fall down drunk before they start smoking; but when they have had all the drink they want, they begin on this perfume. And many smoke the tobacco without drinking too much, and do as has been described until they fall to the ground on their back or side, but without swooning, rather like a man who has fallen asleep. I know that certain Spaniards now use it, especially some of those who have contracted buboes, because they say that while under its effects they do not feel the pain of their disease, and it would seem that the one who does this is like one dead in life, which I think is worse than the suffering they spare themselves, because it is not as though they were cured by it.

Now many of the Negroes that are in this city and in all the island have acquired the same habit, and they raise this plant on the farms and properties of their masters for the purpose described and take the same smokes or tobaccos because they say that when they stop work and smoke tobacco it takes away their weariness.

------------

### No. 21 — THE AGRICULTURAL PROSPECTS OF HISPANIOLA

*(Memorandum of Christopher Columbus, sent to the Spanish Sovereigns, by Antonio de Torres, January 30, 1495)**

You shall say to Their Highnesses, as has been said, that the cause of the illness, so general among all, is the change of water and air, for we see that it spreads to all one after another, and few are in danger. It follows that, under God, the preservation of health depends upon this people being provided with the food to which they are accustomed in Spain, for none of them, or others who may newly arrive, can serve Their Highnesses unless they are in health. And this provision should continue until here a supply can be secured from that which is here sown and planted, I mean from wheat and barley and grapes, towards which little has been done this year, since it was not possible earlier to select a site for a settlement. And directly after it was selected, those few labourers who were here fell ill, and even

*Cited in Jane, *op. cit.*, Vol. I, pp. 82, 84.

if they had been well, they had so few beasts and those so
lean and weak, that it is little that they would have been
able to do.    Nevertheless, they have sown something, mainly
in order to test the soil, which appears to be very wonderful,
so that from this some relief in our necessities may be
expected. We are very sure, as what has been done shows,
that in this country wheat as well as vines will grow very
well.    But it is necessary to wait for the fruit, and if it be
such as the rapid growing of the wheat, and of some few
vines which have been planted, suggests, it is certain that
here there will be no need of Andalusia or of Sicily, and the
same applies to sugar canes, judging from the way in which
some few that have been planted have taken root.    For it is
certain that the beauty of the land of these islands, as well
of the mountains and sierras and rivers, as of the plains,
where there are broad rivers, is such to behold that no other
land on which the sun shines can be better to see or more
lovely.

---

## No. 22 — AGRICULTURAL PESTS

*(Bartolome de las Casas, Historia de las Indias (1559),
Madrid, 1875)\**

Seeing that they were running out of Indians, the
Spaniards began to abandon the mines, for they had nobody
to send there to die, and to look for new sources of profit.
One of these ways was to grow cassia trees, which thrived
so well that it seemed the land was made for them by
Divine Providence and nature's law.... They pinned all their
hopes on cassia.... but just when they were beginning to
enjoy the fruit of their labour.... God sent upon this island
and especially upon the island of San Juan a scourge which,
it was feared, if it grew worse, would depopulate the islands.
This was an invasion of ants.... which could not be stopped
by any human means.    Those in Hispaniola did more damage
than those in San Juan in destroying the trees, while those
of San Juan were more rabid, their sting was more painful
than that of wasps, and at night the only protection from
them was to place the bed over four pans full of water.    In
Hispaniola they ate the trees by the roots, and left them black
and withered, as if they had been struck by lightning.  They
wrought havoc on the orange and pomegranate trees of
which there were large fields in this island, and burned them
all, so that it was pitiful to see them.    In this way many
orchards in this city of Santo Domingo were destroyed....
They relentlessly attacked the cassia trees and.... soon
destroyed and burned them.    I think they destroyed over a

*Op. Cit., Libro Tercero, Cap. CXXVIII, Tomo III, pp. 271, 273.

hundred million of them. It was a pity to see so many rich farms annihilated by a pest for which no remedy could be found....

Some people dug around the trees, as deep as they could, and killed the ants by drowning them in water. At other times they burned them. They found, two or two and a half feet deep in the soil, their nests and eggs, as white as the snow. Every day they burned about one or two pecks, only to find on the following day a larger number alive. The Franciscan priests of La Vega put a stone of corrosive sublimate, weighing about three or four pounds, on a flat roof; all the ants in the house rushed to it, and once they had eaten of it they dropped dead. It seemed as if they had sent a message to all the ants a league and a half away, inviting them to the banquet. I think every single ant came, the roads to the monastery were full of them; finally they climbed up to the roof and after eating of the stone they dropped dead. The roof was as black with ants as if it had been sprayed with coal dust. This lasted as long as the stone lasted, which was as large as two fists or a ball. I saw how large it was when it was first put on the roof, and a few days later it was about the size of an egg. When the priests saw that the stone was of no use at all.... they decided to take it away. Two things amazed them, not without reason: the first was the natural instinct and the strength even of non-sensitive creatures, such as these ants, that they could sense from such a distance, so to speak, or that the same instinct would guide and direct them to the stone; the second, that so small an insect could have such strength as to bite and finally demolish a stone which, before being ground, is as hard as, if not harder than, alum, and almost as hard as a cobble stone.

The Spaniards.... in the city of Santo Domingo decided to seek help from the highest tribunal. They made great processions beseeching Our Lord to free them in His Mercy from so malignant a scourge of their property.... They decided to choose a Saint to intercede for them.... So, one day after the procession, the bishop, the clergy and all the citizens drew lots from the Saints in the Litany.... The luck fell upon Saint Saturnine and, receiving him joyfully as their patron, they celebrated the feast with great solemnity and have done so each year since... The scourge diminished daily, and if it did not disappear completely, it was because of their sins. Now I believe it is all gone, for they have begun to restore some cassia trees, orange trees and pomegranates. I do not mean that they restored those the ants burned down, but that they planted new ones. The cause of this scourge of ants was said by some to be the introduction and planting of plantains.

## (iii) THE SUGAR INDUSTRY

### No. 23—THE RISE AND PROGRESS OF THE SUGAR INDUSTRY OF HISPANIOLA

*(Gonzalo Fernandez de Oviedo y Valdes, Historia General y Natural de las Indias, Islas y Tierra-Firme del Mar Oceano (1535-1557), Madrid, 1851-1855)* *

Now sugar is one of the richest crops to be found in any province or kingdom of the world, and on this island there is so much and it is so good although it was so recently introduced and has been followed for such a short time; and even though the fertility of the land and the abundant supply of water and the great forests that provide wood for the great and steady fires that must be kept up are all so suitable for such crops, all the more credit is due the person who first undertook it and showed how the work should be done.

Everyone was blind until Bachelor Gonzalo de Velosa, at his own cost and investing everything he had, and with great personal effort, brought workmen expert in sugar to this island, and built a horse-powered mill and first made sugar in this island; he alone deserves thanks as the principal inventor of this rich industry. Not because he was the first to plant sugar cane in the Indies, because some time before his coming many had planted it, and had made syrup from it; but, as I have said, he was the first to make sugar on this island, and following his example, afterwards there were many others who did the same. As he had a large plantation of sugar cane, he built a horse-powered mill on the banks of the Nigua River, and brought out workmen from the Canary Islands, and ground the cane and made sugar before anyone else.

But investigating the matter further, I have learned that certain reputable old men, who at present live in this city, say differently, and they maintain that the person who first planted sugar cane on this island was one Pedro de Atienza of the city of Concepcion de la Vega, and that the Mayor of Vega, Miguel Ballester, a native of Catalonia, was the first to make sugar. And they say that he did this more than two years, before Bachelor Velosa; but at the same time they say that the Mayor did very little, and that the source of both the one and the other was the cane of Pedro de Atienza. So, whichever version one wishes to accept, it would seem that the original basis or origin of sugar in this island of the Indies was the cane of Pedro de Atienza, and from these beginnings it grew and multiplied until it became the industry it is today, and each day it increases

*Op. cit., Primera Parte, Libro Cuarto, Tomo I, pp. 218—226. Translation from Ortiz, op. cit., pp. 254—261.

and grows, for although in the last fifteen years certain *ingenios* have failed or deteriorated for reasons I shall set forth in their proper place, others have been perfected. Let us return to Bachelor Velosa and his mill.

As he came to understand the business better, the Comptroller, Christobal de Tapia, and his brother, the Warden of this fortress, Francisco de Tapia, went into partnership with him, and the three of them together established an *ingenio* in Yaguate, a league and a half from the banks of the Nizao River, and some time ago they had a disagreement and the Bachelor sold out his part to the Tapias. Later the Comptroller sold his to Johan de Villoria, who afterwards sold it to the Mayor, Francisco de Tapia, who thus became the sole owner of the first *ingenio* that existed on this island. As in those early days people did not understand as well as they should have the need of great areas of land and accessible water and wood and other supplementary things for such an industry (of which there was not so much as was necessary there), the Mayor, Francisco de Tapia, abandoned that *ingenio* and moved the copper or boilers and equipment and everything he could to another, better location right on the banks of the Nigua, five leagues from the city, where, until he died, the Mayor had a very good *ingenio*, one of the most important in this island.

In order not to repeat over and over again what I shall say now, the reader should bear in mind that what is said of this *ingenio* applies to all others of the same sort, that each of the important and well equipped *ingenios*, in addition to the great expense and value of the building or factory in which the sugar is made, and another large building in which it is refined and stored, often requires an investment of ten or twelve thousand gold ducats before it is complete and ready for operation. And if I should say fifteen thousand ducats, I should not be exaggerating, for they require at least eighty or one hundred Negroes working all the time, and even one hundred and twenty or more to be well supplied; and close by a good herd or two of a thousand, or two or three thousand head of cattle to feed the workers; aside from the expense of trained workers and foremen for making the sugar, and carts to haul the cane to the mill and to bring in wood, and people to make bread and cultivate and irrigate the canefields, and other things that must be done and continual expenditure of money. But it is a fact that the owner of an unencumbered and well-equipped *ingenio* has a fine and rich property, and one that brings in great profit and return to its owner.

So this was the first *ingenio* established in this island, and it should be observed that until sugar was produced on it the ships sailed back to Spain empty, and now they return loaded with sugar, carrying a bigger cargo than they brought out, and a more profitable one....

Another *ingenio*, and one of the best and most important on the whole island, was established by Licentiate Zuazo, who was one of the judges of the Royal Tribunal established in this city by Their Majesties. It is along the banks of the River Oca, sixteen leagues from this city of Santo Domingo, and is one of the fine properties of these parts, and it was left after the days of the Licentiate to his wife, Dona Phelipa, and his two daughters, called Dona Leoner and Dona Emerenciana Zuazo, along with much other wealth and property. And it is the opinion of some who are versed in this industry that this *ingenio* alone, with its Negroes and cattle and equipment and land and appurtenances, is now worth over fifty thousand gold ducats, because it is very well fitted up. And I heard Licentiate Zuazo say that every year he had an income of six thousand gold ducats from this *ingenio*, or more, and that he thought it would bring in much more in the future....

The precentor, Don Alonso de Peralta, of this holy church of Santo Domingo, set up a horse-powered mill in the town of Azua itself, and after his days it was left to his heirs. These mills are not so strong as those powered by water, and are more expensive because instead of the water turning the wheels to grind the sugar, it must be done with power of the many horses required for this work; and this estate went to the heirs of the percentor and to Pedro de Heredia, who is now the Governor of the province of Cartegena on the mainland....

In the town of San Juan de la Maguana, forty leagues from this city of Santo Domingo, there is another important *ingenio* which belongs to the heirs of a resident of the town, whose name was Johan de Leon, and the German company of the Welsers, which bought half of this *ingenio*....

Eleven leagues from this city, along the banks of the river called Cazuy, the late Johan Villorio, the elder, and his brother-in-law, Hieronimo de Aguero, set up a very good *ingenio*. This property was left to the heirs of the two, and also to the heirs of Agostin de Binaido, the Genoese, who has a share in this *ingenio*....

Now summing up the account of these mills and rich sugar plantations, there are on this island twenty important *ingenios* completely installed and four horse-powered mills. And there is the opportunity to set up many others on this island, and there is no island or kingdom among Christians or pagans where there is anything like this industry of sugar. The ships that come out from Spain return loaded with sugar of fine quality, and the skimmings and syrup that are wasted on this island or given away would make another great province rich. And the most amazing thing about these great plantations is that during the time that many of us have lived out here, and of those that have spent over thirty-eight years here, all these have been built up in a short time by our hands and our work for there was not a one to be found when we came out here.

## No. 24—THE PROFITS OF THE SUGAR INDUSTRY IN HISPANIOLA

*(Bartolome de las Casas, Historia de las Indias (1559), Madrid 1875)**

When the Jeronimite friars who were there saw the success with which the Bachelor was carrying on this industry, and that it would be very profitable, in order to encourage others to undertake it, they arranged with the judges of the Tribunal and the officers of the crown to lend 500 gold pesos from the funds of the royal treasury to anyone who should set up a mill, large or small, to make sugar, and afterwards, I believe, they made them other loans, in view of the fact that such mills were expensive....

In this way and on this basis a number of settlers agreed to set up mills to grind the cane with horse-power, and others, who had more funds, began to build powerful water-run mills, which grind more cane and extract more sugar than three horse-powered mills, and so every day more were built, and today there are over thirty-four *ingenios* on this island alone, and some on Sant Juan, and in other parts of these Indies, and, notwithstanding, the price of sugar does not go down. And it should be pointed out that in olden times there was sugar only in Valencia, and then later in the Canary Islands, where there may have been seven or eight mills, and I doubt that that many, and withal the price of an arroba of sugar was not over a ducat, or a little more, and now with all the mills that have been built in these Indies, the arroba is worth two ducats, and it is going up all the time.

## No 25 — STATE AID FOR THE SUGAR INDUSTRY

*(Decree of Charles V, Emperor of the Hapsburg Empire, December 1518)***

I order you to use all diligence to see that the residents of the aforesaid island set up *ingenios* of sugar, and that you assist and favour in every way you can all those who wish to do so, both in lending them funds from our treasury

*Op. cit., Libro Tercero, Cap. CXXIX, Tomo, III, p. 274. Translation from Ortiz, op. cit., pp. 261—62.
** Cited in Ortiz, op. cit., p. 271.

to help them establish these *ingenios*, as well as giving them privilege and use of the lands, and that you do the same with all other residents and settlers, who are willing to work and wish to remain there and build, settle and plant and do such other things as are required for the good and ennoblement and settlement of these lands.

Likewise, because it is my will that in all that can conveniently be done they be relieved and unmolested, and being informed that many of them owe debts to one another, and if these were demanded and collected from them much harm would result and the loss of their property, therefore I charge you that if the persons who owe debts on the aforesaid island cannot conveniently pay them, you arrange with their creditors that, being assured that they will pay them with a certain length of time, they wait for them, and in this you will do me a service.

---

### No. 26—EXEMPTION OF CONSTRUCTION MATERIALS FROM IMPORT DUTIES

*(Decree of Charles V, Emperor of the Hapsburg Empire, 1519)\**

Licentiate Antonio Soriano in the name of this island has reported to me that because the construction of such mills is very expensive, and the materials and machinery required for them brought out from this Kingdom to realms near the aforesaid island cost too much for the people to be able to buy them, and this will prevent this activity from developing further, he implores us to order that the machinery, materials, and other things taken out from this Kingdom for the construction and work of these mills shall not pay tax or other duties, or whatever my pleasure should be. And I, for the reasons set forth, found this good.

---

### No. 27—PROVIDING SUGAR EXPERTS FOR HISPANIOLA

*(Charles V, Emperor of the Hapsburg Empire, to Lopez de Sosa, Governor of Castilla de Oro, August 16, 1519)\*\**

....Our representatives on the island of Hispaniola have written me that on that island there is great need of masters and workmen to set up sugar mills and to manufacture sugar because every day many *ingenios* are being established there, and the place is very well fitted and suitable for this, and I have been informed that in the Canary Islands there are

---

\* Cited in Ortiz, *op. cit.*, pp. 257—276.
\*\* Cited in Ortiz, *op. cit.*, p. 257.

many masters and workmen who would go out to the island if it were not that certain people put obstacles in their way, and because you, while you are preparing to undertake your trip to serve us in that capacity, can do much to attract the aforesaid masters and workmen, and on the way, since you will be stopping at the aforesaid island, you can take them with you there, I am sending you with this the enclosed letters so the governors of those islands may not put any obstacle in the way of their departure, but rather help and favour them in it, and for this reason I order you to present these letters to them, and do everything you can to induce as many masters and workmen to go out to the island as is possible.

---

## No. 28—PROHIBITING ATTACHMENT OF SUGAR FACTORIES

*(Decree of Charles V, Emperor of the Hapsburg Empire, January 15, 1529)\**

We order that there can be no attachment of sugar mills in any part of the Indies, or of slaves or other things necessary for their sustenance and milling, unless it be for sums due to Us, and We allow payment to be made in sugar and products of the mills, nor is the renunciation valid if they make it. And it is also our will that the notaries drawing up contracts and deeds insert no renunciatory clause, under penalty of being suspended from office, and that the officers of the law shall not carry it out.

---

## No. 29—CONDITIONS ON WHICH SUGAR MILLS COULD BE SOLD FOR DEBTS

*(Decree of Charles V, Emperor of the Hapsburg Empire, November 8, 1538)\*\**

There may be attachment of any mill smelting metals or manufacturing sugar if the debt amounts to the full value of the mill.—Our purpose in ordering that there may be no attachment against mills smelting metals and manufacturing sugar, with their slaves, instruments, and machinery, was that they might not cease to prosper for the common good of these kingdoms and of the Indies, because if this were done, the results would be very injurious, and neither the plaintiff nor the defendant would benefit thereby. And

* Cited in Ortiz, *op. cit.*, p. 277.
** Cited in Ortiz, *op. cit.*, pp. 276—279.

because it is necessary to take the claims of creditors into account, we declare and order that if the debt is so large that it amounts to the full value of the mill, with slaves, equipment, and all its fittings, and the debtor has not other property to satisfy the creditor's claims, the whole mill, with slaves and equipment, may be attached in payment of the debt, and the person attaching the property must give guarantees that he will maintain it in working order, as the debtor had it.

---

### No. 30—PUERTO RICAN SUGAR PRODUCTION TOWARDS THE END OF THE SIXTEENTH CENTURY

*(Report of Capt. Juan Melgarejo, Governor of Puerto Rico, to Philip II, King of Spain, January 1, 1582)*\*

There are eleven water mills in the island and one horse-drawn mill, but they make little sugar because they have only a few Negro slaves, and those are old and tired. Every year some die, and once they are all dead this profit, which is the island's chief support today, and which explains why it is not totally abandoned, will come to an end. The annual output of the eleven water mills averages 15,000 *arrobas*\*\* of sugar, but it could be increased to 50,000 and even more if each mill had a hundred slaves. These mills are really settlements, like villages in Spain, because of the beautiful buildings they contain, each slave and overseer having his private house, apart from the "big house", so that the whole looks like a Spanish farmhouse....

---

### No. 31 — THE DECLINE OF THE SUGAR ECONOMY OF PUERTO RICO

*(Report of Don Sancho Ochoa de Castro, Governor of Puerto Rico, 1602)*\*\*\*

The water mills have been totally abandoned. Their owners have turned their attention to the cultivation of ginger and deserted that of sugar. The eight water mills of the island have reached such a pass that last year the production did not even amount to 3,000 *arrobas*, though the island can produce upwards of 10,000 *arrobas*.

On my assumption of the government of the island I found a letter instructing me to give orders for increasing the production of the mills, and the Municipal Council of

\* Cited in Cayetano Coll y Toste, *Boletin Historico de Puerto Rico,* Vol. I, pp. 75—91.

\*\* Approximately 90 *arrobas* are equivalent to one long ton.

\*\*\* Cited in Department of History, University of Puerto Rico, *Antologia de Lecturas sobre la Historia de Puerto Rico,* Tomo I, p. 47, from S. Brau, *Dos Factores de Colonizacion de Puerto Rico,* San Juan, 1908, pp. 11—12.

this city had received a letter to the same effect. . . .I issued an ordinance forbidding owners of mills, either themselves or by their agents, to plant ginger or to turn their attention to anything but the manufacture of sugar. . . .

Last year's ginger crop—which has not yet been com-pletely exported because of a lack of ships — amounted to 15,000 *arrobas*. This could only have been possible by aban-doning the manufacture of sugar, as a result of which the island's trade must be lost, because owing to the overproduc-tion of ginger the price has fallen each year and there are hardly any buyers. . . .

---

*No. 32—THE COMPETITION OF THE SOUTH AMERICAN*
*SUGAR INDUSTRY* . .
*(Thomas Gage, The English-American, A New Survey of the*
*West Indies, London, 1648)\**

Within a mile and a half of this town there is a rich *ingenio* or farm of sugar belonging to one Sebastian de Savaletta, a Biscayan born, who came at first very poor into that country, and served one of his countrymen; but with his good industry and pains he began to get a mule or two to traffic with about the country, till at last he increased his stock to a whole *requa* of mules, and from thence grew so rich that he bought much land about Petapa, which he found to be very fit for sugar, and from thence was encour-aged to build a princely house, whither the best of Guatemala do resort for their recreation. This man maketh a great deal of sugar for the country, and sends every year much to Spain; he keepeth at least threescore slaves of his own for the work of his farm, is very generous in housekeeping, and is thought to be worth above five hundred thousand ducats. Within half a mile from him there is another farm of sugar, which is called but a *trapiche* belonging unto the Augustine friars of Guatemala, which keeps some twenty slaves, and is called a *trapiche* for that it grinds not the sugar cane with that device of the *ingenio*, but grinds a less quantity, and so makes not so much sugar as doth an *ingenio*. From hence three miles is the town of Amatitlan, near unto which standeth a greater *ingenio* of sugar than is that of Savaletta, and is called the *ingenio* of one Anis, because he first founded it, but now it belongeth unto one Pedro Crespo the post-master of Guatemala; this *ingenio* seemeth to be a little town by itself for the many cottages and thatched houses of blackamoor slaves which belong unto it, who may be above a hundred, men, women and children. The chief dwelling house is strong and capacious, and able to entertain a hundred lodgers. These three farms of sugar standing so near unto Guatemala enrich the city much, and occasion great trading from it to Spain.

\* *Op. cit.*, 1946 edition, London (A. P. Newton, ed.), pp. 217—218.

# CHAPTER III

# The White Population Problem

## No. 33—COLUMBUS' POPULATION PROPOSALS

*(Christopher Columbus to Ferdinand and Isabella, King and Queen of Spain, 1493)* *

In the first place, in regard to the Spanish Island: that there should go there settlers up to the number of two thousand who may want to go so as to render the possession of the country safer and cause it to be more profitable and helpful in the intercourse and traffic with the neighbouring islands.

Likewise, that in the said island three or four towns be founded at convenient places, and the settlers be properly distributed among said places and towns....

Likewise, that in each place and settlement there be a mayor or mayors and a clerk according to the custom of Castile.

Likewise, that a church be built, and that priests or friars be sent there for the administration of the sacraments, and for divine worship and the conversion of the Indians.

## No. 34 — ENCOURAGING SETTLERS

*(Decree of Ferdinand and Isabella, King and Queen of Spain, April, 10, 1495)* * *

Any persons who wish to live and dwell in the said Hispaniola without pay, may go and will go freely, and there they will be free, and will pay no duty, and will have for themselves and for their heirs, or for those deriving any right from them, the houses they may build, the lands they may cultivate, and the farms they may plant, for there in the said island they will be assigned lands and places for that purpose by the persons we have put in charge; and those persons who will thus live and dwell in the said Hispaniola without pay, as has been said, will be maintained for a year. We also wish, and this is our will and pleasure, that those who go to the said Hispaniola with permission granted by those whom we have deputed for this purpose, may keep for themselves a third of the gold which they may find and get

*Cited in Bourne, *The Northmen, Columbus and Cabot*, p. 274.
**Cited in Navarrete, *op. cit.*, Tomo II, Num. LXXXVI, p. 197.

in the said island, as long as it is not for exchange, and the
remaining two-thirds will be for Us....; and besides, those
who go with permission may keep all the merchandise and
anything else they may find in the said island, giving a tenth
part of it to Us.... except for the gold of which they will
give us two-thirds....

---

## No 35—STATE AIDED IMMIGRATION

*(Ferdinand and Isabella, King and Queen of Spain to
Christopher Columbus, April 23 and June 15, 1497)\**

....there may go.... with you the number of three
hundred and thirty persons, whom you will select according
to their rank and occupation.... but if you feel that some
of them should be moved by promoting or changing them
from one occupation to another, or from the rank of some
persons to others, you, or whoever has your power, may do
it and will do it according to the manner and form, and at
the time which you deem fit to our service, and to the goodness and usefulness of the said government and business
of the said Indies....

 Item : that when you are in the said Indies, God willing,
you establish.... in Hispaniola another village or fortress
beyond the one on the other side of the island next to the
gold mine....

 Item : that near the said village, or near the one which
is already there, or in some other place which you deem
suitable, there be started and established some farming and
breeding so that the persons.... in the said island may maintain themselves better and cheaper; and in order that this
may be better done, the farmers who will now go to the
said Indies should be given and will be given from the bread
which will be sent there, up to fifty dozen bushels of wheat
for sowing, and up to twenty pairs of cows or mares or
other beasts for farming, and the farmers who thus receive
the said bread will raise it and sow it, and will be obliged
to gather the harvest, and will pay one-tenth of what they
may collect, and the rest they can sell to Christians at the
best price possible, as long as the prices are not too high
for those who buy them, because, if that is the case, you,
our said Admiral, or whoever should have your power, will
moderate and regulate it.

 Item : that the said number of three hundred and
thirty persons who may go to the said Indies shall be paid
and will be paid their salaries at the rates at which up to
now they have been paid, and instead of their usual maintenance, they shall be given and will be given from the bread
which we send there, to each person a *fanega* of wheat per
*Cited in Navarrete, *op. cit.*, Tomo II, Num. CXL, pp. 239—242.

month and twelve maravedis per day so that they may buy other necessary supplies....

Item : that if you, the said Admiral, should see and believe that it is fitting for our service that their number should be augmented over the said three hundred and thirty persons, you may increase it until you reach the number of five hundred persons in all....the said three hundred and thirty persons must be selected by you, our said Admiral... and must be distributed as follows: forty squires, a hundred foot soldiers, thirty sailors, thirty cabin boys, twenty gold washers, fifty farmers and gardeners, twenty officials of all occupations, and thirty women;.... but if it seems to you ....of benefit and convenience to our business to change the said number of persons, reducing the number of officials and putting others in their place, you may do it, as long as the number of persons who will be in the Indies does not exceed three hundred and thirty persons, and not more.

Item : that for the maintenance of the said Admiral, and of your brothers, and other officials who are important persons going with you to the said Indies, and for the said three hundred and thirty persons, and in order to farm and sow and to control the beasts which you shall take there, six thousand six hundred bushels of wheat, and six hundred bushels of barley should and will be taken; which should and will be provided for from the thirds of the bread belonging to us from the Archbishopric of Seville and the Bishopric of Cadiz from last year....

Item: that there will be sent to the said Indies the tools and apparatus which the said Admiral may consider necessary for farming in the said Indies; and likewise, hoes, spades, pickaxes, stone hammers, and levers which would be convenient for the said Indies.

Likewise, that with the cows and mares which are in the said Indies there will be made the number of twenty yokes of cows or mares or donkeys with which they can do farming in the said Indies, as it may seem convenient to the said Admiral.

And likewise, it seems convenient to buy an old vessel in which to carry the supplies and the aforesaid things which may fit in it, because use could be made of its planks, wood and nails for the town which is being built now in the other part of Hispaniola, near the mines; but if it does not seem right to you, the said Admiral, to take the said vessel it shall not be taken.

Besides, there should be taken to the said Indies six hundred bushels of wheat and up to one thousand quintals of biscuit, pending provision for the construction of mills and bakeries, for which purpose there must be taken from here some stones and other mill apparatus.

Item: that there should be taken to the said Indies two tents which will cost up to twenty thousand maravedis.

Item: with respect to the other supplies and provisions which it will be necessary to take to the said Indies for the maintenance and clothing of those who will be there, we believe the following form should be adopted.

That they look for some sincere and reliable persons, who will be charged by you, the said Admiral, to load and carry to the said Indies the said supplies, and other things of great necessity there. for which they shall be given and will be given from the maravedis we have kept for this whatever you think reasonable, and they will let us know when they receive the maravedis, which they will use for the said supplies, which will be loaded and taken to the coast of the said Indies, and going at our risk and at the sea's mercy. Upon arrival there, God willing, they should sell and will sell the said supplies: the wine at fifteen maravedis the *azumbre,** and a pound of salt pork and salt meat at eight maravedis; and the other supplies and vegetables at the price that you and the other Lieutenants may fix for them, so that they may have some profit and will not lose in it, and no harm will be done to the people. From the maravedis which such person or persons may get from the said supplies that they sell, they should give and pay, and will give and pay there to our Treasurer.... in the said Indies, the said maravedis which you had given to them, in order to buy the said supplies, so that with them you will pay the salary of the people....

Item: we should try to send to the said Indies some religious men and clergymen, good persons, so that they will administer the Holy Sacraments to those who will be there, and will try to convert to our Holy Catholic Faith the said native Indians of the said Indies, and will take for them the apparatus and things which are required for the service of the worship of God and for the administration of the sacraments.

Likewise, there should go a physician, an apothecary, a herbist, and some instruments and music should be taken for the entertainment of the people.

---

## No. 36—THE TRANSPORTATION OF CONVICTS

*(Proclamation of Ferdinand and Isabella, King and Queen of Spain, June 22, 1497)**

....we have commanded the loading of certain ships and vessels in which there will go certain people who have been paid for a certain time, and a supply of provisions and

*About 2 litres.
**Cited in Navarrete, *op, cit.,* Tomo II, Num. CXX, p. 249.

supplies for them, and because they are not enough for the development of a town as befits the service of God and ours, if other people do not go to reside and live and serve in them at their own cost, we, wishing to provide for this, for the conversion and settlement as well as for clemency and pity towards our subjects and nationals, issue this our decree.... that each and every male person, and our many subjects and nationals who may have committed up to the day of publication of this decree any murders or any other crimes of whatever nature and quality they might be, except heresy and *lese majeste* or....treason, or perfidy, or sure death, whether caused by fire or arrow, or counterfeiting or sodomy, or stealing of copper, gold or silver, or other things vetoed by Us in our Kingdoms, shall go and serve in person in Hispaniola, at their own cost, as commanded by the Admiral in our name. Those who deserve the death penalty will serve for two years, and those who deserve a minor penalty than death, even though it might be the loss of a member, for a year and will be pardoned for whatever crimes and transgressions of whatever sort and quality and gravity they might be, which they may have done or committed up to the day of the publication of this our Decree, except for the cases aforesaid....

## No. 37 — COLUMBUS' DESCRIPTION OF THE EARLY SETTLERS

### (Christopher Columbus to the Nurse of the Prince Don John, 1500)*

....in the whole of Espanola there are very few save vagabonds, and not one with wife and children.... a dissolute people, who fear neither God, nor their King and Queen, being full of vices and wickedness....

....It is useless to publish such immunities in the Indies; to the settlers who have taken up residence it is a pure gain, for the best lands were given to them, and at a low valuation they will be worth two hundred thousand at the end of the four years when the period of residence is ended, without their digging a spadeful in them. I would not speak thus if the settlers were married, but there are not six among them all who are not on the lookout to gather what they can and depart speedily. It would be a good thing if people should go from Castile, and also if it were known who and what they are, and if the country could be settled with honest people....Now that so much gold is found, a dispute arises as to which brings more profit,

*Cited in Bourne, *The Northmen, Columbus and Cabot,* pp. 373-374, 377-378.

whether to go about robbing, or to go to the mines. A hundred castellanos* are as easily obtained for a woman as for
a farm, and it is very general and there are plenty of dealers
who go looking about for girls; those form nine to ten are
now in demand, and for all ages a good price must be paid.

---

### No. 38—POPULATION AND PROFITS

*(Ferdinand I, King of Spain, to Nicolas de Ovando, Governor
of Hispaniola, October 21, 1507)***

I should like to know why you request that no more
people, even workmen, be allowed to go there until you ask
for them. It is believed here that the more people there are
to work, the greater will be the profit.

---

### No. 39 — THE COLONIAL DEMAND FOR FREEDOM OF MOVEMENT

*(Alonso Zuazo, Judge of Hispaniola, to Cardinal Ximenes,
Regent of Spain, January 22, 1518)* ***

It is necessary to allow people from all parts of the
world to come to this land to populate it freely, and to
grant general permission for this purpose, excluding only
Moors, Jews and reconciled persons, their children and
grandchildren, as prescribed in the ordinance, since such
persons are always evilly disposed, seditious and revolution-
ary in towns and communities.

---

### No. 40—THE SURPLUS POPULATION THEORY IN HISPANIOLA

*(The Jeronimite Commission to Cardinal Ximenes, Regent of
Spain, February 1518)* ****

The admission of many labourers and workmen will ensure the foundation of a population: wheat, vines, cotton
plants, etc., will in time give better return than gold. It
must be proclaimed publicly over there that all natives of

---

*One-sixth of an ounce, or in value about $3.
**Cited in L. B. Simpson, *The Encomienda in New Spain*, University of Cali-
fornia Press, 1950, p. 18.
***Cited in J. A. Saco, *Historia de la Esclavitud de la Raza Africana en el
Nuevo Mundo y en especial en los Paises Americo — Hispanos* (Paris, 1875,
Vols. I and II; Barcelona, 1877-1879, Vols. III and IV), 1938 edition, Coleccion de
Libros Cubanos, Havana, Tomo 1, p. 136.
****Cited in Saco, *op. cit.*, Tomo I, p. 137.

Spain, Portugal and the Canaries are free to go and remain, and that they may carry merchandise and supplies from all ports of Castile without going to Seville. Let his Highness order the surplus population of these realms, etc., to go and colonise these territories.

---

### No. 41—THE  UNDERPOPULATION  PROBLEM

*(Decree of Charles V, Emperor of the Hapsburg Empire, January 15, 1529)\**

The King — Reverend Doctor Sebastian Ramirez, Bishop of Santo Domingo and La Concepcion de la Vega, and our President of the Court of Hispaniola. Friar Tomas de Verlanga, Vicar Provincial of the Dominicans in those parts, on behalf of the Judges, officials and colonists of Hispaniola whom he represented, moved by zeal for the welfare of the island, petitioned us for many things, among them this favour, viz., that there should be a great increase in the population, revenue, etc. This request having been heard by my royal Person on several occasions, as well as by my Council, I have consented to grant the following contract and agreement to the colonists and settlers of the said island.

1. Anyone who undertakes and gives sufficient guarantee for the commencement of a new settlement in the said island, with persons who do not belong to that island or to any other part of the Indies, the said settlement to consist of at least fifty married couples, twenty–five free and twenty–five Negroes, a church and a solid stone presbytery, a priest provided at his expense and who agrees to supply freight and ship stores for all, to build houses for them, to give everyone two cows or oxen, fifty sheep, one mare, ten pigs, two colts, and six hens; to establish a settlement within a year of receiving the land, and to complete it in two more years, building twenty–five stone houses within five years and completing all fifty within ten years, shall be given a site and boundaries for his land by the President of the Court — the site varying in size up to two square leagues, and up to three square leagues if it be more than ten leagues distant from the city of Santo Domingo — without prejudice to the towns and villages previously founded.

2. He shall not be given a site on the harbour nor in any other place where, in the opinion of the President, it may later be to the disadvantage of the Crown.

3. We reserve the forests and trees of Brazil wood, the balsam and drugs which exist in the said limits, because of our contract with other persons in this connection.

\*Cited in Saco, *op. cit.*, Tomo I, pp. 236-239.

4. With the above exceptions, and barring such other precaution as may be necessary to preserve the rights of the Crown, we grant to those who establish settlements as provided above the ownership of the said settlements, with right of succession, civil and criminal jurisdiction, without prejudice to the rights of our sovereignty and those of the Admiral of the Indies.

5. They may establish an inalienable, imperishable and non-transferable right of succession thereto, which may only be rendered null and void by reason of some crime, treason or unnatural sin.

6. We grant them the mines and pearl fisheries in their districts on condition that they pay us a fifth of the returns or the same proportion as the other inhabitants of the island.

7. We grant to the said founders and their successors in the said right of succession the twentieth part of all our profits in the said district.

8. Whatever belongings the first settlers bring into the island for their own use shall be free of all duty on the first occasion.

9. We grant the founder the right to nominate the notary public in his village and the patronage of the benefit or benefits of this office. In each village we also grant the tithes which belong to us in all the Indies by apostolic gift, to assist manufacturing and the clergy.

10. In the deed of ownership, or separately, as they may prefer, we shall create the said founders noblemen and knights, shall give them arms and escutcheon according to their wishes so that they and their descendants and successors may thereafter always be lords, knights and nobles, may use arms, impeach and challenge, accept challenges to combat and duel throughout the Indies.

We entrust the administration of everything, the contract with the settlers, the taking of pledges, etc., the issuance of an order signed with his name, to the President of the Court of Hispaniola.

---

## No. 42 — EMIGRATION TO THE CONTINENT

*(Ramirez Fuenleal, Bishop of Santo Domingo, to Empress of Spain, April 30, 1532)\**

Alvarado is preparing a fleet to go on a voyage of discovery as far as Peru. Very great harm to all that has been discovered results from these expeditions and discoveries, for the people who come to these parts are adventurers in search only of what may be stolen, and as soon as they hear of a new discovery, they scrap their proposal to settle

*Cited in Saco, *op. cit.*, Tomo I, pp. 250-251.

down and make their homes and go off again in the belief
that the land to be discovered is another New Spain. They
die because of the newness of the land.

---

### No. 43 — "MAY GOD TAKE ME TO PERU!"

*(Francisco Manuel de Lando to Charles V, Emperor of the
Hapsburg Empire, Puerto Rico, July 2, 1534)\**

My visit to San German quieted the people who were
all excited about going off to Peru. They are burdened with
debt, especially for slaves whom they bought on credit.
They have mined little gold, and their payments have fallen
due; their property has been attached, and they have been
forced to sell their goods at three-tenths of the purchase
price. Many have taken to the hills.

Crazy over the news from Peru, many have departed
secretly from the numerous little harbours remote from
the main centres of population. Those who remain, even
those with deepest roots in the island, have but a single
thought, "May God take me to Peru". Night and day I keep
watch so that on one should decamp, but I am not certain
that I can restrain the people.

Two months ago I learned that some individuals had
carried off a boat two leagues from this city in order to
leave the island. I sent three boats and twenty horsemen and
there was no end of difficulty in apprehending them because
of the resistance they put up. They desisted only when
three had been killed by arrows, others wounded, and I
appeared on the scene. Some were whipped, the legs of
others were cut off; and I had to overlook some seditious
language from others who had joined them and planned
to await them on Mona Island, two leagues away. If Your
Majesty does not promptly find some remedy, I fear that the
island, even though it may not be totally abandoned, will
remain no more than a wayside inn. It is the entrance and
key to the Indies; it is the first island which the French and
English pirates run into. The Caribs carry off our settlers
and their friends without let or hindrance. If a ship should
come at night, with only fifty men, it would burn and kill
the entire population. I beseech you to grant favours and
privileges to this noble island whose population is now so
depleted that one sees hardly any Spaniards but only
Negroes. . . . I know that some people here have requested
permission to take their Negro slaves to Peru. Your Majesty
should not give permission to go either to them or to the
slaves. . . .

---

*Cited in *Antologia de Lecturas* sobre la Historia de Puerto Rico, Tomo I,
p. 29, from Tapia y Rivera, *op. cit.*, pp. 304-305.

## No. 44 — THE QUALITY OF WHITE IMMIGRANTS

*(Judge Esteve of Hispaniola to Charles V, Emperor of the Hapsburg Empire, 1550)\**

Settlers such as those the Attorney General.... brought over in the capacity of labourers, are of no use. They were barbers, tailors, and useless persons who soon sold the twelve cows and the bull which Your Majesty gave them for their sustenance.... They did not know how to work, and only peopled the hospitals and the cemeteries. There are enough settlers of this kind to spare Your Majesty the necessity of supplying ship stores for more of them.

---

## No. 45 — PORTRAIT OF THE CONQUISTADORES

*(Lopez de Velasco, Geografia y Descripcion universal de las Indias, Madrid, 1571-1574)\*\**

There would be many more Spaniards in those provinces than there now are if permission to go were given to all who want to go there; but ordinarily it has been the general policy to send out from these kingdoms men who hate work and who are of rebellious dispositions and spirits and who are more anxious to get rich quickly than to settle permanently in the country. Not satisfied with being sure of food and clothing, which would never be lacking to anyone in these parts who are moderately diligent in procuring them, whether they be officers or farm hands, or not even that, forgetting their proper place, they raise themselves to a higher level and go about the country, idle vagabonds, making pretensions to offices and allotments of Indians.

---

## No. 46 — SPAIN'S IMMIGRATION AND EMIGRATION POLICY

*(J. Veitia de Linaje, Norte de la Contratacion de las Indias Occidentales, Seville, 1672. English Translation by John Stevens, The Spanish Rule of Trade to the Indies, London, 1702)\*\*\**

2. King Ferdinand, in the year 1511, gave an order for all persons whatsoever, that were subjects of Spain, to be

\*Cited in Saco, *op. cit.*, Tomo II, pp. 28-29.
\*\**Op. cit.*, p. 36.
\*\*\**Op. cit.*, pp. 107-115.

allowed to go over to the Indies without any distinction, or examination, only entering their names, that the numbers might be known.  Afterwards in the years 1518, 1522, 1530, and 1539, several orders passed, which were established as Laws, and direct, that no person reconciled, or newly converted to our Holy Catholic Faith, from Judaism or Mahometanism, nor the children of such, nor the children or grandsons of any that had worn the St. Andrew's Cross of the Inquisition, or been burnt or condemned as heretics, or for any heretical crime, either by male or female line, might go over to the Indies, upon pain of forfeiting all their goods, of an hundred lashes, perpetual banishment from the Indies, and their bodies to be at the King's disposal. In the year 1501, Nicholas de Obando being appointed Governor of the Firm Land, was commanded not to permit any Moors, Jews, heretics, or new converts, to live in that country, except slaves born under Christian masters who are natives of Spain.  Herrera tells us, that Their Catholic Majesties in 1496, granted a pardon to all criminals that would go over to the Island Hispaniola, and the third part of all the gold they got out of the mines, to all persons that would settle there.

3. King Philip II whilst he governed Spain for the Emperor his father in the year 1552, to prevent false informations, ordered, that for the future, the Judges or Commissioners of the India-House, should not suffer any person whatsoever, tho' of such as were allowed, or tho' he had the King's Letter of License, to go over to the Indies, unless they brought certificates from the places where they were born, to make appear whether they were married, or single, describing their persons, setting down their age, and declaring that they are neither Jews nor Moors, nor children of such, persons newly reconciled, nor sons or grandsons of any that have been punished, condemned, or burnt, as heretics, or for heretical crimes, such certificate to be signed by the magistrates of the city, town or place where such persons are born.  In 1559, orders were sent to the Prelates in the Indies, to inquire whether there were any Jews, Moors, or heretics in those parts, and to punish them severely.  And in 1566, all the sons and grandsons of heretics, and new converts, were excluded all places of trust, upon pain of forfeiture of goods, and their bodies to be at the King's disposal.

4. Besides these circumstances mentioned to capacitate persons to go over to the Indies, they are to have His Majesty's leave, or else the President's and Commissioners'; without which, no man, whether native or alien, may pass thither.  The first penalty imposed for breach of this Law, was 100,000 maravedis, that is about 52 1. sterling fine, ten

years banishment for gentlemen, and 100 lashes for mean persons. In the Indies, the Magistrates are directed to apprehend any persons they find are gone over without leave, to imprison them till they can send them back into Spain, upon pain of losing their employments, and forfeiting 50,000 maravedis; that is, 26 1. sterling....

5. Having declared that no persons may go over to the Indies without leave, and whereas the King may grant it to whom he pleases, it remains to show to whom the President and Commissioners may grant leave. They are not only to grant leave to Mestizos, that is Mongrels between Spaniards and Indians, who are brought into Spain, but to oblige them to return, and to furnish them with necessaries, if they have not of their own. They may grant passes to merchants to go over, or return if they came from thence, including married merchants, provided they have leave from their wives, and give 1,000 ducats security to return within three years. To factors, but to them only for three years, tho' they be bachelors, and they are to give security for their return; and this exception to factors makes out, that other bachelors who go over with leave, may stay and inhabit there. To any inhabitants of the Indies, whom they know to be married there, whom they may oblige to go back to their wives. But if they that come from the Indies be not married, excepting merchants, tho' they be born there, they may not return without leave from the King himself. As concerning factors, it is to be observed, that  the President and Commissioners may not only oblige them to return to be accountable to their merchants, but to pay besides the principal, such interest as two merchants shall adjudge, for the time they have delayed returns; and those factors that reside in Spain, and manage for merchants in the Indies, are to be compelled to send the owners their returns without any delay.

6. ....it is the constant practice to give passes, as merchants, to all persons that produce certificates of their having shipped goods to the value of above 300,000 maravedies, that is, between 70 and 80 pounds sterling, as rated, for to pay the King's duties; and strict orders have been given that no passes should be granted to such as pretended themselves to be merchants on account of shipping off some small parcels, alleging they go to keep shops, or set up a trade in those parts.

7. Married women, whose husbands are in the Indies, are permitted to go over to them, and to take along with them a kinsman within the fourth degree of consanguinity, but if the husbands themselves come for their wives, they may not return without the King's leave. In all cases whatsoever, the women are to make the same proofs as the men, as to their qualifications. They that carry over, or send for their wives, are to make sufficient proof that they are such. Married merchants that leave their wives behind, are not compelled to bring certificates as to their qualifications, because they give security to return within three years. All single women are positively forbid going over to the Indies.

8. No person, tho' commissioned by the King for any employment in those parts, being a married man, can go over without his wife; and tho' the President and Commissioners can give leave to merchants, who have their wives' consent, yet they cannot to Governors, or any other Officers, without His Majesty's express dispensation in this case, and the same as to exempting them and their wives from bringing the usual certificates of qualifications, which they must give as well as the meanest person, if they are not exempted by the King. Nor may they go aboard upon the King's Commission, without having his Licence; tho' sometimes, there being no legal obstacle, they have been cleared upon giving security that their pass would come after them from Court. And it is ordered, that the Admirals, and other officers, receive no man, that is commissioned for an employment in the Indies, without a pass from the India-House, tho' he has one from the King. . . .

10. None are to be admitted to go over as servants whose charge is not defrayed by him that names them. Passes, or licences, not made use of when granted, are of no use afterwards; nor any from the King, if they are not presented within two years. Admirals, and other Sea-Commanders, are charged, under the penalty of 1,000 ducats, not to convey over any passengers, as sailors or soldiers; but this does not contradict the order to them, that in case of want of soldiers, they list such passengers as come or go with leave, yet that they give them no pay, but only allowance of provision, to commence eight days before they go aboard.

10.* All passengers are to carry their own provisions, and no Officers to give them their Table. The Admiral is to see all their passes, and to distribute them, to take care

*Sic.

that no masters of ships undertake to furnish their diet; to make them swear they will not stay behind in any port where the fleet shall happen to put in, nor carry any goods ashore before they are searched. All Officers, and beneficed persons, and such as bring over gold or silver that is entered, are to be preferred before others to go aboard the galleons, yet so that they do not encumber themselves with people unfit for service. He that goes over with a licence to reside in any particular town in the Indies, is to make his abode there.... and handicrafts that go over on pretence of following their callings, are to be obliged to perform it....

12. The inhabitants of the Indies may not come to Spain without leave from the Viceroys, Presidents, or Governors of the places of their habitation, in which they are to express the causes of their coming, and whether it is to stay here or return; and if they be agents for any corporation it must be expressed, that they show their commission before the Council within two months after their arrival. The Governors of seaports are forbid granting licences to any persons that are not under their Government, without they bring them from those they belong to; nor is any pass to be given to any that does not make out he is not indebted to the chests belonging to persons departed, or to the King.

12.* Those that pass over to the Indies with leave, are to go aboard the ships that are bound for those ports their licenses mention; and none ought to go aboard the ships from the Canary Islands, without leave from the Council. The inhabitants of those Islands may not settle in the Indies without leave expressly had. There is a particular Officer in the Office of Comptroller of the India-House, who enters all licenses, given to passengers, in books for that purpose. There are no laws but what covetousness breaks through, and therefore some persons have taken out licenses to sell to others, which has been strictly forbid, and both the buyers and sellers ordered to be severely punished, as also those who forge licences. If any married man be found to have gone over under a bachelor's pass, he is to be sent back, and no credit to be given to married men that shall show certificates of their wives being dead, unless they have been passed by the Council.

13. ....the Law says, that from the time the ships sail from the Indies, till they are searched in Seville, no man is to go ashore (but in case it be absolutely necessary, then one is to go in the presence of all the rest) under pain of forfeiture of goods to the Master of the ship: and the persons going ashore, their bodies to be at the King's disposal, and the informer to have the third part of the goods.

*Sic.

14. King Philip the Second, in the year 1560, made an Ordinance to restrain any persons from going to the Indies without license, by which all they shall acquire in those parts is forfeited to the Crown, only one-fifth part for the informer, and that they be secured and sent prisoners into Spain at their own expense: and any effects of theirs brought by them, or sent over, not to be delivered to them or their order, nor to their heirs if they be dead, but to be confiscate to the King. And moreover, the Bull of Pope Alexander VI excommunicates all persons, of what degree or condition soever, that shall presume to go over to the Indies without leave from Their Catholic Majesties.

# CHAPTER IV

# The Problem of Aboriginal Indian Labour

## (i) — THE ABORIGINAL INDIANS

### No. 47—THE CIVILISATION OF THE ABORIGINAL INDIANS

*("Journal of the First Voyage of Christopher Columbus", 1492-1493)\**

#### Friday, 12th of October

....I gave some of them red caps, and glass beads to put round their necks, and many other things of little value, which gave them great pleasure, and made them so much our friends that it was a marvel to see. They afterwards came to the ship's boats where we were, swimming and bringing us parrots, cotton threads in skeins, darts, and many other things; and we exchanged them for other things that we gave them, such as glass beads and small bells. In fine, they took all, and gave what they had with good will. It appeared to me to be a race of people very poor in everything. They go as naked as when their mothers bore them, and so do the women, although I did not see more than one young girl. All I saw were youths, none more than thirty years of age. They are very well made, with very handsome bodies, and very good countenances. Their hair is short and coarse, almost like the hair of a horse's tail. They wear the hair brought down to the eyebrows, except a few locks behind, which they wear long and never cut. They paint themselves black, and they are the colour of the Canarians, neither black nor white. Some paint themselves white, others red, and others of what colour they find. Some paint their faces, others the whole body, some only round the eyes, others only on the nose. They neither carry nor know anything of arms, for I showed them swords, and they took them by the blade and cut themselves through ignorance. They have no iron, their darts being wands without iron, some of them having a fish's tooth at the end, and others being pointed in various ways. They are all of fair stature and size, with good faces, and well made. I saw some with marks of wounds on their bodies, and I made signs to ask what it was, and they gave me to under-

* Cited in Bourne, *The Northmen, Columbus and Cabot*, pp. 110—112, 138, 164, 192, 194—195, 198, 203—204, 224.

stand that people from other adjacent islands came with the
intention of seizing them, and that they defended themselves. I believed, and still believe, that they come here from
the mainland to make them prisoners.... I believe that
they would easily be made Christians, as it appeared to me
that they had no religion. I, our Lord being pleased, will
take hence, at the time of my departure, six natives for
your Highnesses, that they may learn to speak. I saw no
beast of any kind except parrots, on this island....

### Saturday, 13th of October

....They came to the ship in small canoes, made out
of the trunk of a tree like a long boat, and all of one piece,
and wonderfully worked, considering the country. They are
large, some of them holding 40 to 45 men, others smaller,
and some only large enough to hold one man. They are pro-
pelled with a paddle like a baker's shovel, and go at a
marvellous rate....

### Sunday, 4th of November

....He also understood that, far away, there were men
with one eye, and others with dogs' noses who were cannibals, and that when they captured an enemy, they beheaded
him and drank his blood, and cut off his private parts....

### Monday, 3rd of December

....The Admiral assures the Sovereigns that ten
thousand of these men would run from ten, so cowardly and
timid are they....

### Friday, 21st of December

....The Admiral gave them glass beads, brass trinkets,
and bells: not because they asked for anything in return, but
because it seemed right, and above all, because he now
looked upon them as future Christians, and subjects of the
Sovereign, as much as the people of Castile. He further says
that they want nothing except to know the language and be
under governance; for all they may be told to do will be
done without contradiction....

### Saturday, 22nd of December

....As the Indians are so simple, and the Spaniards so
avaricious and grasping, it does not suffice that the Indians
should give them all they want in exchange for a bead or a
bit of glass, but the Spaniards would take everything without any return at all. The Admiral always prohibits this, although, with the exception of gold, the things given by the

Indians are of little value. But the Admiral, seeing the simplicity of the Indians, and that they will give a piece of gold in exchange for six beads, gave the order that nothing should be received from them unless something had been given in exchange....

### Monday, 24th of December

....A better race there cannot be, and both the people and the lands are in such quantity that I know not how to write it. I have spoken in the superlative degree of the country and people of Juana, which they call Cuba, but there is as much difference between them and this island and people as between day and night. I believe that no one who should see them could say less than I have said, and I repeat that the things and the great villages of this island of Espanola, which they call Bohio, are wonderful. All here have a loving manner and gentle speech, unlike the others, who seem to be menacing when they speak. Both men and women are of good stature, and not black. It is true that they all paint, some with black, others with other colours, but most with red. I know that they are tanned by the sun, but this does not affect them much. Their houses and villages are pretty, each with a chief, who acts as their judge, and who is obeyed by them. All these lords use few words, and have excellent manners. Most of their orders are given by a sign with the hand, which is understood with surprising quickness....

### Wednesday, 26th of December

....The Chief.... began to talk of those of Caniba, whom they call Caribes. They come to capture the natives, and have bow and arrows without iron, of which there is no memory in any of these lands, nor of steel, nor any other metal except gold and copper. Of copper the Admiral had only seen very little. The Admiral said, by signs, that the Sovereigns of Castile would order the Caribs to be destroyed, and that all should be taken with their hands tied together.... Now I have given orders for a tower and a fort, both well built, and a large cellar, not because I believe that such defences will be necessary. I believe that with the force I have with me I could subjugate the whole island, which I believe to be larger than Portugal, and the population double.... Still, it is advisable to build this tower, being so far from your Highnesses. The people may thus know the skill of the subjects of your Highnesses, and what they can do; and will obey them with love and fear....

## Sunday, 13th of January

....As soon as they came to the boat, the crew landed, and began to buy the bows and arrows and other arms, in accordance with an order of the Admiral. Having sold two bows, they did not want to give more, but began to attack the Spaniards, and to take hold of them.... the Spaniards attacked the Indians, and gave one a slash with a knife in the buttocks, wounding another in the breast with an arrow.... The Christians would have killed many, if the pilot, who was in command, had not prevented them.... The Admiral regretted the affair for one reason, and was pleased for another. They would have fear of the Christians, and they were no doubt an ill-conditioned people, probably Caribs, who eat men.... he would have liked to have captured some of them....

---

## No. 48—THE CARIBS

### (Dr. Chanca to the Town Council of Seville, 1493)*

....We were enabled to distinguish which of the women were Caribbees, and which were not, by the Caribbees wearing on each leg two bands of woven cotton, the one fastened round the knee, and the other round the ankle; by this means they make the calves of their legs large, and the above-mentioned parts very small, which I imagine that they regard as a mark of elegance; by this peculiarity we distinguished them. The habits of these Caribbees are brutal. There are three islands: this is called Turuqueira; the other, which was the first that we saw, is called Ceyre; the third is called Ayay:** all these are alike as if they were of one race, who do no injury to each other; but each and all of them wage war against the other neighbouring islands, and for the purpose of attacking them, make voyages of a hundred and fifty leagues at sea, with their numerous canoes, which are a small kind of craft with one mast. Their arms are arrows, in the place of iron weapons, and as they have no iron, some of them point their arrows with tortoise-shell, and others make their arrow-heads of fish spines, which are naturally barbed like coarse saws; these prove dangerous weapons to a naked people like the Indians, and may cause death or severe injury, but to men of our nation, are not very formidable. In their attacks upon the neighbouring islands, these people capture as many of the women as they

* Cited in Bourne, The Northmen, Columbus and Cabot, pp. 289—291.
** Generally identified as the three islands of Guadeloupe, Mario Galante and St. Croix, though some claim that the first and third are the two islands which together form Guadeloupe, and identify Ceyre with Dominica.

can, especially those who are young and beautiful, and keep them for servants and to have as concubines; and so great a number do they carry off, that in fifty houses no men were to be seen; and out of the number of the captives, more than twenty were young girls. These women also say that the Caribbees use them with such cruelty as would scarcely be believed; and that they eat the children which they bear to them, and only bring up those which they have by their native wives. Such of their male enemies as they can take alive, they bring to their houses to slaughter them, and those who are killed they devour at once. They say that man's flesh is so good, that there is nothing like it in the world; and this is pretty evident, for of the bones which we found in their houses, they had gnawed everything that could be gnawed, so that nothing remained of them, but what from its great hardness, could not be eaten; in one of the houses we found the neck of a man, cooking in a pot. When they take any boys prisoners, they cut off their member and make use of them as servants until they grow up to manhood, and then when they wish to make a feast they kill and eat them; for they say that the flesh of boys and women is not good to eat. Three of these boys came fleeing to us thus mutilated.

---

## NO. 49—SLAVERY AMONG THE ABORIGINAL INDIANS

*(Tratado que el obispo de la ciudad de Chiapa, D. Fray Bartolome de las Casas, compuso por comision del Consejo Real de las Indias, sobre la materia de los indios que se han hecho en ellas esclavos, Seville, 1552)* *

This word slavery among the Indians does not denote or signify what it does among ourselves. It means only that one is a servant, or someone who is responsible or obliged to help and serve me in some things which I need. So that for an Indian to be a slave of another Indian meant little less than being his son. He had his house, his family, his peculium, his farm, his wife and his children, and he was in enjoyment of his liberty, like the other free subjects who were his neighbours, except when the lord needed to build his house or sow his fields or other similar things.... and all the rest of the time he had to himself and employed it to his own advantage like free persons. Besides which, the treatment which the lords meted out to such servants was very mild and lenient as if they owed them nothing. And thus without comparison they had more freedom than those whom we call in law villeins.

* Cited in J. A. Saco, *Historia de la Esclavitud de los Indios en el Nuevo Mundo, seguida de la Historia de los Repartimientos y Encomiendas,* (Havana, 1883—1892), 1932 edition, Coleccion de Libros Cubanos. Havana, Tomo I, p. 59.

## (ii) — THE SPANISH DILEMMA — CONVERSION OR ENSLAVEMENT OF THE ABORIGINAL INDIANS?

### (a) — THE DILEMMA OF COLUMBUS

### No. 50 — *THE ENSLAVEMENT OF THE ABORIGINAL INDIANS?*

*("Journal of the First Voyage of Christopher Columbus, 1492-1493")\**

#### Friday, 12th of October

....They should be good servants and intelligent, for I observe that they quickly took in what was said to them....

#### Sunday, 14th of October

....these people are very simple as regards the use of arms, as your Highnesses will see from the seven that I caused to be taken, to bring home and learn our language and return; unless your Highnesses should order them all to be brought to Castile, or to be kept as captives on the same island; for with fifty men they can all be subjugated and made to do what is required of them....

#### Monday, 12th of November

....Yesterday a canoe came alongside the ship, with six youths in it. Five came on board, and I ordered them to be detained. They are now here. I afterwards sent to a house on the western side of the river, and seized seven women, old and young, and three children. I did this because the men would behave better in Spain if they had women of their own land, than without them. For on many occasions the men of Guinea have been brought to learn the language in Portugal, and afterwards, when they returned, and it was expected that they would be useful in their land, owing to the good company they had enjoyed and the gifts they had received, they never appeared after arriving. Others may not act thus. But, having women, they have the wish to perform what they are required to do; besides, the women would teach our people their language, which is the same in all these islands, so that those who make voyages in their canoes are understood everywhere. On the other hand, there are a thousand different languages in Guinea, and one native does not understand another....

#### Sunday, 16th of December

....your Highnesses may believe that this island (Hispaniola), and all the others, are as much yours as Castile. Here there is only wanting a settlement and the order to the people to do what is required. For I, with the force I have

* Cited in Bourne, *The Northmen, Columbus and Cabot*, pp. 111, 114, 145—146, 182.

under me, which is not large, could march over all these islands without opposition. I have seen only three sailors land, without wishing to do harm, and a multitude of Indians fled before them. They have no arms, and are without warlike instincts; they all go naked, and are so timid that a thousand would not stand before three of our men. So that they are good to be ordered about, to work and sow, and do all that may be necessary, and to build towns, and they should be taught to go about clothed and to adopt our customs.

---

## No. 51 — OR THE CONVERSION OF THE ABORIGINAL INDIANS?

*("Journal of the First Voyage of Christopher Columbus,"
1492-1493)\**

### Friday, 12th of October

....Presently many inhabitants of the island assembled .... I, that we might form great friendship, for I knew that they were a people who could be more easily freed and converted to our holy faith by love than by force....

### Tuesday, 16th of October

....They do not know any religion, and I believe they could easily be converted to Christianity, for they are very intelligent....

### Tuesday, 6th of November

I hold, most serene Princes, that if devout religious persons were here, knowing the language, they would all turn Christians. I trust in our Lord that your Highnesses will resolve upon this with much diligence, to bring so many great nations within the Church, and to convert them; as you have destroyed those who would not confess the Father, the Son, and the Holy Ghost....

### Monday, 12th of November

....I saw and knew that these people are without any religion, not idolaters, but very gentle, not knowing what is evil, nor the sins of murder and theft, being without arms, and so timid that a hundred would fly before one Spaniard, although they joke with them. They, however, believe and know that there is a God in heaven, and say that we have come from Heaven. At any prayer that we say, they repeat,

* Cited in Bourne, *The Northmen, Columbus and Cabot,* pp. 110, 119, 142—144, 159—160, 198.

and make the sign of the cross. Thus your Highnesses should resolve to make them Christians, for I believe that, if the work was begun, in a little time a multitude of nations would be converted to our faith, with the acquisition of great lordships, peoples, and riches for Spain....

### Tuesday, 27th of November

....After they understand the advantages, I shall labour to make all these people Christians. They will become so readily, because they have no religion nor idolatry, and your Highnesses will send orders to build a city and fortress, and to convert the people....

### Monday, 24th of December

....Your Highnesses may believe that there is no better nor gentler people in the world. Your Highnesses ought to rejoice that they will soon become Christians, and that they will be taught the good customs of your kingdom.

---

### NO. 52 — THE SALVATION OF SOULS?

*(Speech of Christopher Columbus to Ferdinand and Isabella, King and Queen of Spain, at Barcelona, 1493)\**

God had reserved for the Spanish monarch, not only all the treasures of the New World, but a still greater treasure of inestimable value, in the infinite number of souls destined to be brought over into the bosom of the Christian Church.

---

### NO. 53—OR THE ENSLAVEMENT OF CARIBS?

*(Christopher Columbus to Ferdinand and Isabella, King and Queen of Spain, 1494)\*\**

....these cannibals, a people very savage and suitable for the purpose, and well made and of very good intelligence. We believe that they, having abandoned that inhumanity, will be better than any other slaves.

* Cited in T. Southey, *Chronolo..cal History of the West Indies*, London, 1827, Vol. I, pp. 21—22.

\*\*Cited in C. Jane, *Select Documents illustrating the Four Voyages of Columbus*, Works of the Hakluyt Society, Second Series, No. LXV, 1929, Vol. I, p. 92.

## NO. 54—COLUMBUS' PROPOSALS FOR AN ABORIGINAL INDIAN SLAVE TRADE TO EUROPE

*(Memorandum of Christopher Columbus, sent to the Spanish Sovereigns, by Antonio de Torres, January 30, 1495)\**

You shall say to their Highnesses that, owing to the fact that there is here no interpreter, by means of whom it is possible to give to these people understanding of our holy Faith, as their Highnesses desire and also those of us who are here, although every possible effort has been made, there are now sent with these ships some of the cannibals, men and women and boys and girls. These their Highnesses can order to be placed in charge of persons so that they may be able better to learn the language, employing them in forms of service, and ordering that gradually greater care be given to them than to other slaves, so that some may learn from others. If they do not speak to each other or see each other until much later, they will learn more quickly there than here, and they will be better interpreters, although here there has been no failure to do what could be done. It is the truth that, as among these people those of one island have little intercourse with those of another, in languages there is some difference between them, according to whether they are nearer to or farther from each other. And since of all the islands, those of the cannibals are much the largest and much more fully populated, it is thought here that to take some of the men and women and to send them home to Castile would not be anything but well, for they may one day be led to abandon that inhuman custom which they have of eating men, and there in Castile, learning the language, they will much more readily receive baptism and secure the welfare of their souls. Further, among those peoples who have not these habits, great credit will be gained by us when they see that we take and make captive those men, from whom they are accustomed to suffer injury, and of whom they go in such fear that they are terrified at their very name. Assure their Highnesses that here, in this land, our arrival and the sight of the fleet, so under control and beautiful, has given us great authority for the present, and very great security for our affairs in the future. For all the people of this great island, and of the other islands, when they see the good treatment which is meted out to well-doers and the punishment which is inflicted upon those who do evil, will quickly come to obedience so that it will be possible to command them as vassals of their Highnesses. And as already here, wherever a man of them is to be found they not only do willingly all that they are wished to do, but of their own accord set themselves to everything which they understand may please us, their Highnesses may

* Cited in Jane, *op. cit.*, Vol. I, pp. 88, 90, 92.

also be certain that on that side equally, among Christian princes, the coming of this fleet has given them great reputation in many respects, both now and hereafter, which their highnesses will be better able to understand and know than I have power to say.

*Let him be informed of that which has occurred in the case of the cannibals who came here.*

*That is very well, and so it should be done, but let him endeavour, as it may be possible, that they there be converted to our holy Faith, and so let him endeavour in those islands where he may be.*

Item: You shall say to their highnesses that the welfare of the souls of the said cannibals, and also of those here, has induced the idea that the more that may be sent over, the better it will be and in this their highnesses may be served in the following way. That, having seen how necessary cattle and beasts of burden are here, for the support of the people who have to be here, and indeed for all these islands, their highnesses might give licence and a permit for a sufficient number of caravels to come here every year and to carry the said cattle and other supplies and things for the colonization of the country and the development of the land, and this at reasonable prices at the cost of those who transport them. Payment for these things could be made to them in slaves, from among these cannibals, a people very savage and suitable for the purpose, and well made and of very good intelligence. We believe that they, having abandoned that inhumanity, will be better than any other slaves, and their inhumanity they will immediately lose when they are out of their own land. And of these they will be able to take many with the oared *fustas* which it is proposed to build here. It is, however, to be presupposed that each one of the caravels which come from their Highness will have on board a reliable person, who will prevent the said caravels from stopping at any other place or island except here, where the landing and unloading of all the merchandise must be. And further, on those slaves which they carry, their highnesses could levy a duty there. And on this matter you shall bring or send an answer, in order that here the preparations which are necessary may be made with more confidence, if it seems well to their Highnesses.

*As to this, the matter has been postponed for the present, until another voyage has been made there, and let the admiral write that which occurs to him concerning this matter.*

## No. 55—COLUMBUS CALLS THE NEW WORLD INTO EXISTENCE TO REDRESS THE BALANCE OF THE OLD

*(Christopher Columbus to Ferdinand and Isabella, King and Queen of Spain, 1496)\**

We can send from here, in the name of the Holy Trinity, all the slaves and brazil–wood which could be sold. If the information I have is correct, we can sell 4,000 slaves, who will be worth, at least, 20 millions, and 4,000 hundred-weight of brazil-wood, which will be worth just as much. Expenses here may be six millions, so that, at first sight, forty millions would be fine, if it turned out this way. The information seems authentic, because in Castile, Portugal, Aragon, Italy, Sicily, and the islands of Portugal and Aragon and the Canary Islands they need many slaves, and I do not think they get enough from Guinea. Even though they may get enough, one Indian is worth three Negroes.... I went recently to the Cape Verde Islands where the people have a large slave trade, and they are constantly sending ships to barter for slaves, and ships are always in the harbour. I saw that for the worse slaves they asked 8,000 maravedis and the Indians, as I said, are much better slaves, As to the brazil-wood, they need plenty in Castile, Aragon, Genoa, Venice, France, Flanders and England. So that, from these two commodities it seems we can get at least forty millions, if there was not a lack of ships, which I believe, with the help of Our Lord, will not continue if they make a large profit on this trip.... Although they die now, they will not always die. The Negroes and Canary Islanders died at first, and the Indians are even better than the Negroes....

---

### (b) — THE DILEMMA OF THE KING AND QUEEN

## No. 56—THE ESSENTIAL POINT, THE SPREAD OF THE FAITH

*(Ferdinand and Isabella, King and Queen of Spain, to Christopher Columbus, May 29, 1493)\*\**

Christopher Columbus.... has related.... that the people he found in the said islands are people well fitted to be converted to our Holy Catholic Faith, for they have no law or sect. This pleases their Highnesses very much, because in everything the essential point is respect for the service of God our Lord, and the praise of our Holy Catholic

* Cited in Las Casas, *Historia de las Indias*, Libro Primero, Cap. CL, Tomo II, pp. 71—72.
\*\*Cited in Navarrete, *op. cit.*, Tomo II, Num. XLV, pp. 83—84.

Faith. Therefore their Highnesses, wishing that our Catholic
Faith be augmented and enlarged, command and charge the
said Admiral, Viceroy, and Governor, that through all possible means and ways, he shall try and work to attract the
inhabitants of the said island and Terra Firma to conversion
to our Holy Catholic Faith; and to help with the conversion,
their Highnesses are sending over there the learned Father
Buil, together with other religious men, who will make sure
that they be well informed of the things of our Holy Faith,
with the aid of the Indians who have come here, for they
will already know and understand much of our language, and
will try to instruct the others in it as well as possible. In
order the better to ensure this, once the armada has arrived
there, the said Admiral is charged to watch that those who
go in it, and those who will go hereafter, treat the said Indians very well and lovingly, not making them suffer and
encouraging much familiarity and conversation with them,
doing as many good deeds as they can. And likewise, the
said Admiral is graciously to give them some presents from
their Highnesses' merchandise which he has for exchange,
and to honour them much. And in case any person or persons mistreat the said Indians in any way, the said Admiral,
as Viceroy and Governor of their Highnesses, is to punish
him or them severely in virtue of their Highnesses' powers,
with which he is invested for such purpose....

## No. 57—THE BAN ON ABORIGINAL INDIAN SLAVERY IN SPAIN

*(Ferdinand and Isabella, King and Queen of Spain, to Pedro
de Torres, June 20, 1500)\**

You already know how under our command you have in
your power, held under sequestration, some of the Indians
who were brought from the Indies and sold in this City and
its archbishopric and in other parts of Andalucia at the
command of our Admiral of the Indies; we now order that
they shall be liberated, and have commanded the Prefect
Father Francisco de Bobadilla to take them.... to the Indies, and do with them what we have ordered him.

## No. 58—MUTUAL AID

*(Isabella, Queen of Spain, to Nicolas de Ovando, Governor
of Hispaniola, December 20, 1503)\*\**

Whereas the King my Lord and I by the orders we commanded to be given to Nicolas de Ovando.... at the time
he went as our Governor to the islands and the mainland,

* Cited in Navarrete, *op. cit.*, Tomo II, Num. CXXXIV, pp. 287—288.
** Cited in Navarrete, *op. cit.*, Tomo II, Num. CLIII, pp. 346—348.

ordered that the Indian residents and inhabitants of Hispaniola should be free and not subject to servitude. . . .and now I have been informed that due to the excessive liberty which the said Indians have, they run away and avoid association and contact with the Christians; so that, even though the latter are willing to pay them for their daily work, they are unwilling to work, and they go about like vagabonds, and still less can they be reached so that they may be taught and converted to our Holy Catholic Faith, and for this reason the Christians who live and dwell in the said island do not find labour for their farms and for their support, or to help them to mine or collect the gold which there is in the island, which is detrimental to both Christians and Indians. As we wish the said Indians to be converted to our Holy Catholic Faith, and to be taught its doctrines, and because this can be better done by association and dealings between the Indians and the Christians who are in the said island, and by mutual aid so that the said island will be cultivated and populated and its production increased and its gold collected, so that these my Kingdoms and the colonists may profit thereby,. . . I command you. . . . to compel and oblige the said Indians to deal and associate with the Christians of the said island, to work in their buildings in collecting and mining gold and other metals, and to grow food and supplies for the Christian settlers and inhabitants of the said island, each one of them being given for a day's work the wage and food which according to the quality of the soil, the person and his work would seem appropriate to you, commanding each Cacique to be responsible for a certain number of the said Indians, in order that he may require them to go and work where they are needed, and so that on the feast-days and on other appropriate days they may assemble in the places indicated to hear and be taught the faith;. . . . and this they are to do as the free persons they are, and not as slaves; and you are to see to it that the said Indians are well treated, and those who are Christians better than the others, and you are not to agree or allow that anyone shall do them evil or injury or any other offence. . . .

## No. 59 — THE REQUISITION

("*Notificacion e Requerimiento que se ha de hacer a los moradores de las Islas e tierra firme del mar oceano que aun no estan sugetos al Rey Nuestro Senor*" 1509)*

On the part of the King, Don Fernando, and of Dona Juana, his daughter, Queen of Castile and Leon, subduers of the barbarous nations, we their servants notify and make

* Cited in Arthur Helps, *The Spanish Conquest in America and its Relation to the History of Slavery and to the Government of Colonies*, London, 1855, Vol, I, pp. 379—382, The original Spanish will be found in Saco, *Historia de la Esclavitud de los Indios*, Tomo I, pp. 149—153.

known to you, as best we can, that the Lord our God, Living
and Eternal, created the Heaven and the Earth, and one man
and one woman, of whom you and we, and all the men of
the world, were and are descendants, and all those who
come after us. But, on account of the multitude which has
sprung from this man and woman in the five thousand years
since the world was created, it was necessary that some
men should go one way and some another, and that they
should be divided into many kingdoms and provinces, for in
one alone they could not be sustained.

Of all these nations God our Lord gave charge to one
man, called St. Peter, that he should be Lord and Superior
of all the men in the world, that all should obey him, and
that he should be head of the whole human race, wherever
men should live, and under whatever law, sect, or belief they
should be; and he gave him the world for his kingdom and
jurisdiction.

And he commanded him to place his seat in Rome, as
the spot most fitting to rule the world from; but also he permitted him to have his seat in any other part of the world,
and to judge and govern all Christians, Moors, Jews, Gentiles, and all other sects. This man was called Pope, as if to
say, Admirable Great Father and Governor of men. The men
who lived in that time obeyed that St. Peter, and took him
for Lord, King, and Superior of the universe; so also they
have regarded the others who after him have been elected
to the pontificate, and so has it been continued even till now,
and will continue till the end of the world.

One of these Pontiffs, who succeeded that St. Peter as
Lord of the world, in the dignity and seat which I have before mentioned, made donation of these isles and Terra-
Firma to the aforesaid King and Queen and to their successors, our lords, with all that there are in these territories, as
is contained in certain writings which passed upon the subject as aforesaid, which you can see if you wish.

So their Highnesses are kings and lords of these islands
and land of Tierra-Firma by virtue of this donation; and some
islands, and indeed almost all those to whom this has been
notified, have received and served their Highnesses, as lords
and kings, in the way that subjects ought to do, with good
will, without any resistance, immediately, without delay,
when they were informed of the aforesaid facts. And also
they received and obeyed the priests whom their Highnesses
sent to preach to them and to teach them our Holy Faith;
and all these, of their own free will, without any reward or
condition, have become Christians, and are so, and their
Highnesses have joyfully and benignantly received them, and
also have commanded them to be treated as their subjects
and vassals; and you too are held and obliged to do the
same. Wherefore, as best we can, we ask and require you
that you consider what we have said to you, and that you

take the time that shall be necessary to understand and deliberate upon it, and that you acknowledge the Church as the Ruler and Superior of the whole world and the high priest called Pope, and in his name the King and Queen Dona Juana our lords, in his place, as superiors and lords and kings of these islands and this Terra–Firma by virtue of the said donation, and that you consent and give place that these religious fathers should declare and preach to you the aforesaid.

If you do so, you will do well, and that which you are obliged to do to their Highnesses, and we in their name shall receive you in all love and charity, and shall leave you your wives, and your children, and your lands, free without servitude, that you may do with them and with yourselves freely that which you like and think best, and they shall not compel you to turn Christians, unless you yourselves, when informed of the truth, should wish to be converted to our Holy Catholic Faith, as almost all the inhabitants of the rest of the islands have done. And, besides this, their Highnesses award you many privileges and exemptions and will grant you many benefits.

But, if you do not do this, and maliciously make delay in it, I certify to you that, with the help of God, we shall powerfully enter into your country, and shall make war against you in all ways and manners that we can, and shall subject you to the yoke and obedience of the Church and of their Highnessess; we shall take you and your wives and your children, and shall make slaves of them, and as such shall sell and dispose of them as their Highnesses may command; and we shall take away your goods, and shall do you all the mischief and damage that we can, as to vassals who do not obey, and refuse to receive their lord, and resist and contradict him; and we protest that the deaths and losses which shall accrue from this are your fault, and not that of their Highnesses, or ours, nor of these cavaliers who come with us. And that we have said this to you and made this Requisition, we request the notary here present to give us his testimony in writing, and we ask the rest who are present that they should be witnesses of this Requisition.

---

*No. 60 — THE REQUISITION IN PRACTICE*
(Gonzalo Fernandes de Oviedo y Valdes, Historia General
y Natural de las Indias, Islas y Tierra -Firme del Mar
Oceano (1535-1557), Madrid, 1851-1855) *

My Lords, it appears to me that these Indians will not listen to the theology of this Requisition, and that you have no one who can make them understand it; would Your Honour be pleased to keep it until we have some one of

*Cited in Hanke, The Spanish Struggle for Justice in the Conquest of America, University of Pennsylvania Press, Philadelphia, 1949, pp. 33—34.

these Indians in a cage, in order that he may learn it at his leisure and my Lord Bishop may explain it to him....

It appears that they had been suddenly pounced upon and bound before they had learnt or understood anything about Pope or Church, or any one of the many things said in the Requisition; and that after they had been put in chains someone read the Requisition without knowing their language and without any interpreters, and without either the reader or the Indians understanding what was read. And even after it had been explained to them by someone understanding their language, they had no chance to reply, being immediately carried away prisoners, the Spaniards not failing to use the stick on those who did not go fast enough.

### No. 61 — SANCTIONING THE ABORIGINAL INDIAN SLAVE TRADE IN THE CARIBBEAN
*(Contract between Isabella, Queen of Spain, and Cristobal Guerra, July 12, 1503)\**

....to take Indians, men and women, for slaves — which he is to do as nearly as possible with their consent without harming them; and in the same manner he may take monsters and animals of any kind, and all the serpents and fishes he may desire; and all this to belong to him, as has been said, the fourth part being reserved for me.

### No. 62—ENSLAVEMENT OF CARIBS AUTHORISED
*(Proclamation of Isabella, Queen of Spain, October 30, 1503)\*\**

Be it known that the King, my Lord, and I, in order that all the persons who live and reside in the islands and mainland of the Ocean sea should become Christians and be converted to our Holy Catholic Faith, have commanded....that no person or persons.... dare to arrest or capture any.... Indians....to bring them to these my kingdoms or to any other places, or to do any harm or evil to their persons or possessions, under certain penalties prescribed in our decree, and.... since certain persons had brought some Indians from the islands to Spain, we commanded them to be taken and liberated, and they were liberated. Once all this had been done, in order to convince the Indians and encourage them to become Christians so that they would live as rational men, we ordered some of our captains to go to the islands and mainland....and sent with them some religious men to preach and teach them the doctrines of our Holy Catholic Faith, and to persuade them to become our vassals; and while in some of the islands they were welcomed and well received, in the islands of Saint Bernard and "Isla Fuerte", and in the ports of Carthagena, and in the islands

*Cited in Simpson, *op. cit.*, p. 5.
**Cited in Navarrete, *op. cit.*, Tomo II, Appendix, Num. XVII, pp. 478—480.

of Bura, inhabited by a people called Cannibals, they would
not welcome or listen to them, rather they defended themselves with their weapons, and resisted them so that they
could not enter these islands where they live. During this
resistance they killed some Christians, and thereafter they
have....waged war on the Indians who are my vassals,
capturing them to eat them as is their custom; and since I
have been informed that, in the interest of the service both of
God and myself, and of the peace and tranquillity of my
vassals who live in the islands and mainland, these Cannibals should be punished for the crimes they have committed
against my subjects, it behoved me to take appropriate
action: and I commanded my Council to consider the matter;.... accepting with zeal as We do that the Cannibals
should be compelled to adopt our Holy Catholic Faith, they
have been required many times to become Christians and to
be converted and incorporated in the Communion of the
Faithful and under our obedience, and live in security and
treat well their neighbours of the other islands. Not only
have they refused to do so,.... but rather they have tried
and try to defend themselves against being taught the doctrines of our Holy Catholic Faith, and they continually wage
war on our subjects, and have killed many Christians who
have gone to the islands, and being as they are hardened in
their bad habits of idolatry and cannibalism, it was agreed
that I should issue this decree.... I hereby give license and
permission to all and every person who may go at my command, to the islands and mainland of the Ocean heretofore
discovered, as well as to the islands and mainland which
may be discovered hereafter, so that, if the Cannibals still
resist, and refuse to receive and welcome in their lands the
captains and people who at my command go on the said
voyages, and to listen to them to be taught the doctrines of
our Holy Catholic Faith, and become my vassals owning allegiance to me, they are authorised to capture them to take
them to the lands and islands where they live, and to bring
them to these my kingdoms and dominions, and to any other
parts and places they wish, paying us the share that belongs
to us, and to sell them and utilise their services, without
incurring any penalty thereby, because if the Christians
bring them to these lands and make use of their services,
they will be more easily converted and attracted to our Holy
Faith....

## No. 63 — WHO ARE CARIBS?

*(Antonio de Herrera, Historia General de los Hechos de los
Castellanos en los Islas y Tierra Firme del Mar Oceano,
Madrid, 1601-1615)\**

Licentiate Rodrigo de Figueroa, after making diligent

*Op. cit., Decada Segunda, Libro Decimo, Cap. V. Edition of Editorial Guara-
nia, Asuncion del Paraguay, Paraguay, 1945, Tomo III, pp. 334—335

inquiry regarding the Indians who ate human flesh, and the countries inhabited by them, in order that, under the pretext of taking them captive, others should not be captured, issued a decree to the effect that all Indians in the islands not settled by Christians were Caribs, except those of Trinidad, the Bahamas, Barbuda, "Gigantes" and Margarita. He said that all the others were Caribs, savages, enemies of Christianity, who refused to be converted.... And he laid down that, subject to the licences, conditions and instructions which would be issued, it was lawful to invade, capture and make war on the Carib Indians. And he forbade any one to dare to do harm to the Indians in other areas, without an express declaration that they were Caribs, although visits for purposes of trade were allowed. This declaration was very necessary, to avoid the confusion in which the settlers found themselves, over the questions as to who were Caribs, and who were not.

## No. 64 — PROPOSAL FOR AN INTERCOLONIAL CARIB SLAVE TRADE

*(Vasco Nunez de Balboa to Ferdinand II, King of Spain, January 20, 1513)* *

....Those Indians, in certain of the provinces, who eat men, and others at the bottom of the Gulf of Uraba and in the extensive flooded parts near the great river of San Juan and round the gulf, at the entrance of the flat country of the province of Davaive, have no workshops, nor do they support themselves on anything but fish, which they exchange for maize. These are worthless people, and when canoes of Christians have gone on the great river of San Juan, they have come aginst them, and have killed some of our people. The country where the Indians eat men is very bad and useless, and can never at any time be turned to account, But these Indians of Caribana have richly deserved death a thousand times over, for they are a very evil race, and have killed many of our Christians when we lost the ship. I would not make slaves of so bad a people, but would order them to be destroyed, both old and young, that no memory may remain of them. I speak now of Caribana and for twenty leagues inland, the people being evil, and the country sterile and worthless. And it will be serviceable to your Highness to give permission to take these natives to Espanola and the other islands occupied by Christians, to be sold and made profitable, that other slaves may be bought for their price; for it is impossible to keep them even for a day, the country being very extensive, where they can run away and hide. Thus the settlers in these parts, not having Indians secured, cannot work for the ser-

*Cited in Navarrete, *op. cit.*, Tomo III, Seccion Tercera, Num. IV, pp. 367-368.

vice of your Highness, nor extract any gold from the mines. The settlers would also beseech your Highness to grant them permission to bring Indians from Veragua, from a gulf called San Blas, which is fifty leagues from this town, down the coast. Your Highness will be well served in granting this request, because it is a very worthless land, covered with great swamps and forests, and, seen from the sea, it appears to be inundated. So that no profit whatever can be made out of these Indians of Veragua and Caribana, except in this way, by bringing them to Christian settlements, whence they can be taken to Cuba, Jamaica, and other islands inhabited by Christians, to be exchanged for other Indians, of which there are many in those islands. Thus by sending the warlike Indians far from their homes, the natives of these parts will labour well in the islands, and those of the islands here.

---

### No. 65—ENSLAVEMENT OF NATIVES OF USELESS ISLANDS AUTHORISED

*(King Ferdinand II, King of Spain, to Diego Columbus, Governor of the Indies, May 3, 1509)* *

And if by chance they do anything that may merit their being made slaves, I think it will be better to sell them, since in that case as many of the natives of the (useless) islands** can be taken for our service as necessary.

---

### No. 66—THE INDIAN SLAVE TRADE AND THE MIDDLE PASSAGE

*(Bartolome de las Casas, Historia de las Indias (1559), Madrid, 1875)* * *

The Spaniards, seeing that the Indians were dying and declining in numbers in the gold mining industry, on their farms and in other jobs, and concerned only with their worldly loss and the reduction of their profits, they thought that it would be a good idea to replace the natives of Hispaniola who were dying out with Indians from other islands ....they told King Philip....that the Lucayan Islands were full of idle people of whom no use was being made and who would never become Christians there. They asked him to permit the Spanish inhabitants of Hispaniola to equip a few ships in which to bring the Lucayan Indians to the island where they would become Christians and where

---

*Cited in Simpson, *op. cit.*, p. 22.
**The Bahamas,          .
***Op. cit.*, Libro Segundo, Caps, XLIII and XLIV, Tomo II, pp, 346-351,

they would help to mine gold, to the King's advantage.... The King agreed to this (the Council, in its ignorance, being largely responsible for advising him to do so); and he signed the licence, as if rational men were wood cut from trees which it was necessary to bring to Hispaniola for building purposes, or perhaps as if they were herds of sheep or other animals and, even though many might die on the crossing, the loss would be small.

Who would not condemn so great an error of taking away natives of these islands by force to other new lands 100 or 150 leagues away by sea, whether the reason was good or bad, much less when it was to extract gold from the mines (where they would certainly die) for the King or for foreigners whom they had never harmed?.... Even though it was true, which it was not.... that the Indians brought to Hispaniola would be taught and converted to Christianity, God did not want that Christianity at the price of such wickedness.... And, as the final condemnation of this fallacy, the Apostles never took infidels by force from their native land to their own country to convert them....

After King Ferdinand had given his permission....ten or twelve settlers in the cities of La Vega or Concepcion and Santiago contributed 10,000 or 12,000 gold dollars with which they bought two or three ships and hired fifty or sixty men including sailors.... to go and capture the Indians who, confident in the peace and security of their own country, were totally unprepared. These people....surpassed those in all the Indies, and I think in the whole world, in gentleness, simplicity, humility, peaceful disposition and tranquillity and in other natural virtues.... The Spaniards told them the ships came from Hispaniola where the souls of their parents and relatives rested, and that if they wanted to see them they....would take them to it.... With these persuasive and wicked words, they induced those innocent people, men and women, to board the ships.... But on arrival in Hispaniola, when they saw neither their parents nor those they loved, but only tools, such as spades, hoes, bars, and iron sticks and the mines where they soon died, and realising that they had been tricked, some, in despair, killed themselves by drinking the sap of the bitter cassava....

The Spaniards divided them into lots (as many lots as there were individuals who had shares in the ships and expenses), old and young, the sick and the able-bodied.... No more attempt was made in these lots not to separate husband and wife, or father and son, than if they had been brute animals....when some old and sick person fell to anyone's lot, the one who received him said: "Give this old man to the devil; why should I take him? To feed and

bury him? and this sick one, why do you give him to me?
To heal him?".... What man with a heart could endure such
inhuman cruelty? How could those men remember that
commandment which reads, "Thou shalt love thy neighbour
as thyself", when, forgetting that they were Christians and
even men, they treated the Indians in that way? They also
arranged that, in order to meet the expenses incurred and
to pay the wages to the men on the ships, they could sell....
each "piece" for four gold dollars—they called the Indian
a "piece", as if they were dealing with head of cattle....
    I want to relate here what a Spaniard told me in Cuba.
This man had gone from the Lucayos to Cuba (I believe in
an Indian canoe).... He told me how they overcrowded
the ships, sometimes with 200, 300 or 500 people, old and
young, women and children, all of them below deck. To
prevent their escape, they closed the hatchways, and the
Indians were left without light or air. It is very hot below
deck, and besides, since the ships did not carry enough supplies, especially water, of which they had only enough for
the Spaniards....and because also of the lack of food, their
unbearable thirst, the heat, grief and overcrowding (some
being on top of or too close to others), many died and were
thrown in the sea, in such large numbers, that a ship without a compass, map or guide, but only following the track
of the dead bodies, could find its way from the Lucayos to
Hispaniola. These were his words. It was a fact....that
there was not a single ship which went to attack the Indians
of the Lucayan Islands and of the mainland....which did
not throw overboard one-third or one-quarter of those
embarked.

-----

*No. 67 — ENSLAVEMENT OF NATIVES OF LARGER
ISLANDS PROHIBITED*

*(Ferdinand I, King of Spain, to Diego Columbus, Governor
of the Indies, June 15, 1510)\**

    As it is reported that our interests would be best served
if at present no Indians were brought from the Island of
Trynidad as there are Islands much nearer from which they
can be brought and moreover that it is an island of some
size and is said to have gold and that it is at peace and that
trade is carried on with the Indians for pearls and that by
offending these Indians of this Island we should lose the
pearl trade because there are not at present any other
Indians along the whole coast of Tierra-Firme at peace and
that it is well to maintain peace in this Island as the pearl
trade is profitable.
    Therefore I do order you that from now on you shall

*Cited in The Trinidad Historical Society, Publication No. 73, pp, 1-2,

not allow nor permit anyone to take Indians from this said Island and that these said Indians shall always be well treated and preserved.

Furthermore Indians are not to be brought from the islands near to the Island of Sant Xoan nor from the Island of Cuba nor Jamaica since there are other Islands to the north whence Indians may be brought; however if on the Pearl Coast there are Indians who attack those in Sant Xoan and others who serve there not being rebels or against us, then you may grant licences to take them.

Also you should consider whether by making a settlement of Christians in Cuba on the coast, it would be possible to bring Indians from there to gain gold from the mines in Espanola; consider this carefully how it could be done and send me your views.

---

### No. 68 — THE INDIAN SLAVE TRADE FROM THE CONTINENT TO THE WEST INDIES

*(Don Fray Juan de Zumarraga, Bishop-elect of Mexico, to Charles V, Emperor of the Hapsburg Empire, August 27, 1529)* *

As soon as I came to this country.... I was informed that the province of Panuco, of which Nuno de Guzman is governor, had been destroyed and devastated, because the said Nuno de Guzman had taken from it a great number of its free natives and had branded them and sold them in the islands. And, since I wish to learn more about the business—for it seemed to me very harmful and contrary to your Majesty's royal purpose—I have learned and verified that as soon as Nuno de Guzman was received in that province he gave a general license to all its inhabitants to take twenty or thirty slaves (each) for the islands, and this was done. When this trade came to the attention of the merchants and traders of the islands and they saw that it was profitable, they came to the province of Panuco in their own interest, and because Guzman called them, and he himself sent to have ships fitted out for it. And things have come to such a pass that the whole province is dissipated and destroyed. Nine or ten thousand souls have been removed, branded as slaves, and sent to the islands. And truly I think there were more, because about twenty-one ships sailed from there laden....

For this reason so much harm has come to that province, and such has been the astonishment and terror of the natives, that they have decided to adopt as their best remedy, and it has been ordered by their chiefs, to abandon

*Cited in Simpson, *op. cit.*, pp. 217—219.

their villages and fly to the wilderness, and that no one should have intercourse with his wife, so as not to have children to be made slaves of before their eyes and carried away from their country....

All that is known of the fate of the poor Indian vassals of your Majesty who have been taken from this country is that three shiploads of them have sunk, and others have thrown themselves into the sea and drowned; and so would others do if they were not watched and guarded and kept in prison by the Spaniards so that they will not kill themselves. Those who reach the islands, being very weak from hunger and thirst.... and afflicted by the narrowness of their quarters, upon arriving at a land so foreign to their nature, catch diseases and pestilences, and all die. This has been done on the pretext that license for it has been procured from your Majesty, so that merchants may engage in this trade with better will. And, if it is true that your Majesty issued such licenses, for the reverence of God do very great penance for it !

### No. 69—THE NEED OF INDIAN LABOUR

*(Ferdinand II, King of Spain, to Diego Columbus, Governor of Hispaniola, November 12, 1509)\**

....as you know, the greatest need of the island at present is more Indians, so that those who go there from these kingdoms to mine gold may have Indians to mine it with. You can imagine the profit that is being lost.

### No. 70—THE VALUE OF INDIAN LABOUR

*(Ferdinand II, King of Spain, to Diego Columbus, Governor of Hispaniola, June 21, 1511)\*\**

...as you know, all the good of those parts lies in there being a number of Indians to work in the mines and plantations.

### No. 71—THE ROYAL PROFIT FROM INDIAN SLAVERY

*(Ferdinand II, King of Spain, to Juan Ponce de Leon, Governor of Puerto Rico, February 25, 1512)\*\**

You have done me a service by your efforts to pacify the island, and by branding with the letter F on the brow the Indians captured in war, enslaving them, and selling them to the highest bidder, reserving a fifth part of the proceeds for me.

*Cited in Simpson, *op. cit.*, p. 23.
** Cited in Simpson, *op. cit.*, p. 27.
*** Cited in Saco, *Historia de la Esclavitud de los Indios*, Tomo I, p. 156.

## (iii) THE ENCOMIENDA

### No. 72—TRUSTEESHIP: REPORT OF THE ROYAL COMMISSION OF LAWYERS AND THEOLOGIANS, 1512

*(Bartolome de las Casas, Historia de las Indias (1559), Madrid, 1875)* *

Our opinion is as follows: First of all, that, since the Indians are free men and Your Highness and the Queen, may she rest in eternal peace, ordered them to be treated as free men, this should be done. Secondly, that they are to be taught the Holy Faith, as the Pope orders in His Bull and Your Highnesses ordered in your letter; Your Highness should see that all the necessary steps should be diligently taken in this matter. Thirdly, that Your Highness may order them to work, but that the work should be such that it would not be a hindrance to their instruction in the Holy Faith and would be profitable for them and for the state. Your Highness should be served because he is their lord and for teaching them the fundamentals of our Holy Faith and for administering justice to them. Fourthly, that this work should be of such a nature that it is not beyond their capacity, and they should have some free time every day as well as throughout the whole year, as convenient. Fifthly, that they should have their own homes and plots. . . . and that they should be given enough time to till and cultivate these plots in their own way. Sixthly, that they be ordered to associate constantly with the settlers. . . ., because by this contact they would be taught better and more quickly the fundamentals of our Holy Catholic Faith. Seventhly, that they be paid a just wage for their work, not in money but in clothes and other necessaries for their homes.

---

### No. 73 — THE ABORIGINAL INDIAN CODE OF PUERTO RICO

*(Decree of Ferdinand II, King of Spain, Valladolid, January 23, 1513)* **

1. In view of the removal of the Indians from their villages near to those of the Spaniards, all those who hold them in trust will construct for every fifty Indians four huts, thirty feet long and fifteen feet wide, and provide for them three thousand beds of cassava, two thousand of tubers, two hundred and fifty feet of pepper, and fifty feet of cotton to the satisfaction of the inspector, who will see

*Op. cit., Libro Tercero, Cap. VIII, Tomo II, p. 457.
**Cited in Antologia de Lecturas sobre la Historia de Puerto Rico, Tomo I, pp. 24—25, from Tapia y Rivera, Biblioteca Historia de Puerto Rico, pp. 192—196.

to it that half a fanega* of corn is planted and that each Indian is given twelve hens and a rooster, the chickens and eggs being appropriated by the Indians for their own use.

2. The Indians of Puerto Rico are to be removed from their present abode to the new villages with love and flattery.

3. Every Spaniard who holds Indians in trust will build on his plantation a house to serve as a church, to which he will accompany them at dawn and at nightfall to say prayers with them, taking care to correct their errors. The Indians will be given some time off to rest before nightfall, and those who do not attend church will be deprived of this rest period.

4. Those who hold Indians in trust are required to instruct them in matters of the Faith, and every fortnight to examine them to ascertain what they have learned, on pain of a fine of six gold pesos.

5. Where there are four or five villages within the radius of a league, a church will be built in the centre, to which the Indians will come every feast day to hear Mass with those who hold them in trust and to hear the priest's sermon; in the event there is no priest, they will come to hear and say prayers; on pain of a fine of ten pesos on the Spaniard who violates this.

6. If there is any Indian village outside the radius of a league, a church is to be built in it so that the Indians will not be forced to travel a great distance.

7. Bishops who collect tithes from these Indian villages will provide priests to say Mass, hear confessions of those who know Church doctrines and instruct those who do not.

8. A church will be built in the mines wherever there are large numbers of Indians, and all those who work in them will do as those in the settlements are required to do.

9. Those who hold forty or more Indians in trust must instruct one of the boys in reading, writing and matters of the Faith, and since many are in the habit of employing an Indian boy as a page, they will be obliged to instruct him likewise.

10. The priest must visit sick Indians and hear their confession once a year and must go to dying Indians bearing the cross to bury them, all of this free of charge. Those who hold Indians in trust are obliged to bury them when they die, on pain of a fine of four pesos.

11. No Indian must be made to carry loads, except his own belongings when he is being removed from one village to another. If those who hold Indians in trust violate this, they will be liable to a fine of two pesos and to being

*Approximately 1½ acres.

deprived of such Indians for the benefit of the hospital in the village to which they belong.

12. Those who hold Indians in trust must baptise all new-born Indian children within eight days; if no priest is at hand, they are to baptise the children themselves, on pain of a fine of three dollars for failure to do so, the money being turned over to the church where the baptism should take place.

13. Indians are not to be employed in mines for more than five months. At the end of that period they are to rest for forty days, during which time no work is to be assigned to them except bringing their supplies from the woods. During the rest period the gold will be smelted and those who hold Indians in trust will be responsible for instructing them in matters of the Faith.

14. Indians are not to be prevented from performing their ceremonial dances on Sundays and feast days, or on other days after working hours, as experience has taught that this leads to trouble.

15. Those who hold Indians in trust will be obliged to provide for them sufficient bread, tubers and pepper and to give them sufficient food. Besides on feast days they will give each Indian a pound of meat or fish depending on whether it is a meatless day or not, and the Indians will eat it in their huts. They will give them this ration also each day they work in the mines. The penalty for violation is two pesos for each offence.

16. The Indians are to be taught to be satisfied with one wife, and to marry her, according to the laws of the church.

17. The sons of caciques are to be turned over at the age of thirteen to the Franciscan Friars, who will instruct them in reading, writing and matters of the Faith. After four years they are to be returned to those who hold them in trust in order that from them the other Indians may learn the matters of the Faith. They can do this better than we can.

18. Indian women who are more than four months pregnant are not to be sent to the mines or to make beds for food crops. They are to be employed only in light household tasks. This is to be done also for three years after delivery while they are bringing up their children. The penalty for violation of this article is six dollars for each offence.

19. Those who hold Indians in trust are to supply a hammock to each Indian within twelve months, and the inspector is to see to it that this is done and that the Indians do not barter or sell it.

.20. Each Indian is to be paid a gold peso a year for the purchase of clothing; out of this peso the cacique is to receive a real so that he and his wife may be better dressed.

21.  No one is to make use of the services of or to admit into his villages Indians who do not belong to him, on pain of a fine of six pesos for the first offence, twelve pesos for the second, and thirty-six pesos for the third.

22.  In order that the caciques may be better treated, those who had forty Indians are to be given two for their personal service; those who had sixty, three; those who had one hundred and forty or one hundred and sixty, six. These Indians are to work in the service of the cacique and to be employed solely in light tasks and only so that they may not remain idle.

23.  Those who hold Indians in trust are to furnish the inspector information on Indians who have been born, died or came from Hispaniola or elsewhere, on pain of a fine of two ducats for each Indian not reported. The inspectors will keep records of the number and names of Indians held by each settler, and the settlers will give an account to the officials of the gold smelted. The officials will report to us so that we may know whether the Indians are increasing or decreasing.

24.  No one is to whip, beat, or inflict any other punishment on the Indians. Instead they are to report the matter to the inspectors who will punish the Indians. The penalty for violation is five gold pesos.

25.  All those who hold Indians in trust will keep at least one-third of them working in the mines, except the settlers in Cavanna and the new town of Yaquimo which are very far from the mines. These settlers will employ their Indians in making hammocks, rearing pigs, etc.

26.  Those who do not have plantations near to the mines may team up with those who do, so that while some Indians may be put to work in the mines, others will raise food, provided that there is no hiring of Indians, on pain of the penalties mentioned above.

27.  Indians brought from neighbouring islands will be treated like those who are natives of the island, unless they be slaves, who may be treated as their masters please, but with love and gentleness and subject to their being taught matters of the Faith.

28.  To avoid removal of the Indian settlements, we order that, on the death of a Spaniard to whom we granted Indians in trust, or on his being deprived of them because of a crime he has committed, the village should be bought after it has been valued by two persons appointed by the Admiral, Judges of the Court of Appeal and the royal officials.

29.  In each village of the island two inspectors are to be appointed. They will be responsible for the instruction and good treatment of the Indians and for the enforcement of these ordinances.

30.  The Admiral, Judges and officials are to choose the inspectors, as they see fit, provided that they choose them from among the oldest settlers. The inspectors will receive by virtue of their office a few Indians in addition to those allotted to them. But if they are negligent in the performance of their duty, especially with regard to the provision of food and a hammock, they will be deprived even of those they hold in trust.

31.  The inspectors are to inspect the villages, settlements, and mines twice a year, at the beginning and in the middle of the year, once by one inspector and once by the other, so that what the first may miss the other may catch.

32.  Inspectors may not retain on their plantations any runaway or stray Indians, but must deposit them with a trustworthy person so that their owner may recover them when he wishes, on pain of being deprived of one of their own Indians as well as of having to restore the runaway to his owner.

33.  Inspectors are to be given copies of these ordinances signed by the Admiral, Judge and officials, and an instruction by them for their guidance.

34.  The Admiral, Judge and officials will arrange for a biennial impeachment of the inspectors, who are to report on the births and deaths among the Indians in their district during these two years so that we may be advised.

35.  No settler in Hispaniola may be assigned more than one hundred and fifty or less than forty Indians.

---

## No. 74—INSTRUCTIONS TO THE JERONIMITE REFORM COMMISSION

*(Bartolome de las Casas, Historia de las Indias (1559), Madrid, 1875)\**

First of all, the priests must visit the countries themselves, see as much as they can in each island, and find out the number of caciques there are, the number of Indians that each cacique has, and besides the number of other Indians in each island.

Likewise, they are to ascertain how the Indians have been treated up to the present by those who have held them in trust, by the governors, judges and other officers; they are to write down their findings, so that we may take such steps as may be necessary.

Moreover, the priests are to visit the islands, especially Hispaniola, Cuba, San Juan and Jamaica, see the conditions of the land, especially of that close to the mines where the gold is extracted, and consider where settlements can be built, so that it will be easier for the Indians to get to the

*Op. cit.,* Libro Tercero, Cap. LXXXVIII, Tomo III, pp. 123—130.

mines; there should be rivers nearby for fishing and good land to cultivate. Hispaniola is to be visited first, then Jamaica, next San Juan, and finally Cuba.

Settlements must be founded of approximately 300 inhabitants each, and as many houses as may be necessary built.... The cacique's house is to be near the public square and is to be larger and better than the others, for they will all meet there....

These settlements are to be founded where the caciques and Indians wish, so that no hardship should be caused by the removal; they are to be given to understand that this is all done for their welfare, and in order that they may be better treated than heretofore. Those who live very far from the mines are to settle in them and rear cattle and grow cassava, cotton and other crops, from which they are to pay tribute to the King....

Each settlement must have sufficient living space, according to the location, more rather than less, to allow for the increase of population anticipated, by God's will. This space must be divided among the settlers, giving some of the best land to each.... The cacique is to receive as much as four settlers. The rest is to be left for the people as public land, pastures and farms for hogs and other stock....

If the Indians of one cacique are sufficient for a settlement, it shall be founded with them; but if not, the caciques in the vicinity will join in, and each cacique will be the ruler of his own Indians, as usual. The inferior caciques are to obey their superior, as usual, and the principal cacique is to govern the whole village, together with the priest and a Spaniard appointed for that purpose, as is indicated below.

If any Spaniard....wishes to marry a cacique's daughter who will succeed her father for lack of male heirs, this marriage is to take place with the consent of the priest and the Spanish administrator. Once they are married he shall be the cacique and shall be esteemed, obeyed and served as his predecessor... so that in this way all the caciques will be Spanish in a short time and expenses will be greatly reduced.

Likewise....the principal cacique will have the power to punish Indian offenders in the settlements which they govern; and this goes not only for their own Indians, but also for those of the inferior caciques who live in the same village. This extends only to crimes for which the maximum penalty is whipping, and even this punishment is to be imposed only with the consent of the Council and that of the priest or clergyman. All other offences are to be dealt with by the courts....

The municipal officials, as well as the aldermen, constable and others, are to be nominated and appointed by the principal cacique, the priest and the Spanish administrator, and in case of disagreement by two of them.

And for the good government of each village, it is necessary to appoint someone to administer one, two, three or more settlements, according to their size. This administrator is to live in a suitable intermediate place between the villages so as to do his duty well. He is to live in a stone house, outside of the settlement, so that the Indians may not be harmed or angered by contact with his men. He must be a Spaniard who has lived in the Indies, a man of good conscience, who has treated well the Indians given to him in trust; he must be able to rule and govern well and carry out the tasks assigned to him.

The administrator is to visit the village or villages entrusted to his care and arrange with the caciques, especially with the principal cacique in each village, for the Indians to live like civilised people, each one in his house, with his family, and for them to work in the mines, cultivate the land, rear cattle and other stock.... He is not to force them to work more than they are required to, and this is left to his conscience....

To perform his duties he should have three or four Spaniards.... and all the arms necessary. He is not to permit the caciques or Indians to have weapons.... except those needed for hunting. If he needs more assistants, he may have them if he pays them a salary considered fair by the priest. If any Indians wish to live with him, of their own free will, he may not have more than six. He cannot send these Indians to work in the mines; they can serve him only in housework.... and they may leave his service when they wish and return to their settlements.

This administrator, together with the priest, is to do what he can to make the caciques and Indians live like civilised men, making them wear clothes, sleep in beds, and keep the tools and other things given to them; each is to be content with one wife, whom he is not to leave, and the women are to live chastely. The woman who commits adultery and is accused by her husband of it, and the adulterer are to be punished and even whipped by the cacique, with the consent of the administrator and the priest. Likewise the administrator is to take care that the caciques and Indians do not exchange, sell, give away or gamble their possessions, without his permission or the priest's, except for food and alms. They are not to be allowed to eat on the floor. These administrators shall be paid a reasonable salary.... half by Your Highness and the other half by the people entrusted to his care. They must be married men, so as to avoid possible difficulties....

And for the better performance of his duty, he is to write in a book the names of all the caciques and Indians in every house and every village, so that he may know who is absent, or who does not do what he is required to do.

So that the Indians may be instructed in Our Holy Catholic Faith, and well trained in spiritual matters, there must be a priest in every village responsible for instructing them, according to the capacity of each inhabitant, administering the Sacraments to them and preaching to them on Sundays and Feast days. He must make them understand that they have to pay tithes and first fruits to God, the Church and its ministers, because they hear their confessions and administer the Sacraments to them, bury them when they die and pray to God for them. He must make them come to Mass and sit in an orderly manner, with the sexes segregated....

There must be an Indian sacristan, if possible....to serve in the Church and teach the children to read and write until the age of nine, especially the children of the caciques and the other important people of the village, and to speak Spanish....

Likewise, a house is to be built in the middle of the town to serve as a hospital for sick and old people unable to work, and for orphans. For their maintenance they are to cultivate in common a field of 50,000 plots, and weed it when necessary. The hospital staff is to include a married man with his wife who will beg alms for them and from this the couple are to be maintained ....a pound of meat is to be given to each man and woman, as well as to each poor person, in the presence of the cacique or priest, to avoid fraud.

The inhabitants of each village and the men over twenty and under fifty will be obliged to work as follows : one-third are always to be in the mines, and if one falls ill, another is to take his place; they will leave their homes for the mines at sunrise or shortly after, will return home for lunch, have three hours of rest, and then go back to the mines until sunset.... Shifts of two months are to be arranged, or at other intervals as the caciques wish, so that one-third of the men are always working in the mines. Women are not to work in the mines except of their own accord or at their husbands' wish, and if any women do so, they are to be included in the proportion of one-third prescribed for the men....

And since the cacique has much more work and is their ruler, all the inhabitants and workers will be required to give him fifteen days of the year, whenever he wishes it, to work on his farm, without his being obliged to feed them or pay them for it, and the women, children and old men are required to weed his plots as often as may be necessary....

If possible, each village of 300 inhabitants should have

ten or twelve mares, fifty cows, three hundred hogs, and a hundred sows for breeding. These shall be cared for and held in common until the Indians have become accustomed to private property.

There is to be a butcher in the village, who will give two pounds of meat to each household, when the husband is in the village, but only one pound to the wife when the husband is away in the mines. If a man needs more meat for his family, he must get it himself or rear his own stock. On meatless days they must provide their own food. The cacique is always to be given eight pounds of meat. The wives of those working in the mines are to bake some bread for the caciques from their own farms, and send it to him on mares, together with *ajes*, corn, and whatever else the caciques may need.

There is to be a butcher in the mines who will give to each worker a pound and a half or two pounds of meat, as may seem fit. Since there is little fish in that island, it would be well to secure a dispensation for them to eat meat during some days in Lent and on other meatless days. . . .

The gold smelted is to be divided into three parts: one for the King, and the other two for the caciques and the Indians.

From the two-thirds which are to go to the caciques and the Indians they shall pay for the farms and cattle used to establish the settlement and all expenses to be incurred in common. The rest is to be divided equally among the households. . . .

They are to use it to buy the tools and other things needed for mining, and these will be their property and will be written down in a book so that an account may be rendered of it. And from what is left the cacique, the clergyman and the administrator are to buy them clothes, shirts, twelve hens and one rooster for each household, and whatever they may consider necessary, writing it all down so that they may account for everything. And if there is anything still left, it is to be given to an honest person for safe keeping; he is to give an account of it when asked. . . .

Compensation for the Spanish settlers.—The Spaniards are to be compensated in the following different ways: buying farms for them, appointing them administrators of the villages, paying them a miner's salary, giving them permission to mine gold for themselves and for their families, with the obligation to pay only one-tenth of the profit if they are married and have their wives with them, and one-seventh if they are not married, letting them have two or more slaves, half males and half females, so that they may multiply, and those who had Indians in trust and other privileges are to be given some compensation and other rewards in return.

Likewise, it will be of great advantage to them that Your Highness should give them caravels, well equipped with supplies and other necessaries, so that they may go to capture the robust Caribs who eat human beings. They deserve to be made slaves because they have refused to receive our preachers, and they are very troublesome to the Christians and converts to our Holy Faith; they kill them and eat them. They are to divide among themselves and make slaves of those whom they introduce. But the Spaniards are not to go to the other islands and the mainland under the pretext of going to capture Caribs, and there capture the natives, under penalty of death and of confiscation of their possessions.

Another remedy:—The Spaniards who are in the islands will be rewarded if they go to settle the mainland, for those who have grown up in the islands are better suited to the climate of the mainland than those newly arrived from Spain.

And since some of them are in debt to Your Highness and other persons, and they have no way to pay their debts if their Indians are taken away from them, the concession should be made to them that they should not be arrested or imprisoned or restrained if they wish to leave for the mainland and other islands. In order that the settlements should live in a civilised manner, the Indians should be taught trades, such as to be carpenters, stonecutters, blacksmiths, sawyers, tailors and other similar occupations, for the service of the state.

For the time being, this is what should be done for the assistance and preservation of the Indians, until we see from experience what will be the result. But to carry out this policy, a strong man is needed, because the job of taking away the Indians from those who hold them in trust will be very difficult. The priests who go there will see more or less what should be done, and they will have power to add or subtract as they would think best. The old Christians who did harm to the Indians are to be punished by Your Highness' courts, and the Indians are to be witnesses and their evidence accepted, at the discretion of the judge.

---

*No. 75 — DEFENCE OF THE ENCOMIENDA*
*(Memorandum of the Jeronimite Commission to Cardinal Cisneros, Regent of Spain, 1516)\**

If anyone says it is illegal to give the Indians in trust, do not believe it, Your Highness, because it is lawful, provided that the ordinances are obeyed. If the Indians are given their freedom they will relapse into idolatry.

*Cited in Tapia y Rivera, *Biblioteca Histórica de Puerto Rico*, pp. 208—224.

*No. 76 — THE KING'S CONFESSORS OPPOSE THE*
*ENCOMIENDA*

*(Bartolome de las Casas, Historia de las Indias (1559),*
*Madrid, 1875)\**

Item, that sort of ecomienda is contrary to all human
reason and prudence, for no reason and prudence would
suffice to repair the mischiefs in those lands, neither the
reason and prudence in Your Majesty's dominions here, nor
those of all the judges there, even though they were all
angels. As long as the encomienda lasts, no laws would or
will suffice, even though they should be many more than
the *Siete Partidas;* for who will punish the excessive avarice
of the Christians, who having the Indians in their power,
among the wild rocks, where they are seen only by birds
and where within 50 or 60 leagues and more, there is no
court, judge or other Christian to protect them, work them
to death?.... Who is going to weigh the meat which must
be given to the Indians? Who is going to accuse them if
an Indian dies from the blows or whips? You say, my lords,
that the inspectors will make investigations and punish the
guilty; we have already said that being so far away, the
Indians of each lord being located in the mountains and
scattered in different places, what inspectors and what
salaries would suffice? And if there were sufficient inspectors,
which is impossible, who would dare to accuse the settlers?
The Indian would be afraid and he knows that if he com-
plains to the inspector, his owner would roast him; and we
do not have to go as far as the Indies, if we make an inves-
tigation here among us of the life of the inhabitants in
this city, are you going to question the servants of the man
you are going to punish? So Your Lordships can see that
since all those Indians are servants, or better still captives
of those who hold them in encomienda, if they complain
they would not be believed.... If on such estate there were
an angel who did not sleep or eat, or could not be   corrupted by gifts and gold, it would not be humanly possible
to put a stop to all those evils, and in the end Your Lordships will see that the inspector would regard the Spaniard
as a man and maybe as a friend or a benefactor, and the
Indian owned by him as a beast.

Item, that encomienda is contrary to the interest of
the King our lord; first, because it robs him of what makes
him a great lord, which is a large population, which is considered by the Scriptures as the basis of the King's glory
and power....

Item, this encomienda is very harmful to the welfare

\**Op. cit.,* Libro Tercero, Cap. CXXXVI, Tomo III, pp. 297—302.

of the King, our lord, because it takes away from him his just and true title and dominion to those lands.... He who is not lord of any town or does not possess one by inheritance, can become a just lord of one in one of these three ways: first, if the superior of his or that town, as a lawful penalty for evils committed, should put them under the dominion of the person in question, depriving the first lords of it in a lawful way; secondly, if the superior should subject the town to the said prince so that by good deeds, for the temporal and spiritual growth of the town, he would deserve to be lord of it; thirdly, if the town should wish of its own accord and voluntarily to submit itself to the lord. Any prince who without any of these titles possesses and holds dominion over any land, is neither king nor true lord, but a very bad tyrant, for it is obvious that the Pope did not deprive the lords of those lands for crimes, because they were not a danger to the faith, or schismatics, nor would the mere fact that they were infidels suffice to deprive them of their power, especially in lands which were never subject to the Church....

Item, that form of encomienda is contrary to all rules of theology and moral philosophy, which require that the end be preferred to the means and the means be subordinated to the end to be attained; and since our true end is heavenly bliss, and the proper means to attain it are the virtues, and for the exercise of the meritorious virtues life is necessary, and for the conservation of life we need food, and to buy food money is the most remote, useless and unnecessary means, if to this miserable means we subordinate the glory of heaven, the virtues with which we attain it, the life in which they are exercised, the food necessary for it, the worst of it all is that not only do the Indians lose their faith and virtues for gold, but the Christians themselves, as we have seen from experience, become more inhuman and less merciful than the fierce tigers....

Item, this sort of encomienda is against God, Our Lord, ....since there cannot be everlasting salvation without faith, He wants men to have it, and since the faith must come to the soul through the ears He came to preach it.... and to preach it in the whole world he made of his rude disciples wise teachers, enlightened by the Holy Ghost, and before their wisdom all the wise men of the world are left speechless, and for this reason He put in our hands those extensive lands and people. All this is prevented by this wretched encomienda, because, how could the preachers instruct people who are scattered and tired from working?....

Item, this sort of encomienda is against God's Church, because since everybody is occupied in the accursed exercise of mining and not in fertilizing the land so that it should produce natural wealth, there are no tithes from which the good prelates and priests and other ministers can support themselves in order to beget spiritual children for the Church. Thus the Church is not multiplying where it could multiply to the same or greater extent as it is being multiplied throughout the rest of the world....

The first thing.... that should be done to repair the damages is to take away their cause....There have been three causes for all the woes and deaths of these Indians, and they are as follows, excluding the accidental causes: first, excessive work; second, lack of provisions and food; third, discontent with their work and despair of its ever ending. It these are examined, it will be appreciated that they are enough to kill not only physically weak Indians, but strong giants. It is evident that these three evils have been abundantly inflicted upon them, more than their strength could endure; it is left, then, to find a suitable remedy for them.... first, to release them in justice from the oppressive encomienda and hard servitude imposed on them, for it contains much iniquity and damages, and give them their liberty in the following way: that from the people in these islands of Cuba, Hispaniola and others some villages be made of about 200 inhabitants, or according to the nature of the land where they are founded, and that they be assigned a governor, a good and tactful person who is able to instruct them in agriculture, and in cultivating vineyards, vegetable gardens, sugar and other useful crops, and that this individual be paid by the King, our lord, a fixed salary, which shall be taken from the products and profits of the Indians, instead of assigning him a fixed quota, so that it shall not be a third or fourth of what the Indians produce (because if this is done, in order that he may increase his quota, the Indians will work more than they should and he shall reduce the food they need, and the same inconveniences which we have now will arise), but that he shall receive so much per year, so many *castellanos*. He shall order and decide when and what the Indians in his charge should sow and when the crops shall be harvested and how the harvest shall be used for the nourishment of the Indians and that of their wives and children, and he shall sell part of what they sowed to the others who grew no crops, like the officials and those who have their slaves working in the mines, and all the rest shall be carefully kept. Item, that this governor shall determine who shall go to the mines from those who are within his power and at what time of the year, because they say that there are two Augusts, one more fertile than the other, and they could devote themselves to agriculture half the year, and the other half all or most of them could go to the mines. From the gold they shall extract they shall pay the King one-fifth, and from the taxes on their sales they shall pay one-tenth to the Church.... and an account shall be kept of what is left.... from which, first of all, the governor's salary shall be taken out, and the cost of whatever may be necessary for the maintenance of the Indians throughout the whole year, and for the cost of the farming, hammocks and other commodities which the Indians need. At the end of the year, the governor will be obliged to give a complete account, as a steward, of everything that has been collected, provisions as well as other things like gold, and what he has spent, paying from the balance the inspectors which Your Highness sent for this purpose; and all the rest, once the aforesaid things have been paid for, shall be for the said Indians and shall be used, with the approval of the inspectors, in useful things for them, like dresses and jewelry and other things, and in building homes for them, so that, if possible, in the course of time they shall each have his home with its rooms and a chest where they can keep their possessions, and thus they shall be taught to desire private property, to buy jewelry and keep it.... There are many such persons to be found in the Kingdom of Castile who are fit for this responsibility and who will undertake it with goodwill and praise God for it.

This method could be expanded considerably, if it is put in action, and with it all the evils committed in those lands will be avoided, for in this way, the Indians will be completely free, as other peoples, although subject to their governor, which is not contrary to freedom. Item, they will have less work to do, for.... when the governor sees that the product of the Indians' work is for them and not for him, the Indians will not be overworked, and since the profits will be theirs they will not die of hunger.... Item, the Indians themselves, seeing that they are not as exhausted by their labour, and are better fed, will be more content and not as desperate, and seeing that all the product of their labour is for their own advantage, they will be glad to work and will not display the despair and discontent which they have had until now, and work will become a recreation. In this way they will be happier, will multiply, and love those who do them good and they will approach our Holy Faith with great love, seeing that those who live in it receive so many benefits. Before long, instructed and indoctrinated by us, they will become a noble people living in civil society, especially since they are said to be of a gentle and modest nature and capable of and inclined to all virtue, and able to learn and live by themselves, for it was in this way that the other countries were attracted to political society and virtues, like Spain, Germany, and England, which in other times were just as or more barbarous than these Indians....

## No. 77—THE FEUDAL CONCEPT

### (Opinion of the Dominican Fathers, 1544)*

In a well-ordered state it is necessary that there should be rich men, in order that they may resist enemies, and that the poor may live under their protection, as there are in all kingdoms which are well-governed and stable, as in Spain and other kingdoms. And if the Indies are to survive, it is a great error to think that all the inhabitants must be equal, just as neither Spain nor any other kingdom would be preserved if there were not lords and princes and rich men. And in the Indies there can be no rich or powerful men, if they are not given Indian villages in trust, because all the labour on the plantations and farms is performed by the Indians of the villages given in trust to Spaniards, and without them there is no way of making any profit.

## No. 78 — BORROWED GOODS

### (Bernardino de Manzanedo, Emissary of the Jeronimite Commissioners, to Charles V, Emperor of the Hapsburg Empire, 1518) **

One of the principal causes of the depopulation of those parts has been the changes. Since no one has the assurance that he will be able to keep his encomienda Indians, he has used them like borrowed goods, and thus many have perished and are perishing.

## No. 79 — THE DESTRUCTION OF THE INDIANS IN HISPANIOLA

### (Alonso de Zuazo, Judge of Hispaniola, to M. de Chevres, January 22, 1518) ***

In conclusion this is the result of the repartimientos, from the time of the old Admiral to today, When Hispaniola was discovered it contained 1,130,000 Indians; today their number does not exceed 11,000. Judging from what has happened, there will be none of them left in three or four years time unless some remedy is applied.

---

*Cited in Lewis Hanke, La Lucha por la Justicia en la Conquista de America, Buenos Aires, 1949, p. 243.

**Cited in Simpson, op. cit., p. 50.

***Cited in Saco, Historia de la Esclavitud de los Indios, Tomo II, p. 307.

## No. 80 — THE DESTRUCTION OF THE INDIANS IN PUERTO RICO

*(Report of Capt. Juan Melgarejo, Governor of Puerto Rico, to Philip II, King of Spain, January 1, 1582)**

At the time of the division of the Indians which was made when the island was annexed, there were five thousand Indian men and five hundred Indian women, not counting those who were not domesticated and who remained to be distributed. Today there is not a single Indian left, except for a few who were brought from the mainland, about twelve or fifteen. They have all died from illnesses they contracted like measles, colds and smallpox, and because of illtreatment they fled to other islands with Caribs. Those who are left do not live in the town which has been built; some serve as soldiers, others live on their small farms among Spaniards. They do not speak their native language because most of them were born in this island; they are good Christians.

---

## No. 81 THE BAN ON INDIAN SLAVERY: THE CHURCH *(Bull of Pope Paul III, Sublimis Deus Sic Dilexit, June 17, 1537)***

The sublime God so loved the human race that He not only created man in such wise that he might participate in the good that other creatures enjoy, but also endowed him with capacity to attain to the inaccessible and invisible Supreme Good and behold it face to face .... all are capable of receiving the doctrines of the faith.

The enemy of the human race, who opposes all good deeds in order to bring men to destruction, beholding and envying this, invented a means never before heard of, by which he might hinder the preaching of God's word of salvation to the people: he inspired his satellites who, to please him, have not hesitated to publish abroad that the Indians of the West and the South, and other people of whom we have recent knowledge should be treated as dumb brutes created for our service, pretending that they are incapable of receiving the Catholic faith.

We.... consider, however, that the Indians are truly men and that they are not only capable of understanding the Catholic faith but, according to our information, they desire exceedingly to receive it. Desiring to provide ample remedy for these evils, we declare.... that, notwithstanding whatever may have been or may be said to the contrary, the

*Cited in Coll y Toste, *Boletin Historico de Puerto Rico,* Vol. 1, pp. 75—91.
**Cited in Hanke, *The Spanish Struggle for Justice,* pp. 72—73.

said Indians and all other people who may later be discovered by Christians, are by no means to be deprived of
their liberty or the possession of their property, even
though they be outside the faith of Jesus Christ; and that
they may and should, freely and legitimately, enjoy their
liberty and the possession of their property; nor should they
be in any way enslaved; should the contrary happen it shall
be null and of no effect.

By virtue of our apostolic authority, we declare....
that the said Indians and other peoples should be converted
to the faith of Jesus Christ by preaching the word of God
and by the example of good and holy living.

---

## No. 82 — THE BAN ON INDIAN SLAVERY: THE STATE

*("The New Laws for the Good Treatment and Preservation
of the Indians", November 20, 1542)**

....X. As one of the principal things in which the said
*Audiencias* are to serve us is to take very special care about
the good treatment and preservation of the Indians, we
command that they shall always keep themselves informed
of excessss or bad treatment which are or may be committed
by Governors, or by private persons, and of how these have
observed the Ordinances and instructions that have been
given them, which have been made to ensure the good
treatment of the Indians; and in so far as such excesses
have been or may in future be committed, let the said
*Audiencias* take care to remedy, by punishing the
offenders with rigour in conformity with justice....

XI. We decree and command that from now onward,
neither because of war, even though under the category of
rebellion, nor by barter, nor for any other cause in any
other way, may any Indian be made a slave; and we wish
them to be treated as our subjects of the Crown of Spain,
for that they are....

....we direct and command that the *Audiencias*....
shall.... place the enslaved at liberty, unless the persons
holding them as slaves can show a title that they hold and
own them legally....

XII. We order that, for the protection of the Indians,
the *Audiencias* are to take special care that these do not
carry loads; or, if in some parts it cannot be avoided, that
it be done in such a way that the load be not so heavy as
to endanger the life,, health or preservation of the said
Indians, nor be done against their wills, nor unless they are
paid. In no circumstances is such work to be forced on

*Cited in *Documentos Ineditos de las Antiguas Posesiones Espanolas de
Ultramar*, Segunda Serie, Tomo XXIII, Madrid, 1930, pp. 316—322.

them; let those who act otherwise be very severely punished. In this no exception is to be made for any person whatever.

As we have been informed that the pearl fishery has not been conducted with the good order that is desirable, and that it has resulted in the deaths of many Indians and Negroes, we order that no free Indian shall be taken to the said fishery against his will, under pain of death; and let the Bishop and the Judge who may go to Venezuela direct what may appear to them just in order that the slaves employed in the same fishery — Indians as well as Negroes — be protected, and deaths cease. And if it should appear to them that the risk of death cannot be avoided by the said Indians and Negroes, then let the pearl fishery cease; for, as is reasonable, we value much more highly the preservation of lives than the profit which may come to us from the pearls.

As the viceroys, governors and their lieutenants, and our officers, prelates, monasteries, hospitals, religious houses, mints, as well as officers of our revenue, and other persons favoured as officials hold Indians in *encomienda,* and as disorders have arisen in the treatment of those Indians, it is our will and we command that all the Indians they hold and possess shall be promptly placed under our Royal Crown....

We further order that all persons who hold Indians without having a title, but have possessed themselves of them on their own authority, are to give them up and place them under our Royal Crown. As we are informed that other persons, though they hold a title, have been given *repartimientos* in excessive quantity, we order our *Audiencias....* to reduce the *repartimientos* of such persons to fair and moderate proportions, the rest being promptly brought under our Royal Crown, in spite of any petition and appeal that such persons may make. The *Audiencias* are to send an early account of what they have done that we may know how our commands have been obeyed....

The said *Audiencias* shall enquire how the Indians have been treated by the persons who have held them in *encomienda;* and, if it should appear that they ought in justice to be deprived of their Indians, owing to excesses and ill treatment of them, we order that they be promptly so deprived, and that such Indians be placed under our Royal Crown....

We further order and command that from now onward no Viceroy, Governor, *Audiencia,* explorer, or other person whatsoever, has the right to allot Indians in *encomienda* whether by original indenture, transfer, gift, sale, or in any other form or manner, nor by voidance or inheritance; but when a person who owned Indians dies let them be placed under our Royal Crown....

XIII. We order and command that our said Presidents and Judges take great care that Indians who become liberated or unclaimed in any of the above ways be very well treated, and instructed in the doctrines of our holy Catholic faith, and remain, as our subjects, free men. This is to be their principal care and that to which we would have them pay particular attention, and in which they can best serve us....

In addition to the aforesaid we command the said persons who are exploring at our orders to make promptly a valuation of the tribute or service which the Indians in the land discovered should render as our vassals, and let the same tribute be moderate, so that they can endure it, bearing in mind the preservation of these same Indians....

It is our will and we decree that the Indians now alive in the islands of San Juan, and in Cuba and Espanola, both for the present and as long as it shall be our pleasure, be not oppressed with tribute or other royal services, whether of a personal or mixed kind, in excess of what is due from Spaniards who reside in the said islands; but let them be left at their ease that they may the better increase and be instructed in the tenets of our holy catholic faith; and with this object let suitable religious persons be assigned them....

## (iv) THE REVOLT OF THE ABORIGINAL INDIANS

### No. 83—SPAIN'S MILITARY SUPERIORITY

*(Bartolome de las Casas, Historia de las Indias (1559), Madrid, 1875)\**

Since the Admiral perceived that daily the people of the land were taking up arms, ridiculous weapons, in reality, and that their dislike for the Christians was growing, not considering the justice and reason the Indians had for this, he hastened to proceed to the country and disperse and subdue, by force of arms, the people of the entire island.... for which purpose he selected 200 Spanish foot soldiers, the healthiest ones (because many were sick and thin), and 20 men from the cavalry, with many cross-bows, muskets, lances and swords, and another more terrible and frightful weapon against the Indians, besides the horses, was the 20 ferocious greyhounds which, when released and told "at him", in one hour tore each a hundred Indians to pieces; since the people of this island were used to go totally naked from head to foot, one can easily judge what the ferocious greyhounds could do when excited and provoked by those

*Op. cit., Libro Primero, Cap. CIV, Tomo I, pp. 413—414.

who unleashed them on naked bodies or very delicate skins; the effect was greater, indeed, than on tough swine of Carona or deer. This invention began here, excogitated, invented and surrounded by the Devil, and it spread over the entire Indies, and its use will only come to an end when there is no more land in this hemisphere and no more people to subdue and destroy, like other exquisite inventions, most dangerous and harmful to the greater part of the human race, which began here and spread, for the total destruction of these nations... It is also to be noted, that, as the Indians in this island and in many parts of the mainland went naked, and in all other lands their clothing consisted of no more than a thin cotton cloth, one and a half or two yards square at the most; and these (I mean their skins and the cotton cloths) are their defensive weapons in most of these Indies, the cross-bows of the Christians, the muskets of old times and above all the incomparable arquebuses of today are for the Indians incredibly harmful: for there is no need to refer to the swords which today cut a naked Indian in half; the horses, to people who had never seen them and who imagined that man and horse were a single animal, were so terrifying that they buried themselves alive in an abyss, and to their misfortune, after they got to know them, have tangible evidence today in their bodies, houses, towns and kingdoms what they suffer from them or what they feared. It is a fact, that 10 men on horseback, at least in this island (and in all other places in the Indies, unless in the high mountains), are enough to destroy and to despatch with their lances 100,000 men massed against the Christians, in war, without 100 escaping; and this indeed happened in the Vega Real of this island, the terrain of the Vega being as flat as a table....Thus, we cannot use any of our weapons against the Indians which would not be very destructive to them; of their offensive ones against us nothing need be said because, as we said above, the majority are like those used in children's games.

---

### No. 84—TREACHERY IN THE INDIAN RANKS

*(Bartolome de las Casas, Historia de las Indias (1559), Madrid, 1875)*\*

....since the Admiral decided to march over the island with as many Christian troops as he could muster, in order to disperse the Indian bands and subjugate the entire land, the king Guacanagari offered to go with him and to take as many of his own people as possible, to curry favour with and help the Christians, and this he did. It is to be noted here by those who love truth and justice, who are only

\*Op. cit., Libro, Primero, Cap. CII, Tomo I, pp. 404—405.

those free from all passions, and especially temporal interests, that, although for the sake of the Christians and in order that they might remain in the island, the king Guacanagari undertook to curry favour with and help them, and although on the surface it may seem to those who do not penetrate to the heart of the matter that the said Guacanagari was acting well and virtuously, in reality, considering the obligation which, by the law of nature, all men have to the common good and liberty and conservation of their native country and its public state.... this king Guacanagari offended against and violated very much the law of nature, and was a traitor and destroyer of his country and of those of the kings of the island and of the entire nation, and he sinned mortally by helping, supporting, favouring and maintaining the Christians, and therefore all the kings and lords and all the other people of those kingdoms, justly and lawfully turned on him and waged just war against him and his kingdom, as a capital enemy of theirs and the public enemy of all, traitor and squanderer of his country and nation since he helped and favoured and maintained their hosts or public enemies.... harsh people, hard-hearted, strong and strange, who troubled them, disturbed them, illtreated them, oppressed them, placed them in cruel servitude and in the end, wiped them out, destroyed them and killed them, and it was most probable and certain that those strange people, who committed such acts and who gave such proof of their character wherever they went, would establish their roots firmly in the land, and would subvert, destroy and ruin, as they finally did.... all the kingdoms of this island.... and what is more, his own kingdom and his own vassals and subjects—such a traitor to and destroyer of his country and of the whole public state of his kingdom, they could lawfully kill and wage just war against him, and he, if he defended himself, was unjust to them and to the other kings....

---

## No. 85—UNITED FRONT OF THE ABORIGINES

*(Bartolome de las Casas, Historia de las Indias (1559), Madrid, 1875)\**

Another day they went to the mountains to search for the Indians. They reached a village which they found deserted and captured an Indian who told them that three or four leagues away was the village of Mayobanex, and that he was there with a large force ready to fight.... From the mountains they shot with arrows at the Christians and

*\*Op. cit., Libro Primero, Cap. CXX, Tomo I, p. 460.*

wounded some who had no time to put up their shields. The Christians went after them, fired at and killed many of them, and with their swords ripped them up and cut off their arms and legs; many were seized as slaves. The Governor sent one of the prisoners to tell Mayobanex that he did not come to make war on his people, but that he wanted to be friends with him; that he wanted only Guarionex whom he knew Mayobanex was hiding and under whose influence Mayobanex was waging war on the Christians. Therefore, he begged him to surrender Guarionex and that then he would always be his good friend and would always befriend him where his kingdom and people were concerned, but if he did not, he would pursue him with fire and sword until he had destroyed him. It is good to note Mayobanex' answer: "Tell the Christians that Guarionex is a good and virtuous man, who never wronged anyone, as is well known, and is consequently worthy of compassion and should be helped and defended in his hour of need; the Christians, on the contrary, are evil men, tyrants, who come only to usurp other people's land, and know only how to shed the blood of those who never harmed them; therefore, tell them that I neither wish their kindness, nor do I wish to see them, or hear them, that I would rather do with my people what I could to assist Guarionex and destroy them and chase them out of this country."

*No. 86—THE SUPPRESSION OF THE REVOLT*
*(Bartolome de las Casas, Historia de las Indias (1559),*
*Madrid, 1875)\**

They selected their guides very carefully; they arrived at the place where Mayobanex was alone with his wife, children, and a few relatives, totally unprepared; they reached for their swords which, wrapped in palm leaves, they carried on their shoulders, as the Indians carried loads. Mayobanex, terrified, surrendered in order to avoid seeing himself or his wife and children hacked to pieces; they were all, the king, the queen, and the children, bound and taken to the Governor; more fun was made of the captives than can be told. They took them to Concepcion, and put the king in irons and chains, because he had assisted, defended and supported (as he was obliged to by the law of nature, by virtue and pity as well as by his duty to his country) a neighbouring king who found himself in supreme misery and calamity, and inhumanly, against all reason and justice, for what should be praised by Moors and Jews, Gentiles and barbarians, and even more by Christians, they treated

---

*Op. cit.*, Libro Primero, Cap. CXXI, Tomo I, pp. 463—465.

him very badly, and with cruel impiety deprived him of
his kingdom, lordship and liberty.... All the lords and chief
men of the land thought that Mayobanex should be set at
liberty. A number of them decided to come and bring their
presents of bread, game and fish, everything roasted,
because they had no other wealth, and because the Indians
never come to the Christians empty handed, especially if
they have to ask a favour; when they arrived, they begged,
implored and importuned that Mayobanex should be set
free, promising that they would always be obedient and
would serve the Governor and the Christians. The Governor
freed the queen and all the prisoners taken in Mayobanex'
house, children, relatives, and servants, but their tears and
supplications were of no avail as far as Mayobanex was con
cerned. A few days before, the king Guarionex, unable any
longer to live in the rocks and caves and endure his sad
life and especially his hunger, went out to seek food, and
it was impossible to avoid being seen. As people daily came
to visit the king Mayobanex, at the fortress of La Vega or
La Concepcion and bring him food, inevitably the Governor
was informed that Guarionex was in the neighbourhood. He
sent a troop of Spaniards and Indians to look for him; they
found him without much difficulty and brought him back
a prisoner. They imprisoned him in the fortress of La Concepcion, separated from Mayobanex, and kept him there
in irons, chains and fetters, he who ruled over the largest
and best part of this whole island, for no crime committed
by him, without reason or justice.... And so they kept him
in that narrow prison and in that bitter life for three years,
until the year 1502 when he was sent to Castile in irons,
as a result of which he was drowned.... I did not ascertain
the fate of the other good and pious king Mayobanex; I
think he died in prison; when I arrived in this island, he
had been in prison and misery for two years.

---

No. 87—THE UNQUENCHABLE SPIRIT OF RESISTANCE

(Bartolome de las Casas, Historia de las Indias (1559),
Madrid, 1875)*

The cacique Hatuey, seeing that it was useless to fight
against the Spaniards, and having long experience in this
island of their crimes, decided to save himself by flight and
to hide in the brambles. The Spaniards learned from the
Indians whom they captured who he was (because the first
thing they ask for is the lords and chiefs to kill them, as,
once they are dead, it is easy to subdue the rest), many

*Op. cit., Libro Tercero, Cap. XXV, Tomo II, pp. 523—524.

soldiers hurried in search of him so as to capture him, as Diego Velazquez ordered. The search lasted for many days, and they threatened and tortured every Indian they captured alive, so that they would confess where Hatuey was. They said they did not know; they suffered the tortures and denied any knowledge of his hiding place; but finally, they learned where he was, and at last they found him. He was imprisoned as a man who had committed treason.... and was condemned to be burned alive. When they were ready to burn him, and he was tied to the stake, a Franciscan friar urged him as best as he could, to die a Christian and be baptized. Hatuey inquired why should he be like the Christians, who were bad people. The priest answered: "Because those who die Christians go to heaven where they eternally see God and rest". Hatuey then asked him if the Christians went to heaven; and the friar said that those who were good certainly went to heaven. Then, the Indian ended by saying that he did not wish to go there, because the Christians were there.... Thereupon they set fire to the wood and burned him.

## No. 88 — GUERRILLA WARFARE

*(Bartolome de las Casas, Historia de las Indias (1559), Madrid, 1875)*[*]

Some of the few Indians in the island took courage when they saw that Enrique was still a force. An Indian, whom they called the *Ciguayo*, rose in rebellion.... This Ciguayan was a courageous man, although naked as the others. He obtained a lance made of iron from Castile and I believe a sword also..., recruited ten or twelve Indians and with them began to attack the Spaniards in the mines, estates, or country farms, wherever they went, in twos or fours or small groups. He killed all those he found, so that he spread panic, terror and a strange fear throughout the island. No one believed himself safe even in the towns of the interior of the island, and all lived in fear of the Ciguayan. At last, the Spaniards formed a band and pursued him for many days. When they found him, they attacked him. He fought like a mad dog, as if he wore armour from head to toe. Whilst the bitter struggle raged, the Ciguayan retreated into a gorge, and there, while he was fighting, a Spaniard passed a lance half through his body and even then he fought like a Hector. Finally, when he was bleeding and losing strength, all the Spaniards rushed up and put an end to him....

[*]*Op. cit.*, Libro Tercero, Cap. CXXVII, Tomo III, pp. 266—267.

After the Ciguayan's death, another Indian, courageous and strong, rose in rebellion. His name was Tamayo, and with another band which he formed, he continued the work of the Ciguayan, and began to attack all those outside of the towns. He wrought much damage and caused great fear and commotion in this island; he killed many men and some Spanish women and all those he found alone on the estates, leaving not a single person alive, and his whole aim was to steal weapons, lances, swords and all the clothes he could. This was indeed nothing short of a miracle, for though the island contained more than three or four million people, only 300 Spaniards subjugated it and they destroyed three quarters of the inhabitants by war and by a horrible servitude in the mines. At the time of which we are speaking, however, when there were in this island 3,000 or 4,000 Spaniards, and only two Indians for every twelve or fifteen Spaniards, and not together, but separate, one now and the other one later, the Indians made the Spaniards tremble, and they did not consider themselves safe even in their towns. This can only be attributed to the Divine Judgment, which wished to prove to us three things: first that the Indians did not lack courage, or manhood, even though they were naked and very peace loving; secondly, that if only they had weapons like ours, and horses and arquebuses, they would not have been exterminated from the surface of the earth as we exterminated them; thirdly, that that was an indication of the condemnation of such deeds, and of the punishments we shall suffer in the life to come for the heinous sins committed against God and against our fellow-men, if we do not repent in this life.

### No. 89—PASSIVE RESISTANCE

*(Fray Pedro de Cordoba, Vice-Provincial of the Franciscan Friars in Santo Domingo, to Ferdinand V, King of Spain, May 28, 1517)\**

As a result of the sufferings and hard labour they endured, the Indians choose and have chosen suicide; occasionally a hundred have committed mass suicide. The women, exhausted by labour, have shunned conception and childbirth, so that work should not be heaped on them during pregnancy or after delivery; many, when pregnant, have taken something to abort and have aborted. Others, after delivery, have killed their children with their own hands, so as not to place or leave them in such oppressive slavery. These poor people no longer increase or multiply, nor do they bear children, which is a matter of great sorrow.

*Cited in Saco, *Historia de la Esclavitud de los Indios*, Tomo II, pp. 350—351.

### (v) THE PROTECTOR OF THE INDIANS, BARTOLOME DE LAS CASAS

*(Decree of Ferdinand II, King of Spain, September 17, 1516)\**

No. 90 — THE APPOINTMENT OF LAS CASAS

To Bartolome de las Casas, Cleric, a native of Seville and a resident of Cuba in the Indies, *the King and the Queen:*

Inasmuch as we have been informed that you have resided for a long time in those countries, and that hence you are by experience familiar with their affairs, especially those wherein the welfare of the Indians is concerned, and inasmuch as you, by contact with them, have become well acquainted with their customs and manner of living, and whereas we know that you are zealous in the service of God and our own, which makes us hope that you will comply carefully and diligently with our commands and the duties of the charge we hereby give you, and that you will work for the welfare of the souls and bodies of the Spaniards as well as of the Indians; therefore, by these presents we command that you go to the Indies, to Hispaniola, to Cuba, to Porto Rico, to Jamaica and to the Continent, and that you advise, counsel and inform the devout Fathers of St. Jerome, whom we send to reform the Indies, and all other persons, who may co-operate with them, about all the things concerning the liberty, humane treatment and salvation of the souls and bodies of said Indians of the aforementioned Islands and Continent, and that you thence write to us, that you inform us, and that you come to inform us about everything done in said Islands; and in order that you may do everything in a proper manner for the service of Our Lord and our own in the performance of the duties of your office, we hereby give you unreservedly all powers directly or indirectly connected or annexed, ordinarily or extraordinarily necessary to the exercise of your office. And we hereby command our admiral and the judges of the courts of appeal and all other judges in said Islands and Continent, that they respect and cause to be respected this power which we hereby give you, and that they observe and cause to be observed the spirit and the letter of this decree under penalty of our displeasure, and a fine of ten thousand maravedis for each offence.

---

No. 91—LAS CASAS CONDEMNS THE ROYAL POLICY
*(Speech of Bartolome de las Casas to the Emperor Charles V, 1519)\*\**

Most powerful and most high lord and king.

I am one of the oldest immigrants to the Indies, where

\* Cited in Las Casas, *Historia de las Indias*, Libro Tercero, Cap. XC, Tomo III, pp. 135—136.

\*\* Cited in Las Casas, *Historia de las Indias*, Libro Tercero, Cap. CXLIX, Tomo III, pp. 342—344.

I have spent many years and where, I have not read in histories, that sometimes lie, but saw with my own eyes, and, so to speak, came in contact with the cruelties, which have been inflicted on these peaceful and gentle people, cruelties more atrocious and unnatural than any recorded of untutored and savage barbarians. No other reason can be assigned for them than the greed and thirst for gold of our countrymen. They have been practised in two ways: first, by wicked and unjust wars, in which numberless Indians, who had been living in perfect peace in their own homes, and without molesting anybody, were slaughtered. Their countries, that formerly teemed with people and villages without number, have been made desolate; secondly, by enslaving, after doing away with their chiefs and rulers, the common people, whom they parcelled among themselves in *Encomiendas* of fifty or a hundred, and cast them into the mines, where, overwhelmed by incredible labours, they all perish. In coming to Spain I left them behind to die whenever they come in contact with the Spaniards. And, alas! one of the originators of this tyranny was my own father, who thank God, has not now anything more to do with it. At the sight of the injustices and atrocities inflicted upon a people, who had never harmed us, my heart was touched, not because I was a better Christian than anybody else, but because I am compassionate by nature. Hence I journeyed to these realms to inform His Catholic Majesty, your grandfather. I found him in Plasencia, where he kindly granted me an audience, during which I told him the things which I am about to detail to you. He was then on his way to Seville, where he promised me that measures would be adopted to correct the evils. But he died on the way, and my petition as well as his will on behalf of the Indians were frustrated. I next applied to the regents, Cardinal Ximenes and his Eminence the Cardinal of Tortosa. They promptly enacted the necessary legislation to stop the tyranny and the slaughter of so many people. But the persons selected to execute their laws, to root out the poisonous source of so many crimes, and to sow instead the good seed, were found unfit for the task. When I heard that Your Majesty had come to Spain, I hastened to renew my representations to you, and had not your first chancellor died in Zaragosa, a remedy would by this time have been found, and applied. I am to do the same work over again. But I find that the ministers of the enemy of all good are not wanting here about, who endeavour, through their selfish interests, to block my way. Sire, the spiritual interests of your soul excepted, nothing is of greater importance to Your Majesty than the finding of a remedy for these evils, For not one of your European kingdoms or all of them together equal in vastness and greatness your transatlantic possessions. In telling you so, I

feel certain of rendering to Your Majesty as great a service, as mortal vassal has ever rendered to his king. For
so doing I ask no reward or favour, inasmuch as my first
object is not to do a service to Your Majesty. I desire to
speak with all the respect and reverence due to so high
a personage as my king Your Majesty. But, were I not bound
to do so, as liege to my lord, I would not, forsooth, move
to the corner of this room to do you service, if I did not
think and know that, by so doing, I would make a pleasing
offering to God, who is a jealous God, and does not share
with others the honours and glory due to Him by His creatures. For His honour and glory alone, I have undertaken
this self-imposed task. But I know that I cannot take a step
forward without doing, at the same time, an inestimable
service to Your Majesty. That the meaning of my words may
not be misunderstood, I hereby renounce and decline any
favour or temporal reward that Your Majesty might hereafter offer me. And should it come to pass that I, either
personally or through a third party directly or indirectly,
should solicit any favour or reward for my services, I am
willing to be branded as a liar and a traitor to my lord
the king.

The people with whom the New World is swarming
are not only capable of understanding the Christian religion,
but amenable, by reason and persuasion, to the practice of
good morals and the highest virtues. Nature made them free
and they have their kings or rulers to regulate their political
life. The bishop of Darien has told you they are *servi
a natura* because the philosopher said at the beginning of
his *politicus* that *vigentes ingenio naturaliter sunt rectores
et domini aliorum*, whereas the *deficientes a ratione
naturaliter sunt servi*. Between the meaning attributed to
those words by his lordship and that intended by the philosopher, there is as much difference as between heaven and
earth. But granting that the bishop understood him right,
the philosopher was a pagan, who is now burning in hell,
and those of his doctrines only must be followed, which do
not contradict our Christian morals and our Christian faith.
Our holy religion adapts itself equally as well to all the
nations of the world; it embraces them all and deprives
no human being of his natural liberty under pretext or
colour that he or she is *servus a natura*, as the bishop, if
I understand him right, would have you believe. Sire, it
therefore behoves Your Majesty that you banish, at the
beginning of your reign, that gigantically tyrannical system,
which, horrible alike in the sight of God and man, is the
ruin of the majority of mankind. This do, in order that
Our Lord, who died for those people, may bless and prosper
your rule for many days to come.

## No. 92 — LAS CASAS CONDEMNS THE POLICY OF COLUMBUS

*(Bartolome de las Casas, Historia de las Indias (1559), Madrid, 1875)* *

The Admiral thought that he should take to Castile, from this island of Cuba or the mainland...., a few Indians to teach them the Castilian language....

It is a fact that one should endure any toil and danger rather than do such a thing, for, indeed, it was nothing but a violation, tacit or interpretative, of the rules of the law of nature and international law, which state and hold that he who comes simply and trustingly to trade with others, especially if both sides had already trusted each other and traded amicably, should be allowed to return home freely and without impediment, without damage to his person or property. Columbus' action was wrong, the Indians having received the Spaniards in their land and homes so ceremoniously and joyfully, worshipping them as if they were divine, from Heaven.... How would the Admiral have felt if the Indians had forcibly detained the two Christians he had sent into the interior and of what crime would he have thought the Indians guilty? He would certainly have thought that, in order to rescue the two Christians, he might wage just war against them; since the laws and rules of nature and international law are common to all nations, Christians and gentiles, whatever their sect, law, state, colour and condition, without a single difference, the inhabitants of that island had the same right to wage just war on the Admiral and his Christians in order to rescue their neighbours and compatriots. And it adds greatly to the ugliness of this action that the Christians were themselves responsible for the loss of as much authority and prestige as the Indians had credited them with kindness, rectitude and gentleness; and the good intentions of the Admiral are no excuse, no matter how good and beneficial they might later have been, because we must never do a wrong act, however trifling and insignificant it may be, in order that there should spring or be derived from it inestimable advantages.

## No. 93—THE FOUR LORDS AND MASTERS OF THE INDIANS

*(Bartolome de las Casas, Entre los Remedios para.....la Reformacion de las Indias, Madrid, 1543)* * *

It would be just as well to throw the Indians on the horns of wild bulls or to fling them to hungry wolves, lions

*Op. cit., Libro Primero, Cap. XLVI, Tomo I, pp. 232—233.
**Cited in Hanke, *The Spanish Struggle for Justice*, p. 215.

and tigers. The Indians have four lords and masters: Your Majesty, their cacique, the one who holds them in trust, and the planter. The planter is for them a heavier weight than a hundredweight of lead.

---

## No. 94—LAS CASAS CONDEMNS THE POOR WHITES

*(Bartolome de las Casas, Historia de las Indias (1559), Madrid, 1875)**

As they now saw themselves as lords of the native rulers, served and feared by all their people, adult and children, whose flesh trembled before them....the Spaniards more and more forgot their origins, and their arrogance, presumptuousness, luxury and contempt for these most humble people increased. When they got up, though they had neither mules nor horses, they would not walk any distance, but insisted on being borne on the shoulders of the unfortunate Indians if they were in a hurry, or in litters, slung in hammocks, if they were not; and those that carried them, taking turns, had to move swiftly. Accompanying the Spaniards were Indians who carried large leaves to shade them and others who carried goose wings to fan them; I saw many droves of Indians, bound for the mines, loaded down like asses with cassava bread, and many times the men's backs were sore with their burdens like those of beasts. When they reached the Indian villages, the Spaniards would eat and spend what would have been plenty for fifty Indians; the cacique and all the people of the village would have to bring what they had and dance attendance on them. This was not the only way in which they demonstrated their imperiousness and most vain ostentation. They had other trained women servants, in addition to the principal servant, such as the chambermaid, the cook, and others trained for similar occupations. I knew an official organ-maker in those days who had some of these trained maidservants.... It was comical to see the presumption and vanity of the Spaniards, how they esteemed and exalted themselves; those who could not afford a shirt of Castilian linen, cloak, coat, or stockings, but wore only a cotton shirt over another one from Castile, if they could afford even that, and if not, then only the cotton one, with their legs bare, and instead of buskins and shoes rope sandals and leggings....

*Op. cit., Libro Segundo, Cap. I, Tomo II, p. 205.

*No. 95 — LAS CASAS CONDEMNS THE REPARTIMIENTO*
*(Bartolome de las Casas, Historia de las Indias (1559),*
*Madrid, 1875)\**

Thus, the Queen's first and most important wish.... was that the Indians should be taught the doctrines of the Church and converted. As I said before and now reaffirm, during the time Ovando governed this Island, which was about nine years, no more interest was taken in the instruction and conversion of the Indians, and no more action was taken, and no further mention of it made than if the Indians were sticks or stones, cats or dogs....

Ovando dissolved the many large villages there were in this island, and he gave to each Spaniard as many Indians as he wanted; to one 50, to another 100 and to some more and to others less, according to whether each was in his good favour; and in this number there were children and old people, pregnant women, and women who had just given birth, patricians and plebeians, and the very lords and kings of their villages and country. This distribution of Indians.... among the Spaniards was called the *repartimiento*.... From each Indian village many allotments were made, giving a number of Indians to each Spaniard, and with each of these groups he sent the lord or cacique, and he gave the group to the Spaniard whom he wanted to honour and favour most. To those Spaniards, he issued a decree of the *repartimiento* which read as follows: "To you, so and so, are committed in the person of the cacique, so and so, 50 or 100 Indians, so that you might make use of their services, and teach them the fundamentals of our Holy Catholic Faith." Another one read, "To you, so and so, are committed in the person of the cacique, so and so, 50 or 100 Indians, with the cacique himself, so that you may use them in your farms and mines, and teach them the fundamentals of our Holy Catholic Faith".... So that all Indians, children and adults, young and old, men and women... were absolutely condemned to servitude, in which in the long run they died. Such was the liberty which they obtained from the *repartimiento*.

As to the Queen's third point, that the Spaniards should respect the needs of women and children and that husband and wife should be together every night, or at least every Saturday.... Ovando allowed the Spaniards to take the husbands to mine gold, 10, 20, 40 and 80 leagues away, and the women stayed on the plantations or farms, working the soil. They had neither hoes nor oxen, but broke the soil with sticks, sweating in labour incomparably more onerous than that of miners in Castile. The women worked hard for the food they received. They had to dig holes thirty-two inches deep and 12 feet wide, ten or twelve thousand altogether, a hard work even for giants. Their other tasks

*\*Op. cit., Libro Segundo, Caps. XIII—XIV, Tomo II, pp. 249—257.*

were no less onerous; whatever the Spaniards saw was most profitable for them. So that husband and wife were never together, nor did they see each other in eight or ten months, or in a whole year; and when at the end of this period of time they were together again, the men were so tired and exhausted from hunger and work, so fatigued, and the women no less so, that they had no interest in marital relations, and in this way they ceased to bear children. The infant mortality rate was very high, because the mothers, overworked and hungry, had no milk in their breasts; hence, within three months, 7,000 children died in Cuba while I was there. Some mothers drowned their children out of despair; others, as soon as they realised that they were pregnant, took herbs to cause a miscarriage and the babies were stillborn. Since the husbands died in the mines and the women in the farms due to overwork, and the newborn babies due to the lack of milk....they all were bound to die out soon, as they did, and thus, this large, valuable, fertile, although unfortunate island was depopulated. It should be noted that if such things happened throughout the world, and all the human race were not wiped out, it would be a marvel.

As to the Queen's fourth point, that the Indians should work part of the time and not incessantly, and should be treated leniently and humanely, Ovando's decree apportioning them entailed constant work, without rest. If he set any limitations later, which I do not recall, at least it is a fact that they were given little rest.... he allowed cruel Spanish executioners to supervise and direct them.... These people treated the Indians so harshly and with such inhumanity that they seemed to be the ministers of hell, who day and night allowed not a moment of peace and rest. They beat them, slapped them, kicked them, and whipped them, and the Indians never heard a kinder word from them than "dogs". Because of the cruel and harsh treatment they received from the farmers and miners, and the continuous and intolerable tasks that they endured without a murmur, and knowing for certain that they would never survive but would die, as they saw their fellowmen dying, which is what casts the damned in hell into the depths of despair, the Indians began to run away to the mountains where they could hide. Rural constables were appointed to hunt them down and bring them back. In the cities and towns of the Spaniards, Ovando appointed a citizen, the most honourable and prominent, whom he called inspector, and to whom he gave for the office, as if it was a salary, another hundred Indians, apart from those allotted to him during the *repartimiento*....

As to the Queen's fifth point, that the tasks were to be reasonable, etc., these tasks were to mine gold.... which is such, that the men need to be made of iron for this. The saws are moved up and down, the upper part down and the lower part up, digging and breaking rocks and moving stones, and to wash the gold in the rivers the men carry the earth on their shoulders. The washermen stand deep in the water, backs bent.... When the mine is flooded, all the work is done by the men with their arms and large wooden troughs, up and down in order to get the water out. Finally, to appreciate how arduous it is to mine gold and silver, it should be remembered that the greatest penalty the Gentiles imposed upon a martyr, besides death, was to condemn him to mine metals....

At first the Indians were kept working in the mines for six months; then the period was extended to eight.... until they brought all the gold to the smeltery. After it was smelted the King took his share, and the rest was given to the owner of the *repartimiento,* although for many years he never received not even a *castellano,* because he was so much in debt to merchants and other creditors. Because of the many hardships and cruelties they made the Indians suffer in order to mine that damned gold, God consumed it all and no man ever grew rich from it. During the smelting, the Indians who lived in villages two, three or four days' march away were permitted to go home. It may well be imagined how they got home, and what rest they found there, having been eight months away, leaving their women and children alone; if perhaps they had also taken them to the mines, they returned together, husbands and wives, to weep over their unhappy life ! What food would they find when they went to their farms to work and eat, and found them uncultivated and full of weeds, lacking all attention and care? Of those who had come from forty, fifty or eighty leagues away, ten out of a hundred never returned home, but stayed working in the mines and at other tasks until death. Many Spaniards did not hesitate to make the Indians work on Sundays and holidays, and if they were not forced to mine gold, at least they put them to building houses, mending them with straw, collecting wood and other odd jobs. The food they gave the Indians after so much work was *cacabi* bread, which if eaten with enough meat and other things is nourishing, but eaten without meat or fish or other food has little nutritive value. Thus the Indians were fed on *cacabi* bread. The miner killed a pig every week and ate half or more, and for thirty or forty Indians, he cooked a small piece every day from the other half and gave each Indian a small slice, about the size of a nut.... When the miner was eating, the Indians got under the table as dogs and cats do, and if a bone fell on the floor, they picked it up, sucked it, and then crushed it between two stones and what they got from it they ate with the *cacabi*.... (Only the Indians who

worked in the mines got this small slice of pork and the
bones from it, because the men and women who worked on
the plantations, digging and doing other jobs, never knew
.... what it was to eat meat, and ate only *cacabi* and other
roots). There were people in Cuba.... who, out of avarice,
provided no food for the Indians who worked in the fields,
and sent them for two or three days to graze in the country
and to eat the fruits from the trees on the mountains, and
after this.... made them work two or three days more
without another mouthful. In this way, one of them established a farm which was worth 500 or 600 gold dollars or
*castellanos,* and he himself related this in my presence and
that of others as if it were a feat of industry.

As for the Queen's sixth point, that the Indians should
be paid wages commensurate with their work, it may sound
incredible, but I swear it is true, Ovando ordered that they
be paid a daily wage, for their subsistence and for the work
and services they performed, at the rate of three *blancas* *
every two days. Even this wage, however, was not paid, but
half a *blanca* less, since he ordered that each Indian be given
half a gold dollar a year, which is equivalent to 225 maravedis. This wage was paid in kind, in pacotille from Castile....
With 225 maravedis they could buy a comb, a small mirror
and a string of green or blue beads. It is also a fact that
sometimes many years passed, and even this was not paid
to them and little was done for their welfare or to lessen
their suffering, hunger and woes; which were so many, that
they cared about nothing because, starving, all they wanted
was to eat and to find a way out of such a hopeless existence....

As to the seventh command of the Queen, that the
Indians were to be treated as free men, which they were,
and that no harm should be done unto them, that they should
be free to cultivate their farms and to rest and take care of
themselves, etc., it is clear, I believe, from what I have said
that Ovando completely took away their liberty and agreed
to place them under the most cruel and horrible servitude
and captivity that could hardly be believed unless one saw it
with one's own eyes, for the Indians were not free to do anything at all. Even the beasts are free sometimes to graze in
the fields, but the Spaniards did not allow the Indians to do
even this.... they were never free to do anything, except to
go where the cruelty and avarice of the Spaniards sent them,
not as captives, but as beasts, which their owners tied up to
do with as they pleased. When they were allowed to go to
their own towns to rest, they found their women and children dead, and no farm from which to get food.... because
they were not given time to till the soil. Thus their only

*The *blanca* was a copper coin of the value of half a maravedi.

alternative was to scour the country or mountains for herbs or roots and to die there. If they became ill, which frequently happened, due to the many and hard tasks to which they were not accustomed, being very frail people, the Spaniards did not believe them, and without any mercy called them dogs and told them they were shamming sickness in order to avoid work. They also kicked them and beat them, and when they saw that the sickness grew worse and that they could not use the Indians anymore, they allowed them to return to their own villages, twenty, thirty, fifty or eighty leagues away; and for the journey they gave them some roots and *cacabi* bread. Many of these poor people fell in the first stream where they died helpless; others went a little farther, but, in the end, only a few reached their villages. I found some dead by the roadside, and others dying under the trees, and still others groaning in pain and crying out, as best they could: "Hunger! hunger!" This was the liberty and good treatment, Christianity, and freedom from harm which the Indians received under Ovando's rules and orders.

As to the eighth and final injunction of Queen Elizabeth's letter.... that the Indians should associate with the Spaniards (in order that they might be taught the doctrines of the Church and be made Christians....), it was difficult if not impossible for the Indians to become Christians, rather it was pernicious and fatal to them, and it ended in their total destruction. It is clear that no such power was given nor could be given to the Spaniards because the Queen gave this order not for the destruction but for the welfare of the Indians, and Ovando should have taken this into consideration.... It was amazing that even though so many Indians died every eight months and during the smelting from year to year, this wise gentleman did not realise that his orders for the government of the Indians were like a fatal pestilence which decimated them, and he never reformed or abolished his system.... The only change he made in this abuse was as follows: Seeing that the number of the Indians was declining, from deaths in the mines and on the plantations, every eight months or year each Spaniard losing half or a good proportion of his *repartimiento,* the Spaniards themselves.... petitioned him to shuffle the cards, as they put it, and to make a new distribution. To the prominent Spaniards and those in his good graces he gave new Indians to replace those who had died, and since there was not enough cloth for all, many were left without. New distributions were made every two or three years. The Queen never knew of this cruel treatment because she died shortly after she wrote her letter.

*No. 96.—LAS CASAS CONDEMNS THE LAWS OF BURGOS*
*(Bartolome de las Casas, Historia de las Indias (1559)*
*Madrid, 1875)\**

The first article was the one which was most satisfactory
to the Spaniards, once they had been assured that the
Indians allotted to them were theirs in perpetuity. It was to
the effect that all the Indians were to be removed
from their villages where they had been born
and had grown up to other lands near the towns and settlements of the Spaniards which were totally inadequate for
them.... The law ordered that for every fifty Indians those
to whom they had been allotted should build four straw huts
or houses, thirty feet long and fifteen feet wide, on the lands
to which they were removed; should plant 5,000 garden
plots, 3,000 of cassava.... and 2,000 of *ajes*\*\*.... 250 feet
of the pepper used to season what they cooked (if they
cooked anything at all).... half a bushel of corn; and should
give them a dozen hens and a rooster. It should be noted
that less could not have been ordered and provided if the
Indians were sheep or cows; for so many animals, so many
yards and so much pasture....

Another defect of the law.... was that, while it orders
the Spaniards to whom the Indians were allotted to construct
the houses and plant the crops.... in fact the unfortunate
Indians had to construct them by the sweat of their own
brows.... The law was impossible in the light of natural
reason; it ran counter to the customs of the native inhabitants; it was not suited to the time and place; it was superfluous and useless, and it was harmful to and destructive of
the Indians to remove them from their own settlements and
villages. Above all it was made for the benefit and private
interests of the Spaniards and was contrary to the general
and universal welfare of the Indians....

In the second article, the King ordered that the caciques
be removed gently away from their villages to the new
settlements with the least possible harm to them, by coaxing
and persuasion. But what comfort was it to them to be deprived of their power, to see their subjects dead, and to be
sure that they too and what was left of their subjects would
soon die ?

In the third article, it was ordered that every Spaniard
who owned Indians was to construct near to the settlement,
a straw house which was to serve as a church, in which they
would place images of Our Lady and which was to have a
bell to call the Indians to prayer in the evenings as they
came from work and in the mornings before they went to
work. Someone was to go with them to teach them the Ave
Maria, the Pater Noster, the Credo and the Salve Regina;

\*Op. cit., Libro Tercero, Caps. XV and XVI, Tomo II, pp. 482—489.
\*\*A tuber, like the sweet potato.

this person was the miner in the mines and the planter on the plantations or farms. This was to ridicule the Christian faith and religion, for they were to say prayers in Latin or in Spanish, which the Indians understood as much as if they had been said in jargon; it was no more or no less than teaching parrots....

In the following articles, up to the twelfth, it was provided and ordered that within the radius of a league, in a suitable place, a church should be built where the Indians in the vicinity would come to hear Mass. But there was no priest to say it....

By the thirteenth article it was ordered and commanded that the Indians were to work in the gold mines for five months, at the end of which they were to rest for forty days, provided that during that time they cultivated the land from which they derived their subsistence.... This was the rest afforded to those who had worked in the mines for five consecutive months.... This cultivation of garden plots consisted of digging the soil with dried sticks, which served for hoes and spades, not quite as high as the waist and four feet wide....

There was another article which begins thus: "Since the good treatment of the Indians consists for the most part in the food given to them, on which depends the increase of their numbers, we order and command that all persons who own Indians be obliged to give enough bread, tubers and pepper to those who work on the plantations and cooked meat at least on Sundays, Easter and holidays; enough bread and pepper to the Indians working in the mines, as well as a pound of meat daily, with fish, sardines or other nourishing food on meatless days". This is the law which provided for the subsistence of the Indians.... Where could there be more blindness than in ordering that the Indians, who worked on the plantations and farms and who had tasks as hard as or harder than miners in Castile, be given as daily food cassava bread, which was as nourishing as grass; *ajes* which are truffles, and pepper; in a word nothing but grass (it was as much as to say, give them enough straw and hay); and in ordering that on Sundays, holidays, and Easter, they be given a pound of meat, as if it was ordered that they be given new dresses or clean shirts?.... This law also had another defect.... in ordering that on meatless days the Indians were to be given a pound of fish or sardines, and adding " or other foods". It seems as if it was understood that the law was only a matter of duty, because even though there was an abundance of fish in the sea as well as in the rivers, the sole aim of the Spaniards was to amass gold, and not one occupied himself in fishing or....in any other occupation ....Thus, the Indians never saw fish, and much less sardines which had to be brought from Castile. Accordingly, the

Indians in the mines also had to eat roots and herbs on meatless days....

There was another law which ordered that no woman more than four months pregnant was to be sent to the mines or put to work in the fields, but that the Spaniards should.... use them for housework, as well as in baking bread, cooking and weeding. Consider the cruelty and inhumanity: a pregnant woman had to work until her fourth month in the mines and in the garden plots, tasks for giants....until she gave birth she had to work in the home baking bread, which is not an easy task, while weeding the fields is even harder. The injustice of this article, as of all the others, is obvious, and it was unworthy that a royal hand should sign it.

Among the other articles, there were some which ordered that in each town or settlement there should be two inspectors who should visit the Indians twice a year, and who should see that the Indians were not harmed and that the laws were obeyed. The best joke was that one article ordered that Indians were to be allotted to the inspectors besides those they received as settlers. Consider the blindness of the Council and the reverend theologians, who did not realise that the inspectors thereby became a part of the system and would be more tyrannical than the others, as in fact they were.... One of the most important and efficacious reasons for the failure of the many ordinances, cedulas and provisions issued by the King to remedy the woes of the Indians has been that the judges and governors of the Indies have a share and vested interest in the system; and this we have regretted and still regret....

It is necessary here to observe that in framing these laws all the chief Spaniards were present and were consulted. This is obvious, because at that time almost nothing was known about the Indies; cassava, *ajes, axi* or *montones*.... what were hammocks and *areytos,* the Indian dances prohibited by one of the articles.... This clearly proves the blindness or wickedness of the Council, which, in making these laws, consulted the enemies of the Indians, who were interested in their sweat and wretched servitude and who longed eagerly to drain their blood....

Among the other laws made, there was one to this effect: that, in order that the caciques might have servants whom they could order to work for them, if the Indians of a cacique numbered forty and were to be divided among more than one person, two were to be given to him for his personal service; if he had seventy, three; if a hundred, four; and if he had one hundred and fifty, six; but even though he had more than one hundred and fifty, he was not to be given more than six. What greater injustice or disorder could be imagined than to dispossess the natural lords of their subjects, estates and kingdoms.... and from thousands of peo-

ple they used to have, to give them only six persons to serve
them.... The same article states a little further on that the
caciques themselves.... with the six persons assigned to
each, were to go with the Spaniards to whom the majority of
the Indians had been allotted and that they were to be well
treated and not put to work, except in light tasks so that
they should be kept busy, and not become lazy....

## No. 97—THE INDIANS ARE NOT AFRICANS

*(Bartolome de las Casas, Historia de las Indias (1559),
Madrid, 1875)\**

It was indeed amazing to see how blind first the Admiral, and then his successors were, on their arrival, in treating
the native Indians as if they were Africans. But would to
God it had ceased then and that the world was not still
afflicted by it today.

## (vi) THE BATTLE OF THE BOOKS : (a) THE NATURE OF THE ABORIGINAL INDIANS

### No. 98—A PEOPLE STEEPED IN VICE AND BESTIALITY

*(Speech of Fray Tomas Ortiz before the Council of the
Indies, 1512)\*\**

They ate human flesh, and were addicted to it more
than any race of men. They had no system of justice. They
went about naked, and lacked all shame. They were like
stupid asses, half-witted and without feeling, and thought
nothing of killing themselves or others. They did not speak
the truth, unless it was to their advantage. They were inconstant, did not know the meaning of counsel, were ungrateful
and fond of novelty. They gloried in being drunk, and made
wine from different fruits, roots and grains; they got drunk
on fumes and on certain herbs, which made them lose their
senses. They were bestial in their vices. Youth showed no
obedience or courtesy to age, nor children to their parents.
They were incapable of learning the doctrines of the Faith,
and were quite incorrigible. They were treacherous, cruel,
and vindictive, enemies of religion, and never forgave a
wrong. They were arrogant, thieves, liars, and of little intelligence. They kept neither faith nor order; husbands were not
loyal to their wives, or wives to their husbands. They were
sorcerers, fortune tellers, and necromancers. They were
cowardly, like the hare, dirty, like pigs; they ate lice, spiders

*\*Op. cit.,* Libro Segundo, Cap. XXVII, Tomo II, p. 296.
*\*\*Cited in Herrera, op. cit.,* Decada Tercera, Libro Octavo, Cap. X, Tomo
V, pp. 31—32.

and raw worms, wherever they found them. They lacked human art and skill; and when they forgot the teachings of the Faith which they had learned, they said that those things were for Castile and not for them, and that they wished to change neither their customs nor their gods. They wore no beard, and if any grew one, they tore it off. Towards the sick they showed no pity, and although they. were neighbours or relatives, they robbed them when dead or took them to the mountains to die, with a little bread and water each. The older they got the worse they were; up to the age of ten or twelve, it seemed, they had some manners and virtue, but thereafter they became like brute animals. In short, God never created a people more steeped in vice and bestiality, without the admixture of goodness or good breeding. They should be regarded.... as men of little skill and art; and those who had had dealings with them had learned that from experience.

---

### No. 99—THE HAPPIEST PEOPLE IN THE WORLD, IF ONLY THEY KNEW GOD

*(Bartolome de las Casas, Coleccion de Tratados, (1552–1553), Buenos Aires, 1924)\**

God created all these numerous Indian peoples very simple, without evil or duplicity, very obedient and loyal to their rulers. To the Christians for whom they work they are most humble, patient, peaceable and orderly, bear no grudge, are not bellicose, vicious or quarrelsome, show no rancour, hatred or desire for revenge. They are also the most delicate and frail.... people in the world, the least capable of enduring toil and the most susceptible to sickness. No children of princes or lords brought up amongst us in luxury and refinement are more delicate than they, even though there may be some among them of peasant stock. They are also very poor people, who neither own or wish to own worldly goods. I believe that they would be the happiest people in the world, if only they knew God.

---

### No. 100—THE INDIANS ARE "LITTLE MEN"
*(Juan Gines de Sepulveda, Democrates alter, Madrid 1547)\*\**

It does not appear to me to be contrary to justice or to Christianity to allot some Indians to honourable, just and prudent Spaniards to work in the cities or fields.... so that they may be taught just and human ways, and introduced to

---

*Cited in Hanke, *The Spanish Struggle for Justice*, p. 96.
\*\*Cited in Hanke, *The Spanish Struggle for Justice*, pp. 122—123; Hanke, *La Lucha por la Justicia*, p. 335; Fernando Ortiz, *El Engano de las Razas*, La Habana, 1946, pp. 214—215.

and imbued with the Christian religion. . . . These peoples require, by their own nature and in their own interests, to be
placed under the authority of civilized and virtuous princes
or nations, so that they may learn from the might, wisdom
and law of their conquerors, to practise better morals,
worthier customs, and a more civilized way of life. . . . The
Indians are as inferior to the Christians in these characteris-
tics as children are to adults, as women are to men. They are
as different from Spaniards as cruel people are from mild
people, as monkeys from men.

Compare then those blessings enjoyed by Spaniards of
prudence, genius, magnanimity, temperance, humanity, and
religion with those of the little men in whom you will scarcely find even vestiges of humanity, who not only possess no
science but who also lack letters and preserve no monument
of their history except certain vague and obscure reminis-
cences of some things on certain paintings. Neither do they
have written laws, but barbaric institutions and customs.
They do not even have private property. . . .

How can we doubt that these people — so uncivilized,
so barbaric, contaminated with so many impieties and ob-
scenities — have been justly conquered by such an excellent,
pious, and most just king as was Ferdinand the Catholic,
and as is now Emperor Charles, and by such a most humane
nation and excellent in every kind of virtue ?

---

## No. 101 — ALL THE PEOPLES OF THE WORLD ARE MEN
### (Bartolome de las Casas, Historia de las Indias (1559), Madrid, 1875)*

All the peoples of the world are men. . . . all have understanding and volition, all have the five exterior senses
and the four interior senses, and are moved by the objects
of these, all take satisfaction in goodness and feel pleasure
with happy and delicious things, all regret and abhor evil.

---

## No. 102 — THERE ARE NO BACKWARD RACES
### (Bartolome de las Casas, Apologetica Historia, Madrid, 1547)**

No nation exists today, nor could exist, no matter how
barbarous, fierce, or depraved its customs may be, which
may not be attracted and converted to all political virtues
and to all the humanity of domestic, political, and rational
men.

*Cited in Hanke, *The Spanish Struggle for Justice*, p. 125.
**Cited in Hanke, *The Spanish Struggle for Justice*, p. 125.

No. 103 — "IT REPENTETH ME THAT I MADE THEM"

(Gonzalo Fernandez de Oviedo y Valdes, Historia General y
Natural de las Indias Islas y Tierra-Firme del Mar Oceano,
(1535-1557), Madrid, 1851-1855)*

All the Indians of these islands were allotted by the
Admiral in repartimientos and encomiendas to all the settlers
who came to live in these parts; and in the opinion of many
who saw what happened and speak of it as eye-witnesses,
the Admiral, when he discovered these islands, passed sentence of death on a million or more Indians, men and women, of all ages, adults and children. Of this number and of
those since born, it is believed that there do not survive today, in this year, 1548, 500 Indians, adults and children, who
are natives and the offspring or stock of those he found on
arrival. The majority of those in the islands today have been
brought by the Christians from other islands or the mainland to serve them. As the mines were very rich, and the
greed of the settlers insatiable, some of them worked the
Indians to excess, others did not give them as much food as
they ought; in addition to this, the Indians are by nature
idle and vicious, disinclined to work, of a melancholy disposition, cowardly, base, prone to evil, liars, forgetful and
inconstant. Many of them, by way of amusement, poisoned
themselves so as not to work, and others hanged themselves,
whilst so many epidemics broke out, especially smallpox over
the whole island, that in a short time the Indians were wiped
out.

A large part of the blame for the death of these people was
also attributed to the transfers of the Indians made by the
governors and distributors. Transferring them from master to
master and from lord to lord, or taking them away from an
avaricious master to hand them over to one more avaricious,
obviously led to and were instrumental in the disappearance
of this people, and this explains why.... the Indians died.
Matters reached such a pass that not only were the Indians
allotted to settlers, but they were given also to noblemen
and favourites, persons in the good graces of and close to
the King, members of the Royal Council of Castile and the
Indies, and others. This was indeed intolerable, for although
they were noblemen and men of conscience, perhaps their
overseers and factors who dealt with their Indians overworked them.... And as they were agents and ministers of
men in high favour, no one dared to interfere with them
even when they did wrong. Certainly no Christian would
envy the wealth which was thus procured. But this was not
the complete reason for the final disappearance of the In-

*Op. cit., Libro Tercero, Cap. VI; Libro Quarto, Cap. III, Tomo I, pp. 142—146,
199.

dians. God permitted it because of the sins of the immode-
rate Christians who enjoyed the sweat of the Indians' toil
only because they did not help the Indians with his teachings in such a way that they should know God. Nor did the
Spaniards cease to add to this, for the divine permission
which excluded the Indians from the earth, the great, heinous and enormous sins and abominations of these savage and
bestial people; in regard to whom that terrible and just sentence of the sovereign and eternal God is truly meet and
just: "....It repenteth me that I made them".... From
which I infer that God in his mysterious way had forgotten
those Indians for a long time, and when he remembered
them...., seeing that the wickedness of man on earth was
great, and that all the thoughts of his heart were inclined to
evil, agreed to wipe them off the face of the earth, allowing
only a few innocent ones, and especially children who had
been baptized, to be saved, and all the others to pay for it.

Indeed, as all those who know these Indies (or parts
of them) affirm, there are no provinces of the islands or
mainland which the Christians have seen up to the present,
in which the Indians have not been or are not sodomites,
besides being all idolaters; they have many other vices, so
ugly that many of them are too obscene to be listened to
without loathing and shame, nor could I write about them
because of their great number and filthiness. Apart from
the two which I have mentioned these people had many
abominations and transgressions and different faults, besides
being most ungrateful, of poor memory and limited ability.
And if there is any good in them, it is when they are on
the threshold of adolescence; but once they enter it, they
become subject to many faults and vices, many of them
abominable....

All this has been discussed and argued by many clergymen and scholars....and many prelates and great men in
Spain have thoroughly thrashed out this matter, to assure
the conscience of the Kings about the treatment of these
Indians, and also to find a remedy in their minds both for
their salvation as well as for their maintenance and preservation. Many special royal commands and provisions have
been issued to the governors and administrators of justice
and their officials, but in my opinion none have been of any
avail to stop the destruction of these unfortunate people in
these islands....I do not wish to blame any of those who
have been there for this; but I know that what the Dominican
friars said was contradicted by the Franciscans, who took
the view that what they advocated was best; and what the
Franciscans advised the Dominicans denied, being sure they
were right. And thus, as time elapsed, the Franciscans came
to defend the views which the Dominicans had originally

held; and what the Franciscans had at first praised, they later rejected and then the Dominicans approved it. So that both held the same opinions at different times, but they continued to differ on everything; what I mean is that the opinions entertained by one group were never endorsed by the other at the same time. One can appreciate how difficult it was for those who listened to understand this question or to decide which side the layman should take who had to choose what was best for his conscience, seeing that the opinions held in the preceding year were considered bad in the following year, and what was then bad was later praised. This was not only a dangerous predicament for those newly converted to the faith, but it made even pure Christians hesitate; since they saw that some friars would not confess those who did not release the Indians, while other clergymen of the contrary opinion confessed them and administered the Sacraments to them.

I am narrating what I saw with my own eyes. I wish thereby to call to account or to blame not so much the many good clergymen past and present in this island and the Indies as the unhappiness and misfortune of the Indians themselves....God does nothing unjust, and would not permit such grievous things only for mysterious reasons of his own. Nor is it to be imagined that all the clergy, or some of them, did not work for the reformation and security of the consciences of the Christians and to avoid the disappearance of the Indians....And now that they have been wiped out, these clergymen, with the experience they have of what has happened, can better decide and determine what needs to be done with the other Indians who are still to be subdued in those numerous kingdoms and provinces of the mainland. For my own part, I do not absolve the Christians who have grown rich from or enjoyed the labour of these Indians, if they illtreated them or did not work actively for their salvation....

---

## No. 104—OVIEDO'S "GOSSIP"

*(Bartolome de las Casas, Historia de las Indias (1559), Madrid, 1875)\**

Oviedo writes as if he had witnessed everything he says about these islands, and not as one who had lived in Santo Domingo for many years, which is about the same as if he had written while living in Seville. All that he saw and took part in was the tyrannies and destructions which took place on the mainland during the five years he

*Op. cit., Libro Tercero, Caps. CXLII — CXLVI, Tomo III, pp. 322–336.

spent there... We do not doubt that he witnessed those
evils to which he contributed, but all that he says is to
the detriment of the Indians and in excuse and justification
of the cruelties, ambition and covetousness of the Spaniards.
Therefore, everything he wrote about, except Darien, was
what he heard from the sailors to or desolators of these
lands, who told him only what he wanted to hear, that is, "We
conquered, we subdued those dogs who defended such and
such a province, we enslaved them, we distributed the land,
we threw them in the mines". But if they had told him: "We
killed thousands of them, we threw them to the dogs who
tore them to pieces, we put the knife to everybody's throat,
men and women, old men and children, we filled the huts
with people and then burned them alive," little of this, we
may be sure, will be found in Oviedo's *History*. But, if they
told him that the Indians were idolaters, and sacrificed ten
men, which they exaggerated to ten thousand, and if they
attributed to them abominable vices which they could not
have known of unless they themselves were participants in
or accomplices of them, his *History* will be full of this....

What I believe from Oviedo's writings and gossip is
what he says about the trees and herbs of Hispaniola, for
these have been and are seen by all those who wish to see
them, and the same goes for those of the mainland....But
everything he says about the Indians in this island....
especially with regard to the unnatural vices which he
ascribed to them, is false; and we know this from the diligent investigations we made in the past, long before Oviedo
thought of coming to the Indies*....What more can he
say, even if it were true, in defamation of this whole new
world (where there are so many nations), and misleading
the old world where his history is read? If it is a mortal
sin to vilify someone, and the offender is obliged to make
restitution for the harm done, how did Oviedo sin and how
much restitution would he have to make for defaming so
many people, so many countries full of human beings whom
he never saw or heard, accusing them of such horrible sins?
As a result of this defamation the Indians were led to hate
and despise everything Christian, while the Spaniards who
came to these lands killed the Indians in war as if they
were killing bugs, and committed so many cruelties against
these naked and defenceless people which they would not
have committed against tigers, bears or lions, and which
tigers and other wild animals, even though hungry, would
not have done to other beasts.... The only thing he can
say about them is that they were all more or less corrupted
by idolatry, for there was no one to teach them of the true
God. Oviedo should stop to think how his ancestors and
the whole world lived before the Son of God came down

*Las Casas here cites Oviedo's strictures, some of which are presented in
No. 103 above.

to earth to dispel the darkness of ignorance, bringing with Him the Word of the Gospel....

It will still be useful to reply to each defect that Oviedo falsely attributes to the Indians and for which he excludes almost all of them from every hope of conversion and salvation.... With respect to his accusation that they were sodomites, this has been proved to be false.... He says they are ungrateful.... How blind or malicious was Oviedo, to accuse the people of this land of ingratitude when it was Oviedo and his men who destroyed them and took their land, and when, but for the Indians and their humaneness and kindness in serving, feeding, and saving them from many dangers, they would all have died! And what gratitude and reward have the Spaniards shown by depopulating the land and exterminating so many millions in this island, in the other islands and in the eighteen thousand leagues covered by the mainland....

Oviedo adds that he does not think God would punish and destroy the Indians unless they were to blame, and except for their vices and idolatry. This sinner does not realize that those who destroyed them will suffer a much greater punishment in hell for, being Christians, they should have brought them to God by their good example....

Oviedo says that these people were naturally lazy, vicious and disinclined to work; we have already dealt with the accusation that they are vicious, but we wish to add the hope that God may not consider the vices and sins of the Spaniards, excluding matters of faith, more abominable and more deserving of eternal damnation than those of the Indians. With regard to the laziness of the Indians, we understand why it is so. They are naturally delicate, like the children of princes, as a result of the region and climate in which they live and of other natural factors.... In addition, they were always naked, and this made them more delicate; besides, they ate very little and most of their food lacked nutritive value. Notwithstanding these facts they lived and multiplied, and they must have multiplied to an astonishing extent, for we found many populous villages, and very little effort was needed for them to obtain in abundance all that was necessary. Their leisure time, once they had satisfied their needs (for they did not kill themselves working to make a fortune and increase their estate), was spent in decorous exercises, like playing ball, which was very tiring, or dancing and singing (where they recited all their history and past events). Since they had no idols, they had no sacrifices or religious ceremonies, and therefore, there was hardly any sign of idolatry among them.... The time left from agriculture, housework, and fishing, was spent in handicrafts.... Thus, they were not as idle as Oviedo claims....

They had no defects or vices, for the truth was that

they led more virtuous lives than the Spaniards....there-
fore Oviedo should rather praise them than vilify them. He
adds that they are of a melancholy disposition, regarding
as a vice what was merely natural and not a sin.... He says
they are base cowards; men are not base for being humble,
peaceful and gentle as they were....They had certain habits
which seemed wrong to the Christians and are a little
indecent, like sitting down to urinate and breaking wind in
the presence of other people.... But you will not find an
Indian sharing another man's wife or any other woman but
his own; the same cannot be said of the Spaniards who
came to these lands. That they are cowards is not exactly
a vice but something natural, and this cowardice springs
from kindness and noble feelings, from unwillingness to
harm or be harmed; cowardice is a vice when a virtuous
act should be performed, and when, for fear of death or
injury, you do not resist evil. For example, if a man sees
his people suffering servitude or death, and he does not
help, or fight, or die if necessary to defend them, or if for
fear of those dangers he commits a sin or acts contrary to
virtue, then cowardice is a vice. In this case, many of these
people, naked, lacking the many and powerful weapons of
the Spaniards, and especially their horses, when they saw
they were being oppressed and killed in their work from
the injuries and injustices they suffered as well as in the
wars against the Spaniards, their oppressors and destroyers,
they resisted and fought so courageously that, even though
they had their bellies ripped open by swords, were tripped
by the horses, and speared by men on horseback (each
one killed 10,000 of them in one hour), lions or the bravest
men in history could not have shown greater courage. And
we should ask Oviedo, who boasts that he was a captain
on the mainland who stole and enslaved men to kill them
in his mines, what became of Francisco Becerra, Juan de
Tavira, Vasco Nunez and many others who were killed by
the Indians in combat. In the wars between the Indians and
the Spaniards, naked Indians performed feats which proved
their courage.... Their misfortune was that they lacked
guns and horses, because if they had had them to defend
themselves from such ruthless enemies, not so many of them
would have perished, nor would those who destroyed them
sing their own praises, nor would Oviedo vilify them as he
has done....

Oviedo also says that the Indians....have poor
memories. He is wrong in this as he is in everything else,
and also contradicts himself. It is well known that all Indians
have good memories, for they remember everything that
happened many years ago, as if they had it written down.
(And I cite Oviedo himself in proof of this, for he says....

that the Indians' songs were a history or an account of past events, of war as well as peace, so that by these songs they should not forget their heroic deeds. They remember these songs better than if they had them written down in books, and in this way they recite genealogies, the woes they have suffered, and especially, their famous victories in battle, etc. These are his own words. Then, they do not have poor memories, as Oviedo says). It seems obvious also from what they memorize of the Christian doctrine, that ten men with good memory could not memorize in twenty days what they memorize in one day....

Oviedo also says that the Indians are liars. Would to God he and his men had not frequently lied to the Indians and had not been the cause of the lies the Indians told to them.... The reason for the lies the Indians told and tell the Spaniards where they have not yet been destroyed is the oppression, horrible servitude and cruel tyranny with which they were and are illtreated, because they could not escape more illtreatment and grief except by lying and pretending, so as to please the Spaniards and appease their implacable fury. And in this connection....there are many sayings of the Indians which are worth consideration. When the Spaniards asked the Indians (and this happened more than once), if they were Christians, one Indian answered: "Yes, sir, I am already somewhat of a Christian, for I have learned a little how to lie; soon I shall be an expert liar, and I shall be a real Christian...."

Oviedo tells the truth when he says that many Indians killed themselves; but that it was a pastime, that is something he made up.... To prove this, Oviedo should tell us whether he ever heard that the Indians killed themselves as a pastime before the Spaniards came to these lands and oppressed them....people who did not know the true God believed that when you die you pass to another life where the souls eat, drink, sing, dance and have enough corporal rest. And why should we be surprised that, suffering so much in this life, they should wish and strive to leave it and to go and enjoy the other life?....

Oviedo says elsewhere that God must have a reason to permit the destruction of the Indians, and no doubt He will soon wipe them off the face of the earth because of their many crimes, for they are incorrigible, and learn nothing from punishment, lenient treatment or advice, etc.... No matter how Divine Justice lets them suffer, punishing them in this life, and may seem to abandon them, leaving them as victims of our insatiable covetousness, if any of them have been predestined to enjoy Divine Goodness, something a Christian should not doubt, nothing will stop them from enjoying eternal life after death. And then perhaps,

after we have treated them so cruelly, God will vent His
anger on us, for our violence and tyranny, and will move
other nations to do to us what we did to them, and in the end
destroy us as we destroyed them. Perhaps those whom we
so despised will exceed our people in number at the right
hand on the day of    judgment.   This possibility    should
frighten us day and night.

The reason for the ruin and destruction of the Indians,
says Oviedo, is their disloyalty, their indifference to punishment, lenient treatment, good advice, and that they are
naturally impious, and without shame.... He talked as if he
was referring to a piece of furniture in his home, which he
had turned inside out, when he had only dealt with them
for five years, and knew only those from the province of
Darien.... All he had done was attack, rob, kill, capture,
and throw them to work in the gold mines and at other
tasks, where they died from hunger, fatigue and cruel afflictions. And even them....he handed them over to a cruel
butcher, a servant of his, who was told to put them to
work.... Oviedo paid no more attention to them than if
they were ants or bedbugs. How could Oviedo know that all
these people (including those of this island, to whom he
refers, and of the other parts of the Indies which he never
saw) had bad thoughts and were perverts? (And if he
should say that others who had dealings with them had
told him so, we would give them the same answer we give
him, that since they only sought to kidnap, capture and kill
these people, we would give them the same credit that we
give to false witnesses.) In order to understand better what
he says, that they learn nothing from punishment, leniency
or good advice, Oviedo should indicate to us whether they
were punished, coaxed and advised so that they would come
and listen to the preaching of the Gospel, and give up their
vices and sins, or whether it was because they ran away
from the gold mines.... If Oviedo could only see the results
of the preaching of the Gospel which the Divine Providence
daily reaps at the hands and from the industry of His servants, among the people whom the cruel knife of the Spaniards has not yet wiped off the face of the earth, as it has
in these islands and many areas of the mainland, who leave
their false gods whom they adored out of ignorance, and
give up their other vices and are converted with faith and
devotion to believe in the true God, Redeemer of the world;
if he could see how they improve and how clearly they
profit from that improvement, he would not vilify so many
people....He could have heard from   trustworthy   people
while in Santo Domingo, where he lived for many years,
after there were no Indians left in the island, how in New
Spain, Peru and other provinces, where there were clergy

to instruct them, the Indians did profit inestimably from their teachings....it would be useful if he would tell us whether during the five years he spent in Darien and the twenty or thirty he lived in Hispaniola....he saw the faith being preached and the Christian doctrine being taught to any Indians?....The poor fellow says that it has been forty-three years since the Christians first came to these lands, and during this time the Indians should have already understood something so important as the salvation of their souls. But even if they could live to be two hundred years....they would be killed and destroyed before they heard anything about their salvation.

---

## No. 105—"I RETRACT EVERYTHING I SAID"

*(Deathbed declaration of Fray Domingo de Betanzos to Antonio de Causeco, Notary Public of the King of Spain, in Valladolid, September 13, 1549)\**

I say that I, Domingo de Betanzos, friar of Santo Domingo, have frequently, in discussing matters relating to the Indians, spoken of their defects, and I have submitted to His Majesty's Council of the Indies a signed memorial dealing with these defects, in which I said that the Indians were beasts, that they had sinned, that God had condemned them, and that they would all perish. Great scandal may have resulted from this and the Spaniards may have taken advantage of it to commit more evils and injury on the Indians and kill more of them than they might have if they had not known of this memorial.... Because I am ill and it may be Our Lord's wish that I recover and because I wish to make such reparation as I can to ease my conscience, I now swear and beseech the Royal Council of the Indies and implore all who who see or hear in the Indies, Spain or elsewhere, not to give any credence to anything which I have spoken or written against the Indians and to their detriment. I do not remember having done so, but if I, did, I say that I am a man, and as such liable to err, and I believe that I erred through not knowing their language or because of some other ignorance....I retract everything I said.... It grieves me that I cannot retract my statements in person before the Council of the Indies and before the whole world if it were necessary, and I revoke and nullify all the offensive and scandalous statements in the memorial, and everything that I said in it or elsewhere to the detriment of the Indians and contrary to the salvation of their souls and the welfare of their bodies I hereby revoke.

*Cited in Hanke, *La Lucha por la Justicia*, pp. 122-123.

## No. 106—"AMERICA IS A RICH AND BEAUTIFUL WHORE"

*(Francisco de Quevedo, La Hora de Todos y la Fortuna con Seso, 1636)\**

....Observe that America is a rich and beautiful whore. The Christians say that Heaven punished the Indies because they adored idols; and we Indians say that Heaven will punish the Christians because they adore the Indies.

## No. 107 — THE REVENGE OF THE INDIANS

*(Francisco de Quevedo, El Entrometido y la Duena y el Soplon, 1628)\*\**

There came the devil of tobacco and the devil of choco-late, who, although I had my doubts about them, I never regarded as complete devils. They told me they had avenged the Indies against Spain, for they had done more harm by introducing among us those powders and smoke and choco-late cups and chocolate-beaters than the Catholic King had ever done through Columbus and Cortes and Almagro and Pizarro. For it was much better and cleaner and more honourable to be killed by a musket ball or a lance than by snuffling and sneezing and belching and dizziness and fever; the chocolate-bibbers idolize the cup that they raise on high and adore and go into a trance over; the tobacco addicts are like Lutherans: if they take it in smoke, they are serv-ing their apprenticeship for hell; if in snuff, for catarrh.

## No. 108—NEW WORLD UTOPIA: AN ENGLISH ATTACK ON SPANISH POLICY

*(Sir Thomas More, Utopia, London, 1516)\*\*\**

...For this same Raphael Hythloday... His patrimony that he was born unto, he left to his brethren (for he is a Portugal born) and for the desire that he had to see, and know the far countries of the world, he joined himself in company with Amerigo Vespucci, and in the three last voyages of those four that be now in print and abroad in every man's hands, he continued still in his company, saving that in the last voyage he came not home again with him. For he made such means and shift, what by entreatance, and what by importune suit, that he got licence of master Amerigo (though it were sore against his will) to be one of the twenty-four which in the end of the last voyage were left in the country of Gulike. He was therefore left behind for his mind sake, as one that took more thought and care for travelling than dying.... But after the departing of

*\*Cited in Ortiz, Cuban Counterpoint, Tobacco and Sugar, p. 211.*
*\*\*Cited in Ortiz, Cuban Counterpoint, Tobacco and Sugar, pp. 210—211,*
*\*\*\*Op. cit., Oxford edition, 1952, pp. 3—4, 48, 76, 80, 99, 139.*

master Vespucci, when he had travelled through and about
many countries with five of his companions Gulikians, at
the last by marvellous chance he arrived in Taprobane, from
whence he went to Caliquit, where he chanced to find certain
of his country ships, wherein he returned again into his
country, nothing less than looked for....
 ....When I consider with myself and weigh in my mind
the wise and godly ordinances of the Utopians, among whom
with very few laws all things be so well and wealthily
ordered, that virtue is had in price and estimation, and yet,
all things being there common, every man hath abundance
of everything....
 The island of Utopia containeth in breadth in the middle
part of it (for there it is broadest) two hundred miles....
 ....No household or farm in the country hath fewer
than forty persons, men and women, besides two bondmen,
which be all under the rule and order of the good man, and
the good wife of the house, being both very sage and dis-
creet persons.... For they dividing the day and the night
into twenty-four hours, appoint and assign only six of those
hours to work....
 ....For the magistrates do not exercise their citizens
against their wills in unneedful labours. For why? In the
institution of that weal public, this end is only and chiefly
pretended and minded, that what time may possibly be
spared from the necessary occupations and affairs of the
commonwealth, all that the citizens should withdraw from
the bodily service to the free liberty of the mind, and gar-
nishing of the same. For herein they suppose the felicity
of this life to consist....
 ....In this hall all vile service, all slavery, and drud-
gery, with all laboursome toil and business, is done by
bondmen....
 ....And seeing they be all thereof partners equally,
therefore can no man there be poor or needy....
 ....For this cause they keep an inestimable treasure.
But yet not as a treasure: but so they have it, and use it, as
in good faith I am ashamed to show: fearing that my words
shall not be believed. And this I have more cause to fear,
for that I know how difficult and hardly I myself would
have believed another man telling the same, if I had not
presently seen it with mine own eyes....For whereas
they eat and drink in earthen and glass vessels, which indeed
be curiously and properly made, and yet be of very small
value: of gold and silver they make commonly chamber
pots, and other like vessels, that serve for most vile uses,
not only in their common halls, but in every man's private
house. Futhermore of the same metals they make great
chains, with fetters, and gyves wherein they tie their bondmen. Finally whosoever for any offence be infamed, by

their ears hang rings of gold, upon their fingers they wear rings of gold, and about their necks chains of gold, and in conclusion their heads be tied about with gold. Thus by all means that may be they procure to have gold and silver among them in reproach and infamy. And therefore these metals, which other nations do as grievously and sorrowfully forge, as in a manner from their own lives: if they should altogether at once be taken from the Utopians, no man there would think that he had lost the worth of one farthing....

For they marvel that any man be so foolish, as to have delight and pleasure in the glistering of a little trifling stone, which may behold any of the stars, or else the sun itself. Or that any man is so mad, as to count himself the nobler for the smaller or finer thread of wool, which self-same wool (be it now in never so fine a spun thread) did once a sheep wear: and yet was she all that time no other thing than a sheep. They marvel also that gold, which of the own nature is a thing so unprofitable, is now among all people in so high estimation, that man himself, by whom, yea and for the use of whom it is so much set by, is in much less estimation than the gold itself....

They neither make bondmen of prisoners taken in battle, unless it be in a battle that they fought themselves, nor of bondmen's children, nor to be short, any man whom they can get out of another country, though he were there a bondman. But either such as among themselves for heinous offences be punished with bondage, or else such as in the cities of other lands for great trespasses be condemned to death. And of this sort of bondmen they have most store.

For many of them they bring home sometimes paying very little for them, yea most commonly getting them gratis. These sorts of bondmen they keep not only in continual work and labour, but also in bands. But their own men they handle hardest, whom they judge more desperate, and to have deserved greater punishment, because they being so godly brought up to virtue in so excellent a commonwealth, could not for all that be refrained from misdoing. Another kind of bondmen they have, when a vile drudge being a poor labourer in another country doth choose of his own free will to be a bondman among them. These they handle and order honestly, and entertain almost as gently as their own free citizens, saving that they put them to a little more labour, as thereto accustomed. If any such be disposed to depart thence (which seldom is seen) they neither hold him against his will, neither send him away with empty hands....

....And though no man have anything, yet every man is rich....

## No. 109 — THE NOBLE SAVAGE: A FRENCH ATTACK ON SPANISH POLICY

*(Michael de Montaigne, "Of Coaches" (1585-1588) and "Of Cannibals" (1578-1580), Paris)* *

**Our world has lately discovered another. . . . as large, well peopled, and fruitful as this whereon we live, and yet so raw and childish, that we yet teach it its *a, b, c;* 'tis not above fifty years since it knew neither letters, weights, measures, vestments, corn, nor vines; it was then quite naked, in the mother's lap, and only lived upon what she gave it. . . . I am greatly afraid that we have very much precipitated its declension and ruin by our contagion, and that we have sold it our opinions and our arts at a very dear rate. It was an infant world, and yet we have not whipped and subjected it to our discipline by the advantage of our valour and natural forces; neither have we won it by our justice and goodness, nor subdued it by our magnanimity. Most of their answers, and the negotiations we have had with them, witness that they were nothing behind us in pertinency and clearness of understanding; the astonishing magnificence of the cities of Cusco and Mexico, and, amongst many other such like things, the garden of that king, where all the trees, fruits, and plants, according to the order and stature they have in a garden, were excellently formed in gold, as in his cabinet were all the animals bred upon the land and the sea of his dominions; and the beauty of their manufactures, in jewels, feathers, cotton, and painting, gave ample proof that they were as little inferior to us in industry. But as to devotion, observance of the laws, goodness, liberality, and plain dealing, it was of main use to us that we had not so much as they; for they have lost, sold, and betrayed themselves by this advantage.

As to boldness and courage, stability, constancy against pain, hunger, and death, I should not fear to oppose the examples I find amongst them, to the most famous examples of elder times, that we find in our records on this side of the world. For as to those who have subdued them, take but away the sleights and artifices they practised to deceive them, and the just astonishment it was to those nations to see so sudden and unexpected an arrival of men with beards, differing in language, religion, shape, and countenance, from so remote a part of the world, and where they had never heard there was any habitation, mounted upon great unknown monsters, against those who had never so much as seen a horse, or any other beast, trained up to carry a man or any other loading; shelled in a hard and shining skin, with a cutting and glittering weapon in his hand against them,

* Cited in The Complete Works of Montaigue, London, pp. 693-697, 152—157.
** "Of Coaches".

who, for the wonder of the brightness of a looking-glass or a knife, would truck great treasures of gold and pearl; and who had neither knowledge nor matter with which, even at leisure, they could penetrate our steel; to which may be added the lightning and thunder of our pieces and arquebuses, enough to frighten Caesar himself, if surprised with as little experience of them; against people naked, except where the invention of a little quilted cotton was in use; without other arms, at the most, than bows, stones, staves, and bucklers of wood; people surprised, under colour of friendship and good faith, by the curiosity of seeing strange and unknown things; take but away, I say, this disparity from the conquerors, and you take away all the occasion of so many victories.   When I look upon that invincible ardour wherewith so many thousands of men, women, and children have so often presented, and thrown themselves into inevitable dangers, for the defence of their gods and liberties; that generous obstinacy, to suffer all extremities and difficulties, and death itself, rather than submit to the dominion of those by whom they had been so shamefully abused; and some of them choosing rather to die of hunger and fasting than to accept of nourishment from the hands of their so basely victorious enemies; I take it that whoever would have attacked them upon equal terms of arms, experience, and number, would have had as hard. and perhaps a harder, game to play, than in any other war we have seen.

Why did not so noble a conquest fall under Alexander, or the ancient Greeks and Romans; and so great a revolution and change of so many empires and nations fall into hands that might have gently made plain and smooth whatever was rough and savage amongst them, and have cherished and assisted the good seeds that nature had there produced; mixing not only with the culture of land and the ornament of cities, the arts of this part of the world, in what was necessary, but also the Greek and Roman virtues, with those that were originals of the country! What a particular reparation had it been to them, and what a general good to the whole world, had our first examples and deportment in those parts allured those people to the admiration and imitation of virtue, and had begot betwixt them and us a fraternal society and intelligence! How easy had it been to have made advantage of souls so innocent, and so eager to learn; having for the most part naturally so good capacities! Whereas, on the contrary, we have taken advantage of their ignorance and inexperience, with the greater ease to incline them to treachery, luxury, avarice, and towards all sorts of inhumanity and cruelty, by the pattern and example of our manners; whoever put at so high a price the benefit of merchandise and traffic? So many cities levelled with the ground, so many nations exterminated, so many millions of people fallen by the edge of the sword, and the richest and most beautiful part of the world turned upside down for the traffic of pearls and pepper! Mechanical victories! Never did ambition, never did political animosities engage men against one another, in such horrible hostilities and calamities. . . . God did meritoriously permit that all this great plunder should be swallowed by the sea in transportation, or by civil wars, wherewith they devoured one another, and the most of the actors in it were buried upon the place, without any fruit of their victory. . . .

. . . . *I find that there is nothing barbarous and savage in this nation, by any thing that I can gather excepting that everyone gives the title of barbarism to everything that is not in use in his own country; as, indeed, we have no other level of truth and reason than the example and idea of the opinions and customs of the place wherein we live. There is always the perfect religion, there the perfect government, there the perfect everything. This nation are savages, in the same way that we say fruits are wild, which nature produces of herself, and by her own ordinary progress; whereas, in truth, we ought rather to call those wild whose natures we have changed by our artifices, and diverted from the common order. . . .

These nations then seem to me to be so far barbarous, as having received but very little form and fashion from art and human invention, and being consequently not much remote from their original simplicity. The laws of nature govern them still, not as yet much vitiated with any mixture of ours; nay, in such purity that I am sometimes troubled we were no sooner acquainted with these people, and that they were not discovered in those better times, when there were men much more able to judge of them than we are. I am sorry that Plato and Lycurgus had no knowledge of them; for, to my apprehension, what we now see in those natives does not only surpass all the images with which the poets have adorned the golden age, and all their inventions in feigning a happy state of man, but moreover the fancy, and even the wish and desire of philosophy itself. So native and so pure a simplicity as we by experience see to be in them, could never enter into their imagination, nor could they ever believe that human society could have been maintained with so little artifice. Should I tell Plato that it is a nation wherein there is no manner of traffic, no knowledge of letters, no science of numbers, no name of magistrate, nor political superiority; no use of service, riches or poverty; no contracts, no successions, no dividends, no properties, no employments, but those of leisure; no respect of kindred, but in common; no clothing, no agriculture, no metal, no use of corn or wine; and where so much as the

* "Of Cannibals".

very words that signify lying, treachery, dissimulation, avarice, envy, detraction, and pardon, were never heard of —how much would he find his imaginary republic short of this perfection? . . . .

They have wars with the nations that live farther within the mainland, beyond their mountains, to which they go naked, and without other arms than their bows and wooden swords, pointed at one end like the head of a javelin. The obstinacy of their battles is wonderful; they never end without great effusion of blood; for as to running away, or fear, they know not what it is. Everyone for a trophy brings home the head of an enemy he has killed, which he fixes over the door of his house. After having a long time treated their prisoners very well, and given them all the luxuries they can think of, he to whom the prisoner belongs invites a great assembly of his kindred and friends, who being come, he ties a rope to one of the arms of the prisoner, of which at a distance, out of his reach, he holds the one end himself, and gives to the friend he loves best the other arm, to hold after the same manner; which being done, they two, in the presence of all the assembly, dispatch him with their swords. After that they roast him, eat him amongst them, and send some chops to their absent friends; which nevertheless they do not do, as some think, for nourishment, as the Scythians anciently did, but as a representation of an extreme revenge. . . . Having observed the Portuguese, who were in league with their enemies, to inflict another sort of death upon any of them they took prisoners, which was to set them up to the girdle in the earth, to shoot at the remaining part till it was struck full of arrows, and then to hang them; they who thought those people of the other world (as men who had sown the knowledge of a great many vices amongst their neighbours, and were much greater masters in all kind of malignity than they), did not exercise this sort of revenge without reason, and that it must needs be more painful than theirs, began to leave their old way and to follow this. I am not sorry that we should here take notice of the barbarous horror of so cruel an act, but that, seeing so clearly into their faults, we should be so blind to our own. I conceive there is more barbarity in eating a man alive than when he is dead; in tearing a body that is yet perfectly sentient, limb from limb, by racks and torments, in roasting it by degrees, causing it to be bit and worried by dogs and swine (as we have not only read, but lately seen, not amongst inveterate and mortal enemies, but amongst neighbours and fellow-citizens, and, what is worse, under colour of piety and religion), than to roast and eat him after he is dead. . . .

We may, then, well call these people barbarous, in respect to the rules of reason; but not in respect to ourselves, who, in all sorts of barbarity, exceed them. Their

wars are throughout noble and generous, and carry as much
excuse and fair pretence as this human malady is capable
of; having with them no other foundation than the sole
jealousy of valour. Their disputes are not for the conquests
of new lands, those they already possess being so fruitful
by nature as to supply them, without labour or concern, with
all things necessary, in such abundance that they have no
need to enlarge their borders. And they are moreover
happy in this, that they only covet so much as their natural
necessities require; all beyond that is superfluous to them.
Men of the same age generally call one another brothers,
those who are younger, sons and daughters, and the old men
are fathers to all. These leave to their heirs in common
this full possession of goods, without any manner of
division, or other title than what nature bestows upon her
creatures in bringing them into the world. If their neighbours pass the mountains, and come to attack them, and
obtain a victory, all the victors gain by it is glory only, and
the advantage of having proved themselves the better in
valour and virtue; for they never meddle with the goods of
the conquered, but presently return in their own country,
where they have no want of any necessary; nor of this
greatest of all goods, to know how to enjoy their conditions
happily, and to be content. And these in turn do the same.

---

### (h) SPAIN'S TITLE TO THE INDIES

*No. 110—THEORY OF SPANISH IMPERIALISM*

*(Matias de Paz, "Concerning the Rule of the King of Spain
over the Indies", 1512)\**

1. Whether Our Most Christian King may govern these
Indians despotically or tyrannically.
  Answer : It is not just for Christian Princes to make
war on infidels because of a desire to dominate or for their
wealth, but only to spread the faith. Therefore, if the inhabitants of those lands never before Christianized wish to listen
to and receive the faith, Christian Princes may not invade
their territory. Likewise, it is very convenient that these infidels be requested to embrace the faith.
2. Whether the King may exercise over them political
dominion.
  Answer : If an invitation to accept Christianity has not
been made, the infidels may justly defend themselves even
though the King, moved by Christian zeal and supported by
papal authority, has waged just war. Such infidels may not

*Cited in Hanke, *The Spanish Struggle for Justice*, pp. 27—28

be held as slaves unless they pertinaciously deny obedience to the prince or refuse to accept Christianity.

3. Whether those who have required heavy personal services of these Indians, treating them like slaves, are obliged to make restitution.

Answer : Only by authorization of the Pope will it be lawful for the King to govern these Indians politically and annex them forever to his crown. Therefore those who have oppressed them despotically after they were converted must make appropriate restitution. Once they are converted, it will be lawful, as is the case in all political rule, to require some services from them — even greater services than are exacted from Christians in Spain — so long as they are reasonable — to cover the travel costs and other expenses connected with the maintenance of peace and good adminis-tration of those distant provinces.

---

## NO. 111—ROYAL CENSORSHIP

*(Charles V, Emperor of the Hapsburg Empire, to Prior of San Esteban Monastery in Salamanca, November 10, 1539)\**

I have been advised that certain friars have discussed and disputed in their sermons and dissertations our rights to the Indies, islands and mainland.... Discussion of such matters without our knowledge and without first advising us of it, besides being very prejudicial and scandalous, may lead to many difficulties to the disservice of God, disrespect of the Holy See and the Vicar of Christ, and detriment of our royal sovereignty over these kingdoms. We have decided therefore to require you, and we hereby require and com-mand you, that without any delay you summon the scholars and friars in question who have discussed this matter, either in sermons, dissertations, or in any other way, publicly or privately, and make them swear to the time, place, and in whose presence they have discussed this matter, either in substance or in minutes and memorials, and whether they have given copies to other persons, churchmen or laymen. And you will send their declarations and their writings on the subject, leaving them not a single copy in their posses-sion, with a memorial signed by you, to Fray Nicolas de Santo Tomas.... And you will order them, on your behalf and ours, that at no time in the future, without an express licence from us, are they to discuss or preach about or dis-pute this subject, or have any written statement thereon printed....

*Cited in Hanke, *La Lucha por la Justicia*, pp, 374—375,

## No. 112—SPAIN'S JUST TITLE TO THE INDIES

### (Francisco de Vitoria, De Indias, Madrid, 1540)*

1. The Spaniards have the right to travel in the countries in question and to live there, provided they do no harm to the natives and the natives do not seek to prevent them ....in which case the Spaniards may justly wage war against them....this would be the first title which the Spaniards might have for seizing the provinces and sovereignty of the natives.

2. The Spaniards have the right to preach and declare the gospel in barbarian lands. If war were necessary to achieve this just end, it should be waged with moderation and a sense of proportion.... and with an intent directed more to the welfare of the aborigines than to their own gain .... This would be a second lawful title whereby the Indians might fall into the power of Spain.

3. If the Indian princes attempt to force any of the converted aborigines to return to idolatry, this would constitute a third title.

4. The Pope may give converted Indians to a Christian sovereign and dethrone infidel rulers, with or without petition from the Christians. This would be another title by which Spain might acquire just sovereignty over the New World.... the Pope may, in the interest of the Faith and to avoid danger, exempt all Christians from obedience and submission to infidel rulers.

5. The Spaniards may intervene and dethrone rulers, if necessary, to rescue innocent people from an unjust death, such as cannibalism.

6. True and voluntary choice by the Indians of the Spaniards as rulers would be a sixth title.

7. The Spaniards could justly take up the cause of allies and friends....

8. The Spaniards might assume the burden of a mandate to fit the natives for admission to the international community upon a basis of equality.... it might be maintained that in the natives' own interests the sovereigns of Spain might undertake the administration of their country, providing them with prefects and governors for their towns, and might even give them new lords, so long as this was clearly for their benefit.

*Cited in Hanke, La Lucha por la Justicia, pp. 377—378; and The Spanish Struggle for Justice pp. 151—152.

*No. 113—THE SPIRITUAL WELFARE OF THE INDIANS*

*(Fray Tomas de Torre, Prior of the Dominicans, Speech to the Municipal Council of Guatemala, 1545)\**

I marvel. Gentlemen, that you are so ill-informed as not to know that we came from Spain to this province solely for the welfare of the Indians, and that we in our labours are not concerned with profit and advantage for you, our countrymen.... whom we may call flesh of our flesh and bone of our bone.... The welfare which we desire and hope to bring to the Indians is not a temporal welfare, because we think not of gold or silver, but it is.... their spiritual welfare, instruction in the holy, Catholic doctrine approved and made known by the most learned men in the world, whom, by the mercy of God. our Spain possesses, and in particular the distinguished University of Salamanca and the convent of San Esteban in that city; the scholar Fray Francisco de Vitoria, who is at present residing there, would do honour to an entire world. It is this doctrine, then, which we bring from such distant lands, like the merchant's grain of wheat ...., and it is this which we have begun to scatter, publish and make known in the sermons which my colleagues and I have preached in this city, and which you, gentlemen, from concern with your worldly affairs and respect of your fellowmen, do not wish to hear. It is for this reason that it was obligatory on us to go among the Indians, a savage and barbarous people who, as erroneous opinions hold, are not to be included in the species of man.

---

*No. 114—THE VALLADOLID INQUIRY*

*(Domingo de Soto, Speech to the Judges at Valladolid, August 1550) \*\**

The purpose for which Your Lordships are gathered together here.... is, in general, to discuss and determine what form of government and what laws may best ensure the preaching and extension of our Holy Catholic Faith in the New World;.... and to investigate what organisation is needed to keep the peoples of the New World in obedience to the Emperor, without damage to his royal conscience, and in conformity with the Bull of Alexander.

\*Cited in Hanke, *La Lucha por la Justicia*, p. 380,
\*\*Cited in Hanke, *The Spanish Struggle for Justice*, p. 118.

## No. 115—LAS CASAS VERSUS SEPULVEDA

*(Bartolome de las Casas, Speech to the Judges at Valladolid.*
*1550)\**

The Doctor (Sepulveda) founds these rights upon our superiority in arms, and upon our having more bodily strength than the Indians. This is simply to place our kings in the position of tyrants. The right of those kings rests upon their extension of the Gospel in the new world, and their good government of the Indian nations. These duties they would be bound to fulfil even at their own expense; much more so considering the treasures they have received from the Indies. To deny this doctrine is to flatter and deceive our monarchs, and to put their salvation in peril. The doctor perverts the natural order of things, making the means the end, and what is accessory, the principal.... He who is ignorant of this, small is his knowledge, and he who denies it is no more of a Christian than Mahomet was.... To this end (to prevent the total perdition of the Indies) I direct all my efforts, not, as the doctor would make out, to shut the gates of justification and annul the sovereignty of the Kings of Castile; but I shut the gate upon false claims made on their behalf, and I open the gates to those claims of sovereignty which are founded upon law, which are solid, strong, truly Catholic and truly Christian.

---

## No. 116—THE CONDEMNATION OF SPANISH RULE IN THE INDIES

*(Bartolome de las Casas, La Solucion a las doce dudas*
*Madrid, 1564) \*\**

1. All infidels, no matter what their sect or their sins against natural or divine law, justly hold jurisdiction over those things which they acquired without prejudicing anyone else.

2. There are four classes of infidels, and the Indians fall in the fourth class, among those who have never previously been subjected to a Christian ruler, or have never done any harm to Christians. Infidels in this category may not be justly molested nor may any king or emperor wage war on them.

3. The sole reason for the Papal donation was the conversion of the Indians.

*Cited in Hanke, *The Spanish Struggle for Justice*, p. 121,
\*\*Cited in Hanke, *La Lucha por la Justicia*, pp. 408—409,

4. When this donation was made, the Pope did not claim to deprive the native kings and lords of the Indies of their estates, jurisdiction, honour or dignities.

5. The King of Spain must pay for the expenses of the conversion and cannot compel the Indians to contribute unless they wish to do so.

6. The kings and villages of the Indies must consent to the sovereignty of the kings of Spain and to the Papal donation to make both valid.

7. The first arrival of the Spaniards, in 1492, and all their acts since that date have been evil and tyrannical.

8. At least from 1510 to the present year, 1564, there has not been nor is there today any man in all the Indies who has kept or keeps his word or who may be excused for not doing so with respect to four matters: first, the wars waged by the Spaniards on the Indians all over the Indies; second, the invasions or discoveries which have taken and are taking place daily; third, buying and selling as slaves prisoners captured in these wars; fourth, the articles imported and sold to those who waged the wars, such as arquebuses, gunpowder, crossbows, and above all horses, which have been more destructive to the Indians than any other weapon.

---

## No. 117—THE DEFENCE OF SPANISH RULE IN THE INDIES

*(Francisco de Toledo, Viceroy of Peru, to King of Spain, 1573)\**

1. Your Majesty is the legitimate ruler of this Kingdom, and the Incas are tyrannical usurpers.

2. Your Majesty may appoint caciques over the Indians at your will and pleasure and as you see fit, for a limited or indefinite period, with or without jurisdiction, without paying attention to rights of succession; and this would be one of the most important measures for the spiritual and temporal government of the Indians, because the caciques will always be what they have been, in their virtues as well as their vices.

3. In the light of Your Majesty's legitimate sovereignty over this kingdom, and if it is agreeable to good government, Your Majesty may give and bestow the land on Spaniards for a limited or indefinite period, without those scruples hitherto raised, which lightly affirm that the Incas were legitimate kings and the caciques native lords; that is all false. . . .

4. As Your Majesty is the real ruler of this kingdom,

---

*Cited in Hanke, *La Lucha por la Justicia*, pp. 415—416; *The Spanish Struggle for Justice*, p. 167. This was a summary of a formal inquiry instituted by the Viceroy.

and as there are no legitimate heirs of the Inca tyrants, all the mines, minerals and agricultural wealth, all the idols and treasures in the tombs, the lands and livestock reserved for the service of the Incas, and which are not private property, justly belong to Your Majesty as King and lord as if it was property which was vacant, unowned, and, so to speak, derelict.

5. It is the duty of Your Majesty, as legitimate ruler, to tutor and defend the native Indians of this kingdom, and, as their tutor, given their weak reason and rude understanding, Your Majesty must devise laws for their conservation and require them to obey these laws, even though they are or appear to be inconsistent with their liberty.

---

### (vii) THE OPINION OF THE SPANISH SETTLERS AND PLANTERS

#### No. 118—THE CONQUISTADORES AND THE ENCOMIENDA

*(Antonio de Herrera, Historia General de los Hechos de los Castellanos en las Islas y Tierra Firme del Mar Oceano, Madrid, 1601-1615)* \*

A council was held in Barcelona, and was attended by prominent members of the King's Councils and other clergymen, who for several days discussed the question of the treatment of the Indians.

On behalf of the conquistadors and soldiers it was argued : "That consideration should be given to rewarding them for the toils they had endured, the hunger, the dangers they had run of losing their life and of being eaten by the savages, and other cruelties, hardships and sufferings which no nation in the world ever endured, in order to extend its religion and the empire of its prince, his arms, language and customs, undertaking such long voyages with such constancy and at so little expense to the Royal Treasury. And that if the King had acted favourably towards them, without busying himself with other undertakings, they would have discovered and conquered much more, without thought of fatigue, vigil, death, without fears of being so distressed by hunger, that they ate one another, or of heat or cold, going naked, without necessary weapons, against such a large number of men. And that these people are savages, steeped in idolatry, who sacrifice human beings, eat human flesh, and deal with the devil. They practise sodomy and have many wives; their vice is drunkenness, they go about naked and know no shame, and have other vices.... And if the Spaniards did not live among them, keeping them in sub-

\*Op. cit., Decada Quarta, Libro Sexto, Cap. XI, Tomo V, pp. 316—317.

jection, to incline them to the holy preaching of the Gospel, with good advice, so that by such contact they should learn Spanish customs and civil society, teaching them farming methods, so that they might profit by them, and if the Spaniards did not make use of human labour but of beasts, whence results, as is well known, the profit to all Europe, enriching Italy, France, Germany and other countries, there would be no gain, nor would the teaching of the clergy bear any fruit among them. Going alone to preach to them, without anyone to protect them or assure their safety, the clergy were killed and sacrificed by the Indians, some publicly, others secretly, and it was impossible to ascertain who did it so that they might be punished. And if the Indians were not given in *encomienda*. . . . the Spaniards would not be able to support themselves; for how could they support themselves on the King's or anyone else's pay? It was clear that they would have to abandon the country and the progress made in religion and civil society would be lost; besides, even though the Spaniards might withdraw to towns by themselves, to live on farming and tillage, and they too could live in a state of nature, since the country, by the grace of God was not sterile or desert and did not deserve to be forgotten, they would not have undertaken such long and dangerous voyages and endured so much without hope of reward; and it was clear that if they left the Indians to themselves, the Indians would inevitably forget the Faith and return to their vices, for the reasons given, and others, and the King would lose the country.

---

*No. 119.—THE SETTLERS AND THE ENCOMIENDA*
(*Report of the Jeronimite Commission to Cardinal Cisneros, 1516*)*

1. The Indians are vicious, especially in their lust, gluttony and laziness; they take more pride in going off to the woods and eating roots, spiders and other filth than in the Spanish way of life.

2. If they were set at liberty, they would revert to their nakedness, idolatry and superstitions, and would forget all they have been taught. They lack the capacity for living, without tutelage, like Christian Spaniards; the cleverest among them is more stupid than the humblest peasant in Spain; so that liberty would be pernicious to their bodies and souls. They were already set at liberty by command of the Catholic Sovereigns, and experience taught us what has been said above, besides which they rebelled and the suppression of the revolt was an arduous task and it was necessary again to give them in trust to the Spaniards.

*Cited in Tapia y Rivera, *Biblioteca Historica*, pp. 208—224. This report is based on the evidence of thirteen witnesses, the oldest and most eminent inhabitants of Hispaniola.

3. Opinions differ as to whether it is wise to remove them from their villages and settle them close to the Spanish towns. The majority are in favour of this for their bodily and spiritual welfare, because they will be better taught the doctrines of the Church, will learn to live like Christians and rational beings.... and they will not have to move as often, while the Spaniards will be relieved of the expense of sending each time for them. Thus although the Indians may not like this, they should be compelled to do it for their own good.

Some believe that they should be settled close to the Spaniards and given good lands for their corn fields, chickens, etc., but that under no circumstances should this be done against their will, because many of them would commit suicide by drinking the cassava sap or in other ways, as they have done before for matters of no consequence, merely on hearing that it was planned to remove them; and certainly the old folks, if uprooted, would die from the change. Therefore it will be necessary to dissemble with some of them, to give presents to others, and to win their goodwill by treating them well so that they may come voluntarily.

One witness says that, even though they are willing to come, their removal should not be permitted because it would really be fatal for them. In addition a large part of the country would be depopulated and no one would be able to travel across the island because of the lack of food and roads in such depopulated areas.

4. There is a similar difference of opinion as to whether their removal would be more conducive to their salvation. There are no clergymen or priests to teach them in their settlements, which are for the most part small and poor. They die without the Sacraments and without being urged to repent their sins, and their children are not taught the doctrines of the Church until the age of twelve or fourteen when they begin to work for the Spaniards. In the light of these considerations, the majority are in favour of their removal; but others believe that the change would be most harmful to them and that it would be preferable to send priests to teach them in their settlements, where they would willingly accept the doctrines.

5. As to whether it is wise to continue to give them in trust, as at present, or whether it will be better to appoint a governor to look after them (as Casas proposes), or whether they should be set at liberty, the consensus of opinion is that they should continue as they are, but that the allotments of Indians should, as far as possible, be made perpetual, taking all possible precautions to assure them good treatment, reduction of hours, more food and higher wages.

Only one witness says that, if they are set at liberty, their numbers would increase, whilst, if given in trust, as at present, they will all die in a short space of time, irrespective of how many more ordinances are promulgated.

6. In the event that they were again to be given in trust, there should under no circumstances be a general distribution....the Indians allotted to Your Highness and to absentees should be taken away, and be divided up among the married settlers who are men of conscience, who would treat them well and intend to establish their domicile in the country.

---

## No. 120—"I HAVE COME TO TAKE THEIR GOLD"

*(Fray Bernardino de Minaya, Memorial to Charles V, Emperor of the Hapsburg Empire, n.d.)* *

We proceeded to the coast of Peru, finding deserted villages wherever the Spaniards had passed; and after travelling a few days greatly in need, we reached Pizarro.... They wanted to ship the Indians assigned to their service to be sold in Panama in return for wine, vinegar and oil. When I learned of this I advised them....that His Majesty the Emperor had ordered that the Indians should not be enslaved even though they were the aggressors....I told Pizarro that....God had made the Indies known in order that souls should be won for the Faith, and that this was the aim of the Pope and the Emperor....and that it was in order that the Indians should be brought to a knowledge of God and not be robbed and despoiled of their lands that they were given in trust to the Catholic Sovereigns, as is stated in the Bull of Pope Alexander granting the Indies to Spain. Pizarro replied that he had come from Mexico to take their gold away from the Indians, and that he would not do what I asked. And thus I bade him farewell with my companions, although he pleaded with me not to go, and offered me my share of the gold which they had obtained in the villages. I told him that I wanted no part of any illgotten gold, and that I did not wish by my presence to countenance such robbery.

*Cited in Hanke, *La Lucha por la Justicia*, pp. 114—115, The date of the memorial, as suggested by the reference to the Emperor's order against the enslavement of the Indians, is probably after 1528 or after 1530.

## No. 121—LAS CASAS, THE TROUBLE-MAKER

*(City Council of Guatemala to Charles V, Emperor of the Hapsburg Empire, September 19, 1543)* *

It is affirmed by some that the source of this cruel sentence** is one Fray Bartolome de las Casas. We are greatly astonished, unconquered Prince, that a matter of such antiquity, initiated by your grandparents, weighed by so many hands, considered by such good and clear minds so well versed in law and so abundant in good will, should be reversed by a friar unread in law, unholy, envious, vainglorious, unquiet, not free from cupidity (for all of which clear proof can be offered), and, above all else, a troublemaker, so much so that there is no part of the Indies from which he has not been expelled; nor can he be suffered in any monastery; nor is he given to obeying anyone; and for this reason he never tarries....

(They beg His Majesty not to condemn them without a hearing)... unless that religious is a prophet or he has learned what he knows through inspiration—which he has not, or even through experience. He says that he has been in these parts thirty-odd years; but thirty of them he spent in Espanola and Cuba, where the Indians were soon finished, and where he did his share in finishing them, and he might have told the truth about what happened (there).

....We say this not to speak evil of him; we say it, because he is not competent to give testimony of the Indies, which are New Spain (for the rest are not called Indies), and in this New Spain, which he saw from the roads over which he passed, there is much doctrine among the natives, and knowledge of God and the King and, for the time they have been taught in the doctrine, they greatly exceed all the kingdoms and seigneuries of Your Majesty. We are astounded to hear such things from that religious.

## No. 122 — THE COLONIAL OPPOSITION TO LAS CASAS

*(Fray Tolibio de Motolinia to Charles V, Emperor of the Hapsburg Empire, January 2, 1555)* ***

Las Casas says that everything the Spaniards have here is illgotten, even though they have obtained it by trade, and even though there are many farmers and mechanics and others who have earned a living by their sweat and industry. And that it may be better understood, Your Majesty should know that five or six years ago, as he says, I was ordered by Your Majesty and your Council of the Indies to

*Cited in Simpson, *op. cit.*, pp. 230—231.
**The New Laws of 1542.
***Cited in Simpson, *op. cit.*, pp, 235—237, 242,

collect certain MS *confesionarios* that Las Casas had left here in the Indies; and I gave them to Don Antonio de Mendoza, your viceroy, and he burned them, because they contained false and scandalous statements. Now in the last ships that have arrived in New Spain the said *confesionarios* have come printed and have caused no little uproar and scandal in this country, because many times in them he calls the conquerors and encomenderos and merchants, tyrants, robbers, violators, rapers, and bullies. He said that they have always tyrannised and today are still tyrannising over the Indians. He also says that all the tributes of the Indians are and have been taken unjustly and tyrannically. If such is the case Your Majesty's conscience were in a pretty state, for Your Majesty has half or the majority of all the more important provinces and towns of New Spain, and the encomenderos and conquerors have only what Your Majesty will give them. And (he says) that all the Indians they have should be assessed more moderately and that they should be well treated and cared for—as by the grace of God, almost all are today—and that they should be taught doctrine and given justice—and so it is done. But, nevertheless, Las Casas says all the above and more, and moreso his principal insults are directed against Your Majesty; and he condemns all men of law of your council, calling them many times unjust and tyrannical. He also insults and condemns all those who are or have been in New Spain, ecclesiastics as well as laymen, and the presidents and *audiencias* of Your Majesty. Certainly the Marquis del Valle and Bishop Don Sebastian Ramirez and Don Antonio de Mendoza and Luis de Velasco, who is governing now with the oidores, have ruled and governed and are governing very well both Spaniards and Indians.

Truly, for the few canons that Las Casas has studied, he presumes a great deal, and his disorder seems very great and his humility small, and he thinks that everyone is wrong and that he alone is right, for he says the following words literally: "All the conquerors have been robbers and rapers, and most of them more notorious for evil and cruelty than ever men were, as is now manifest to all the world".

"All the conquerors", he says, without excepting any. Now Your Majesty knows the instructions and commands carried by those who go on conquests, and that they labour to keep them, and that they are of as good a life and conscience as Las Casas, and of greater rectitude and piety. I am astonished that Your Majesty and those of your councils have been able so long to suffer such an ill-humoured, unquiet, importunate, noisy, trouble-making fellow, as turbulent in his religious habit as he is ill-mannered, insulting, harmful, and restless. I have known Las Casas for

fifteen years before he came to this country. Once he
started out for the land of Peru but, unable to reach his
destination, he stopped in Nicaragua, staying there for only
a short time. Thence he went to Guatemala, and stayed
there even less; and afterwards he was in the province of
Oaxaca, and did not stay there either, as elsewhere. Then,
when he came to Mexico he stopped at the monastery of
the Dominicans and immediately tired of it, and again took
to wandering and going about in his trouble-makings, always
writing accusations and about other peoples' lives, seeking
out the evils and cruelties that the Spaniards had committed
throughout this land so as to exaggerate and magnify the
evils and sins that have been committed. And in all this
he was more zealous and just than the other Christians, and
more than the religious, and here he hardly concerned himself with religion!....

It is not just for Las Casas to say that the service
of the Christians oppresses them unbearably, and that the
Spaniards think less of the Indians than they do of their
beasts, and even less than the dung of the town square....

---

## No. 123—THE COLONIALS AND THE NEW LAWS

*(Memorial of the Attorneys of New Spain to Charles V,
Emperor of the Hapsburg Empire, June, 1545)\**

We, the *procuradores* of New Spain, affirm that it is
necessary....that for what touches upon the service of God
and of Your Majesty and the good of the natives of those
parts and the perpetuity of them and of the Spaniards who
reside in them, the Indians who are in them shall be given
in perpetuity...

And all those who have reported, collecting and
exaggerating ill-treatments of Indians, have kept quiet about
the many good treatments and good works that have been
done and are done in New Spain every day, which, in compensation, exceed the bad ones of past times....Thus, for
the measure of perpetuity, what was committed many years
ago by individual persons, perhaps with reason and necessity, ought not to be taken into consideration, for if we
look at what is committed in Spain in one year, if it were
reported jointly, much more scandal would be aroused than
by all which....may have been done for gain in the Indies
in many years....

Many others could be given why there cannot be
perpetuity unless Indians are awarded, for there would be

*Cited in Hanke, *La Lucha por la Justicia*, pp. 233—234.

no one to cultivate the land or practise trades or work on farms, so that there might be profits. Nor will the Spaniards apply themselves to it unless they know that they are to have Indians in perpetuity. Intercourse with the Spaniards increases trade, but there cannot be Spaniards except in the way we have said. From these, great riches have come and are still drawn every day, which have been drawn, not from what the Indians give, but from what the Spaniards who have Indians have secured.

---

### No. 124—"LET IT BE OBEYED BUT NOT ENFORCED"

*(Tratado que el Obispo de la Ciudad Real de Chiapa, D. Fray Bartolome de las Casas, o Casaus, compuso por comision del Consejo Real de las Indias sobre la materia de los indios que se han hecho en ellos esclavos, Seville, 1552)* [1]

Never, up to the present, have the Spaniards obeyed any command, law, order or instruction which the Catholic Kings of the past issued, or a single instruction of His Majesty relating to the wars or to anything which had been decreed for the good of the Indians; and I stake my life that not a single instruction has been obeyed. In proof of this, study the commissions of inquiry into the acts of all former governors, the evidence which some adduced against others, and the investigations which have hourly been made even in this court, and Your Highness will find that there has not been nor is there a single governor (except for the Viceroy D. Antonio and the Licentiate Cerrado today, and the Bishop of Cuenca D. Sebastian Ramirez among those now dead) who has conducted himself like a Christian, or who has feared God or obeyed God's law or the King's, and who has not been a destroyer, robber and unjust murderer of all that branch of the human race.

*Cited in Saco, *Historia de la Esclavitud de los Indios*, Tomo I, pp. 185—186.

# CHAPTER V

# Negro Slavery and the Slave Trade

---

## (i) THE RATIONALISATION OF THE NEGRO SLAVE TRADE AND SLAVERY

### No. 125 — THE PRESERVATION OF THE INDIANS: LAS CASAS

*(Bartolome de las Casas, Historia de las Indias (1559), Madrid, 1875)\**

In view of the intention of the clergyman Casas and since the clergy of Santo Domingo did not want to give absolution to those who owned Indians, if they did not set them free, some of the Spaniards in this island told Las Casas that if he would get them a license from the King allowing them to bring a dozen Negro slaves from Castile, they would grant the Indians their freedom. Remembering this, Las Casas urged in his memorials that the Spanish settlers should be allowed to bring approximately a dozen Negro slaves, because with them they could maintain themselves in this land and would free the Indians. (The advice that a license should be given to bring Negro slaves to these lands was first given by Las Casas, ignorant of the injustice with which the Portuguese capture and enslave them; when he realized it, he would not have recommended it for anything in the world, because he considered them to be unjustly and tyrannically enslaved, and the reasons valid for the Indians were also valid for the Negroes). The advice and measures proposed by Las Casas, in order that the Spaniards would live in these lands without owning Indians, from which it follows that the Indians were to be given their freedom, pleased the High Chancellor and Cardinal of Tortosa, Adriano, who later became Pope, because he was informed of everything, and all the other Flemish councillors who learned of it. The clergyman was asked how many Negro slaves he believed should be brought to these islands. He answered that he did not know. A decree was therefore sent by the King to the officials of the House of Trade of Seville, to meet and determine what number they thought was convenient; and they answered that for these four islands — Hispaniola, San Juan, Cuba and Jamaica — they believed that at the present time 4,000 Negro slaves would be enough.

*\*Op, cit., Libro Tercero, Cap, CII, Tomo III, p, 177,*

*No. 126 — THE PRESERVATION OF THE INDIANS : THE JERONIMITES*

*(The Jeronimite Fathers in Hispaniola to Cardinal Ximenes, Regent of Spain, January 18, 1518)\**

Moreover, since newly imported Negroes may be introduced into these islands, in order to secure those of the calibre we know is needed for this part of the world, would Your Highness have authority granted us to fit out vessels in this island to go to Cape Verde Islands and the Guinea Coast to fetch them, or have permission given to some other person from those kingdoms to bring them hither. Indeed, Your Highness, if this concession be granted, apart from the fact that it will be a great benefit to the populations of these Islands and a source of income to Your Highness, it will ensure that these Indians, your vassals, are cared for and assisted in their work and enabled to pay greater attention to the care of their souls and the multiplication of their race.

*No. 127 — THE PRESERVATION OF THE INDIANS: THE DOMINICANS*

*(Antonio de Herrera, Historia de los Hechos de los Castellanos en las Isla y Tierra-Firme del Mar Oceano, Madrid, 1601-1615)\*\**

As the monks of the Dominican Order continued to emphasise the necessity of relieving the condition of the Indians.... it was ordered that, since the labour of one Negro was more valuable than that of four Indians, every effort should be made to bring to Hispaniola many Negroes from Guinea.

*No. 128—NO NEGROES, NO SUGAR*

*(Gonzalo Fernandez de Oviedo y Valdes, Historia General y Natural de las Indias, Islas y Tierra-Firme del Mar Oceano (1535-1557). Madrid, 1851-1855)\*\*\**

There are so many Negroes in this Island\*\*\*\* as a result of the sugar factories, that the land seems an effigy or an image of Ethiopia itself.

\*Cited in Saco, *Historia de la Esclavitud de la Raza Africana*, Tomo I, p. 142.
\*\**Op. cit.*, Decada Primera, Libro Noveno, Cap, V, Tomo II, pp. 188—189.
\*\*\**Op. cit.*, Primera Parte, Libro Quinto, Cap. V, Tomo I, p. 255.
\*\*\*\*Hispaniola.

## No. 129 — THE DEVELOPMENT OF THE COLONIES

*(Bartolome de Las Casas to the Council of the Indies, January, 20, 1531)\**

The remedy in so far as the Christians are concerned is certainly this: that His Majesty be good enough to lend each one of these islands\*\* five or six hundred Negroes, or as many as appear to be sufficient at present, to be distributed among the settlers who only have Indians now.... they should be given credit for three years, the Negroes being mortgaged for the said debt. At the end of that period His Majesty will be repaid, his land peopled and his income considerably increased....

One of the causes, Gentlemen, which have contributed to the ruin of this land and the fact that the increase of its population was not greater at least in the last ten or eleven years, is the failure to grant permission freely to all those who wished to do so to introduce Negroes. I sought and obtained this favour from His Majesty.

## No. 130—THE DEVELOPMENT OF HISPANIOLA

*(Attorneys of the City of Santiago de Cuba and the Towns of Puerto Principe and Sancti Spiritus in Hispaniola to Charles V, Emperor of the Hapsburg Empire, 1542)\*\*\**

Here the chief urgency is Negroes. We pray licence for each citizen to bring over male and female Negro slaves free of all duty.

## No. 131 — THE DEVELOPMENT OF CUBA

*(The City of Santiago de Cuba to Charles V, Emperor of the Hapsburg Empire, April 10, 1537)\*\*\*\**

Your Majesty already knows that the native Indians are very much on the decline, and, as the most lasting arrangement is the introduction of Negroes, we entreat you to permit the colonists to bring over two or three hundred of these without payment of licence, but paying duty only at the rate of seven and a half per cent.

\*Cited in Saco, *Historia de la Esclavitud de la Raza Africana,* Tomo I, pp, 168—169,

\*\*The four Greater Antilles.

\*\*\*Cited in H. H. S. Aimes, *A History of Slavery in Cuba,* 1511 to 1868, New York, 1907, p. 11.

\*\*\*\*Cited in Saco, *Historia de la Esclavitud de la Raza Africana,* Tomo I, p. 277.

## No. 132—THE DEVELOPMENT OF PUERTO RICO

*(Diego de Salamanca, Bishop of San Juan, to Philip II, King of Spain, April 6, 1579)\**

The fundamental reason for the deterioration and decline of this island is the lack of slaves to work in the sugar mills and to mine the gold as they used to. The yield of the gold was so high that the fifths of Your Majesty were worth more than twenty–five thousand ducats.... This has stopped not because the gold is exhausted but because there are no slaves to mine it; but if large numbers were imported for this purpose the Royal Treasury would profit greatly thereby and this poor island would regain the title of Puerto Rico, which was given to it originally and now belongs to it in name only....

## No. 133 — THE DEVELOPMENT OF TRINIDAD

*(Dr. Salcedo de Merva to Philip III, King of Spain, January 31, 1618)\*\**

He stated that a short while ago trees of cacao had been found in the Island of Trinidad. In order to develop this discovery he suggested that 300 pieces of slaves should be sent to that Island of whom two-thirds should be men and one-third women.

## No. 134 — THE WELFARE OF THE SPANIARDS

*(Judge Hurtado of Hispaniola to Charles V, Emperor of the Hapsburg Empire, April 7, 1550)\*\*\**

Negroes are essential in the Indies since Spaniards do not work there. All Spaniards who go there immediately become gentlemen, and as they are too poor to buy Negroes at 150 pesos, the country is depopulated. It is requested that the price be fixed at 100 pesos.

## No. 135 — THE WELFARE OF THE NEGROES
*(Alonso Zuazo, Judge of Hispaniola, to Cardinal Ximenes, Regent of Spain, January 22, 1518)\*\*\*\**

Indeed, there is urgent need for Negro slaves, as I have written to inform His Highness, and in as much as Your

*Cited in Coll y Toste, *Boletin Historico de Puerto Rico*, Vol. XI, pp. 204—205.
**Cited in The Trinidad Historical Society, Publication No. 190.
***Cited in Saco, *Historia de la Esclavitud de la Raza Africana*, Tomo II, p. 19.
****Cited in Saco, *Historia de la Esclavitud de la Raza Africana*, Tomo I, pp. 143—144.

Lordship will see that part of my letter to His Highness, I shall not repeat it here, except to say that it is urgent to have them brought. Ships sail from these islands for Seville to purchase essential goods such as cloth of various colours as well as other merchandise, which is used as ransom in Cape Verde whither the goods are carried with the permission of the King of Portugal. By virtue of the said ransom, let ships go there and bring away as many male and female Negroes as possible, newly imported and between the ages of fifteen to eighteen or twenty years. They will be made to adopt our customs in this island and they will be settled in villages and married to their women folk. The burden of work of the Indians will be eased and an unlimited amount of gold will be mined. This is the best land in the world for Negroes, women and old men, and it is very rarely that one of these people die.

## No. 136 — THE PROFIT TO THE KING

*(The Jeronimite Fathers in Hispaniola to Cardinal Ximenes, Regent of Spain, June 22, 1517)* *

As we have already stated at length in writing, it is essential that Your Lordship give instructions for the granting of a general permit to these islands, in particular to this island, and to San Juan, to introduce newly imported slaves, since experience has shown their great value in assisting the Indians, if these must remain vassals, or in helping the Spaniards, not to mention the great profit which will accrue to His Highness from their sale. We entreat Your Lordship to be good enough to grant this request, especially as people here are importuning us on this question and we see that they are right.

## No. 137—THE PROFIT TO THE TREASURY

*(Report of Capt. Juan Melgarejo, Governor of Puerto Rico to Philip II, King of Spain, January 1, 1582)* **

If Your Majesty would be so kind as to order one thousand Negroes to be brought to this island and sold to the settlers, in a very short period of time they will be paid for and the settlers will become rich and the Royal Treasury will benefit considerably.

*Cited in Saco, *Historia de la Esclavitud de la Raza Africana*, Tomo I, pp. 141—142,

**Cited in Coll y Toste, *Boletin Historico de Puerto Rico*, Vol. I, pp. 75—91.

## (ii) — THE ORGANISATION OF THE NEGRO SLAVE TRADE

### No. 138 — THE ROYAL MONOPOLY
*(Decree of Ferdinand II, King of Spain, August 18, 1518)*\*

Our officials who reside in the city of Seville in our House of Trade of the Indies; Know ye that I have given permission, and by the present do give it, to Lorenzo de Gorrevod, Governor of Bresa, member of my Council, whereby he, or the person or persons who may have his authority therefor, may proceed to take to the Indies, the islands and the mainland of the ocean sea already discovered or to be discovered, four thousand Negro slaves both male and female, provided they be Christians, in whatever proportions he may choose. Until these are all taken and transported no other slaves, male or female, may be transported, except those whom I have given permission up to the present date. Therefore, I order you to allow and consent to the Governor of Bresa aforesaid or the person or persons aforesaid who may have his said authority to transport and take the four thousand slaves male and female, without molesting him in any way; and if the said Governor of Bresa or the persons aforesaid who may have his authority should make any arrangements with traders or other persons to ship the said slaves, male or female, direct from the isles of Guinea and other regions from which they are wont to bring the said Negroes to these realms and to Portugal, or from any other region they please, even though they do not bring them to register in that House, they may do so provided that you take sufficient security that they bring you proof of how many they have taken to each island and that the said Negroes male and female have become Christians on reaching each island, and how they have paid the customs duties there, in order that those taken be known and be not in excess of the aforesaid number. Notwithstanding any prohibition and order that may exist to the contrary, I require you and order you in regard to this not to collect any duty in that House on the said slaves, but rather you are to allow them to be taken freely, and this my decree shall be written down in the books of that House.

_____

### No. 139—THE ASIENTO
*(J. Veitia de Linaje, Norte de la Contratacion de las Indias Occidentales, Seville, 1672. English Translation by John Stevens, The Spanish Rule of Trade to the Indies, London, 1702)*\*\*

1. Among the first Ordinances made for the better government of those large provinces, conquered in the Indies,

\*Cited in E, Donnan, *Documents Illustrative of the History of the Slave Trade to America*, Carnegie Institution of Washington, 1930—1935, Vol. I, pp. 41—43.

\*\**Op. cit.*, pp. 155—161.

one was the prohibiting the carrying thither any men or
women slaves, white, black, mixed, or mulattos, but most
particularly such as were of Barbary, of the race of Moors,
Jews, or mulattos; for which last, the 'penalty over and
above their being brought back and forfeited to the King,
which is general to all, is 1000 pieces of eight fine, to be
equally divided between the King, the Judge, and the
informer; and if it be a mean person that has not where-
withal to pay, to receive an hundred lashes.

2. Few years after the discovery of the Indies, it
appeared the Indians were not able to go through with the
labour of the mines, tillage, and other employments, and
therefore the aforesaid Ordinance was dispensed with, and
leave given to carry some slaves, provided they were blacks,
excluding all sorts of Barbary slaves, mulattos, and among
the blacks, those they call Gelofes, from the town of Gelofe,
these being accounted haughty and mutinous.

3. The Emperor Charles the V. having ordered that
no converted Moors or their children should go over, the
Council of the Kingdom of Mexico informed King Philip the
II. that there were several Moriscoes of the Kingdom of
Granada gone over with licences, whom they looked upon
to be as dangerous as those of Barbary. His Majesty thanked
them for the advice, and commanded them to be immediately
sent over into Spain, as well the slaves as those that were
free, notwithstanding any licences they might have.

4. In the Year 1550, an order was sent to the India-
house, directing the Commissioners, not to permit any
Levant blacks to go over to the Indies, because some of
them were of a Moorish race, or at least conversant with
them; and therefore it was not convenient such people tho'
of the Guinea race, should go over to a country where the
Holy Faith was planting.

5. It is also forbid to carry to the Indies blacks that
speak Spanish, taking them to be such, who have been a
year in Spain or Portugal, because they debauched the
ignorant, stirring them up to be mutinous and disobedient
to their masters; yet this seems to be made void by another
order of 1570, directing leave to be given to carry over
married blacks, provided their wives went with them, and
that their masters make oath that they are married, for
there is no doubt they could speak Spanish, if they had
wives and children. As concerning slaves marrying, the
laws of Spain are ordered to be observed, and that tho'
they marry with their masters' consent, they shall remain
slaves.

6. There are many more Ordinances concerning the
blacks in the Indies, forbidding the men the carrying of any
weapon, and their women the wearing of gold, silk, veils or
pearls; the men being out in the night, or having any Indians

to serve them. That the blacks and mulattos, who are free, live with masters that are well known; and that they pay such duty to the King, as answers to that the vulgar sort pays in Spain. Much more might be said concerning the punishment of runaway blacks, whom they call Cimarrones, the care prelates are commanded to have of instructing them in the Faith, and many other particulars, but that it belongs not to the subject matter of this book.

7. In process of time, as the labour of the mines, and tillage increased, there came to be a greater scarcity of labouring people, which enhanced the price of blacks, caused greater numbers to be carried over, and in Spain they paid 30 ducats a head for the licence to carry them, besides 20 royals of a duty they called Aduanilla, or the little Custom; they that could not pay the money down, gave bond to pay 40 ducats in the Indies, for the 30, and 30 royals for the 20. These duties were for the Crown of Castile, besides which there was another for that of Portugal, and for the landing in the Indies. Which duties by degrees ran so high, that there were undertakers, who contracted for the whole cargoes of blacks, and the revenue arising by them was looked upon as so safe, that it was appropriated as an hereditary fund. These contracts for carrying over blacks to the Indies were made by outcry, the fairest bidder taking place in the same manner as was used in farming the customs and other duties. The first undertaker of this sort we meet with was Peter Gomez Reinel, who contracted for nine years, to carry over every year 4,250 Blacks, supposing 3,500 of them would come thither alive, whereof 2,000 were to be conveyed to such ports, as the Council should appoint. The articles agreed upon with him were 46, which being the foundation of all contracts made ever since, I will give an abridgment of them as follows :

8. That only the contractor be allowed to carry over, sell, and give licenses for blacks for nine years, to the number of 4,250 every year and for as many as he did not ship off, besides paying the duty, he should forfeit 10 ducats a head, yet so that what he fell short of delivering alive one year, he might deliver the next. That 2,000 should be delivered where the King should direct, giving notice 15 months before; and he should be obliged to stay with these 20 days after proclaiming his arrival in the ports. That he might carry 600 every year up the river of Buenos Ayres, whilst it was not found inconvenient, but was very soon, and no discount to be allowed him, in case this article were not fulfilled. That the undertaker might sell his blacks in the Indies, as he could agree with the buyers. Several penalties to be imposed on those that should carry blacks without leave. Judges are appointed as conservators of this trade, the manner assigned of searching ships, that they may

carry no blacks. The undertakers allowed to sail single, without being obliged to stay for the flotas, and to choose such vessels as they thought fit, excepting Easterling and Dutch hulks; all the men to be Spaniards and Portugueses.

9. The undertaker to pay 100,000 ducats a year for the duties belonging to the Crown of Castile; to give 150,000 ducats security; the blacks that were designed for Peru not to stay in the Firm Land; an open office to be kept at Seville and Lisbon, to sell licences to any that would buy, not exacting above 30 ducats for each: that he should be obliged to trust as long as the Council should appoint; that His Majesty should have liberty to farm the Trade of S. Thomas, Cabo Verde, Angola, Mina, and any other in Guinea, yet so that the third and fourth parts, belonging to the Crown of Castile, should go to the undertaker; that the ships, sailing from Castile, within the time limited by the contract should be received in the Indies, tho' they came thither after it was expired. That the Council might give to the number of 900 licences; that no contract should be made to the prejudice of the undertaker; that he should recover his due, as if it were the King's revenue; that of any blacks sent by stealth, there should the 30 ducats and 20 royals be recovered, the rest to be equally divided between the Judge, the undertaker and the informer; the same to be understood of such as were not entered, or put into the wrong ports. That the undertaker might keep factors in the Indies, but that they should not be allowed to trade there, nor carry any more than the necessary provisions and clothing for the blacks; and if anything remained, they might not sell it upon pain of death and forfeiture of goods.

10. Their factors were allowed arms defensive and offensive; all the produce of the contract was to be entered and remitted to the India-House, and pay duties; no blacks to be passed without his or his agent's hands; the Judges of the goods of persons decreased, were forbid meddling with those of their factors that died; that certain laws should not extend to the undertaker; that there should be oath made before the Council, how many slaves had been carried over.

---

## No. 140 — THE OPPOSITION TO MONOPOLY
*(Opinion of the Council of the Indies, to Charles V, Emperor of the Hapsburg Empire, June 19, 1552)**

(The consequences** would be) either to extract very little gold and silver to the prejudice of the interests of settlers in the Indies and of the royal dues or to put Indians

*Cited in Saco, *Historia de la Esclavitud de la Raza Africana,* Tomo II, pp, 37—38,

**Royal Order of May 23, 1552, permitting licences for the transportation of Negro slaves from Portugal, Cape Verde, Guinea and elsewhere,

in the mines; to tie Your Highness' hands so that they cannot render assistance to the people of the Indies and other private persons who are greatly in need of it; to break the laws and navigation ordinances of these kingdoms; to enable those persons to make a profit of three million on a hundred thousand ducats; to cause His Majesty to lose perhaps a hundred thousand ducats annually and the Indies to be ruined. Could you in conscience permit this ruin for the sake of a hundred ducats which are now offered ?

---

### No. 141—THE CONTRABAND SLAVE TRADE

*(Judge Esteve of Hispaniola to Charles V, Emperor of the Hapsburg Empire, 1550)\**

If the registers show one hundred, two hundred enter illegally, and, if they are caught, they say they are on another's permit. While they are on the vessels, no matter how many are travelling, they cannot be taken up as strays. There is fraud even in searching the ships. The Attorney-General should be advised of this.

---

### No. 142—THE GOODS IN THE SLAVE TRADE

*(Antonio de Berrio, Governor of Trinidad, to Council of the Indies, January 1, 1593)\*\**

The grant is also made me of 500 licences for Negroes free from all dues belonging to His Majesty. All this will be negotiated at the same time and what is necessary at present is to associate me with some trader who is not a buccaneer but has courage and wealth and that he should bring a great quantity of articles for barter, hatchets, which must be good, billhooks, knives, amber and glass beads, taguache ware and no other because neither turquoise nor coral are profitable; trumpets, some needles, cloaks, bells, small mirrors and some large and very good ones for the Chiefs. This is necessary at the present time because if the country cannot be conquered for a great while, it would perish directly, I mean to say in less than a year; but 10,000 Castilian ducats may be invested in this merchandize and in future when I have money, I want you to invest it and 50,000 ducats will be little to invest in these trifles and for others besides I am taking 500,000 ducats. May God bring us to that time.

*Cited in Saco, *Historia de la Esclavitud de la Raza Africana*, Tomo II, p. 28.
**Cited in The Trinidad Historical Society, Publication No. 16, p. 8. (Spelling corrected)

You may assure the traders who may wish to come to Trinidad and pledge them my word as a Castilian gentleman that they will be rewarded and that I shall endeavour that that city may be called the city of truth in contrast to Margarita which, in respect of those who govern it, is called the city of falsehood.

## No. 143—THE DEMAND FOR SLAVES

*(Ferdinand I, King of Spain to a Royal Official in Hispaniola, June 21, 1511)* \*

I do not understand why so many Negroes have died: take good care of them.

## No. 144—SUPPLY AND DEMAND

*(Royal Officials of Hispaniola to Charles V, Emperor of the Hapsburg Empire, March 30, 1550)* \*\*

The price of Negroes has increased considerably, for they alone, and not the Spaniards, work. On behalf of all the Indies, we request a general reduction of the price and permission for Indians from Portuguese Brazil to enter this island.

## (iii) NEGRO SLAVERY

## No. 145—SPAIN'S CODE NOIR

*(Ordenanzas para el cabildo y regimiento de la villa de la Habana y las demas villas y lugares de esta isla que hizo y ordeno el ilustre Sr. Dr. Alonso de Caceres, oidor de la dicha Audiencia real de la cuidad Santo Domingo, visitador y juez de residencia de esta Isla, January 14, 1574)* \*\*\*

49. No tavern-keeper may sell wine to Negro slaves. But since many slaves who work for wages which they bring to their masters whom they support thereby, and those Negroes travel far to work, and sometimes need to drink wine, the tavern-keepers may allow them to drink not more

---

*Cited in Saco, *Historia de la Esclavitud de la Raza Africana*, Tomo I, p. 105.
**Cited in Saco, *Historia de la Esclavitud de la Raza Africana*, Tomo II, p. 27.
***Cited in Instituto Panamerica de Geografia y Historia, *Contribuciones a la Historia Municipal de America*, Mexico, D.F., 1951, pp. 89—93, 97.

than half a pint in their taverns....but are not to allow them to take it out in a jar or vessel; the Negroes must drink it in the tavern. Any tavern-keeper who sells wine to Negroes in any other way is subject to a fine of two ducats for the first offence....for the second offence, the penalty will be double, while for the third offence he shall pay double and may lose his licence as a tavern-keeper. Any person who sells wine will be subject to this penalty, even though he may be a merchant who has imported it from Castile and sells it in his own home.

50. No one may employ a Negro to sell wine. Nor may a free Negro woman sell it, nor a tavern-keeper, unless he is a trustworthy person, without a licence from the Municipal Council. Anyone who sells wine without a licence, and who employs a slave to sell it will be fined two ducats....

52. No Negro slave may carry swords, knives or other weapons, even though he is in the company of his master, except when he accompanies his master at night....or goes to the field with him during the day, on pain of confiscation of the weapons for the first offence, and for the second, besides confiscation, 20 lashes in the pillory or at the prison gate. The hooked knives, points, stripping knives and other weapons which the Negro herdsmen and field Negroes carry may not be taken away from them, nor will they be punished for carrying them if they are on their way either home from the field or to the field from home.

53. Free Negroes, of whom there are many in this town who are citizens and officials, and, because this is a port, if it is their turn to keep watch, are authorised to own and carry arms, unless for some reason the authorities forbid any of them to carry them.

54. Many citizens hire Negroes to work for wages. Such Negroes are employed in different occupations, and go about like free men, working at what they please, and at the end of the week or month they hand over their wages to their masters. Others run lodging houses to board travellers, and have in such houses their own Negro women. It frequently happens that such Negroes, when they know that a fleet or a ship is leaving, hide and run away with the linen they are given to wash and with other articles given to them for safe keeping, until the departure of the fleet or ship, knowing that the passenger cannot stay on shore but must depart, and they keep these articles. Others keep the tools which are given to them for their work. There are other problems as well. We therefore order that no one may hire out a Negro man or woman, or set them up in a house to earn their own keep, or to take in lodgers....without first notifying the Municipal Council which must issue a licence for it. The Council will not issue a licence unless the person binds himself before the notary

to pay in full, without any lawsuits, all damages which may be done by such Negroes....and for all the clothes and other articles which such Negroes may receive....

55. No Negro slave may have a hut of his own to sleep in, even though he is hired out for wages; he will sleep in his master's house. The huts cannot be rented out, nor can their master give them to the Negroes, on pain of the hut being confiscated from the slave to whom it was given as his own and who sleeps in it, even though he is the master's own slave, or from the slave to whom it is rented out....unless the master had set up the hut or house with a licence from the Municipal Council....

56. No Negro slave may stay outside the home of his master or of the person whom he is serving at night after curfew, unless he is sent on an errand by his master or by the person whom he is serving; under the penalty that any slave caught outside his home after curfew will receive thirty lashes....For this reason, the bell should be rung each night at least for a quarter of an hour, two hours and a half after it gets dark....

57. No white person or Negro may allow a Negro slave to spend the night in his house, subject to a fine for the first offence of three ducats.... and imprisonment foi ten days; for the second offence, both punishments will be doubled; and for the third offence he will be exiled from this town for one year.

58. Some persons shelter fugitive and runaway slaves on their plantations or ranches, give them food, employ them for several days, and frequently buy them from their masters saying that they are ready to buy them at their own risk, if they find them, and the owners, since the slaves have run away and they do not know where they are, sell them for less than they are worth, and there are other frauds and deceits. We therefore order that no person may shelter and feed a runaway slave on his plantation or ranch, nor may any planter or overseer shelter, feed or employ him, on pain of being proceeded against as a receiver or concealer of stolen goods, and of being obliged to pay the slave's master all the wages that the slave may have earned from the day he employed him until he is restored to his master, even though he escapes; and if the slave is not recovered, he must pay the owner the price of the slave. And so that no one may claim ignorance, saying that the slave was not a runaway, and that it is the custom in the country to give food and shelter to any passing slave, it must be understood that a runaway is any slave who stays on any plantation or ranch for more than one day....

59. Any planter and overseer may and must appre-

hend any fugitive or runaway Negro, without penalty or
slander, and then take him to the judge; and if he does
not have the means of doing this, he must inform the slave's
master and the authorities that he has imprisoned the slave
in the stocks which are required to be kept on the plantations
or ranches.

60. Many people avail themselves of the services of
their slaves and do not feed and dress them. The result is
that such slaves go and steal food from the neighbouring
plantations and, due to such ill-treatment, rise up in revolt
and run away. We accordingly order all those who have
Negroes on their plantations, ranches, pig farms or other
places, to give them enough to eat for the work they perform, and, in addition, two pairs of trousers or coarse
undershirts, at least once every year, and not to punish
them excessively or cruelly. To supervise the enforcement
of this ordinance and ascertain how the slaves are treated,
the mayors of this town are required to visit the ranches
and plantations, one during the month of March and the
other during the month of October, to obtain information
about the treatment of the Negroes, and whether they have
been given food and clothes; and if they find bad Negroes,
who disturb the others, they are to order their masters to
have them sold outside the island.

61. Many people treat their slaves with great cruelty,
whipping them brutally, larding them with different kinds
of resin, burning them, and inflicting other cruelties from
which they die. The slaves are so intimidated and punished,
that they kill themselves, or throw themsleves into the
sea or run away, or rise up in rebellion, and one has merely
to say that the master killed his slave, and no proceedings
are instituted against him. Therefore anyone who treats his
slave with such cruelty and excessive punishment will be
compelled by the authorities to sell the slave, and he will
be punished in the light of the excesses committed.

62. Many Negroes run away to the mountains and
crags, and only occasionally are the deserters and rebels
caught by the overseers, planters and swineherds. We therefore order and command that any planter, overseer, cowherd
or other person who apprehends a runaway Negro within
two leagues from this town, shall be paid by the master
of the slave four ducats; if the slave is apprehended further
away, within twenty to forty leagues, twelve ducats; and
if the slave is apprehended more than forty leagues away,
fifteen ducats....

80. For the imprisonment of rural runaways and the
punishment of slaves on the plantations or ranches, it is
mandatory for owners of plantations with huts and of
ranches and pig farms to keep stocks, to which end they are

hereby given the necessary licence, and owners who do not keep stocks will be fined one ducat....

---

## No. 146 — THE DANGER OF MALE SLAVES

*(Ferdinand I. King of Spain, to Don Pedro Suarez de Deza, Bishop of La Concepcion de la Vega, Hispaniola, September 27, 1514)\**

In order to complete the church sooner, you may send over ten slaves. You say that they approve of Negro slaves over there, and that, it is necessary that their number should be increased at present: not young men, however, since there seems to be a great number of these, and it might lead to trouble.

---

## No. 147 — THE ADVANTAGE OF MARRIED SLAVES

*(Ferdinand I, King of Spain, to Miguel Pasamonte, Treasurer of Hispaniola, April 1514)\*\**

Female slaves will be provided, who, through marriage with the male slaves, will make the latter less eager for revolt, and the number of runaways will be reduced to a minimum, as you say.

---

## No. 148 — HOW TO HANDLE NEGRO REBELLIONS

*(Alonso Zuazo, Judge of Hispaniola, to Cardinal Ximenes, Regent of Spain, January 22, 1518)\*\*\**

It is idle to fear that the Negroes may rebel: there are widows living calmly in the Portuguese islands with as many as eight hundred slaves: everything depends on how they are governed. I found that on the arrival of some Spanish-speaking Negroes others fled to the hills: I whipped some, cut off the ears of others, and there were no further complaints.

---

## No. 149 — FEAR OF NEGRO REBELLIONS

*(Audiencia of Hispaniola to Charles V, Emperor of the Hapsburg Empire, July 23, 1546)\*\*\*\**

On account of the habit of the Negroes to rise up in revolt, the settlers dare not give their slaves an order except

---

*Cited in Saco, *Historia de la Esclavitud de la Raza Africana,* Tomo I, p. 128.
\*\*Cited in Saco, *Historia de la Esclavitud de la Raza Africana,* Tomo I, p. 128.
\*\*\*Cited in Saco, *Historia de la Esclavitud de la Raza Africana,* Tomo, I, p. 144.
\*\*\*\*Cited in Saco, *Historia de la Esclavitud de la Raza Africana,* Tomo II, pp. 5—6.

in the gentlest manner. And now the position is greatly improved. The emancipation of the Indians who were held as slaves has been greatly felt on the mainland. For this and other reasons, the attorneys are leaving. To sustain the war with the Negroes and the siege of their strongholds, excise and duty were levied, to which the clergymen have always contributed. Now they are claiming exemption.

---

## No. 150 — THE NEGRO DANGER IN HISPANIOLA:
## A WARNING

*(Alvaro de Castro, Archdeacon of Hispaniola, to Council of the Indies, March 26, 1542)\**

The Negroes are already doing business and trading among themselves to an extent involving great value and cunning, and, as a result, big and notable robberies are being committed on all the farms in the country. There is not a Negro in this island, newly imported though he may be, who does not rob each day, a little or a great deal, as the case may be. Some steal to pay for the day's work which they have agreed to give their masters, the value of which is a tomin a day, some to give to the female slaves, others in order to wear clothing and shoes. Night and day they rob and steal anything in the country, including gold to be melted. These thefts are concealed with the assistance of two or three hundred Negroes called "fences", who go about the city seeking to make profits, as I have said.... and to pay the daily wage in exchange for each day, or month or year, that they are at large and travel about the island. They take away stolen goods for sale and carry and conceal all that they are accustomed to conceal in the interior. Indeed, the Negroes of this city flaunt such wealth in gold and clothing and are so comfortably off that, in my opinion, they are freer than we are.

I have spoken many times to the Court about putting a stop to this, for if the Negroes wish to rebel outright, one hundred of them are sufficient to conquer the island, and twenty thousand Spaniards would not suffice to bring them to subjection. The island is large and well wooded, and they are warlike and expert at hiding out in the forests.

*Cited in Saco, *Historia de la Esclavitud de la Raza Africana*, Tomo I, pp, 301—302,

## No. 151 — CHRISTIANITY A DEAD LETTER

*(Father Daimen Lopez de Haro, Bishop of San Juan, Report of a Diocesan Synod, San Juan, April 30 - May 6, 1645)\**

The Bishop strongly recommends that when cargoes of Negro slaves arrive in the harbour, priests should immediately be assigned to instruct them in the Christian Faith and to teach them the doctrine of the Church in order to baptize them, and also to see to it that the Negroes hear Mass and go to confession and communion. A dead letter! Those who went to the slave camp were the officials of the Royal Treasury with the portable furnace and the coals to brand the slaves and collect the eight pesos of duty which the King derived from the slave trade. The slave trader took good care to inform the Bishop, through the merchant agent, that the Africans had already been baptized, some in Ethiopia and others in the Cape Verde Islands. The Bishop accepted this and advised that if there was any doubt, they should be baptized again in the parish where the mill to which they had been assigned was located, leaving it to the conscience of those who bought them if they did not do this.

"That does not bother me!" say those soulless sceptics, dealers in mahogany flesh; and the hard-hearted buyer echoes it.

---

## (iv)—THE ATTITUDE TO NEGROES, SLAVERY AND THE SLAVE TRADE

### No. 152—THE REPENTANCE OF LAS CASAS

*(Bartolome de las Casas, Historia de las Indias (1559), Madrid, 1875) \*\**

Las Casas soon repented his advice; and he blamed himself for his oversight, because as he later saw and ascertained.... the enslavement of the Negroes was as unjust as that of the Indians, and it was not a wise solution to advise the importation of Negroes in order that the Indians might be set free, even though he thought they were lawfully captured. He was not certain that his ignorance and goodwill would excuse him in God's eyes. There were then in Hispaniola about ten or twelve Negroes who belonged to the King and who had been introduced to build the fortress at the mouth of the river. But....so many others were imported that more

*Cited in Coll y Toste, *Boletin Historico de Puerto Rico*, Vol, XIII, pp, 1—3,
\*\**Op. cit.*, Libro Tercero, Cap. CXXIX, Tomo III, pp. 275—276.

than 30,000 Negroes have been brought to this island and
more than 100,000, I believe, to all the Indies. This was
of no benefit to the Indians and they were not set free....
As the number of sugar mills increased daily (the water
mills needing at least eighty slaves and the animal-drawn
mills about thirty or forty), the need to import Negroes to
work in them also increased and so did the profits from the
King's duties. The consequence was that the Portuguese,
who had long been carrying on their man-stealing in Guinea
and unjustly enslaving the Negroes, seeing that we had such
need of slaves and paid a good price for them, redoubled
their efforts to steal and capture them in all possible ways,
bad and wicked. In like manner the Negroes, seeing in their
turn how desperately they are sought and wanted, fight unjust wars among themselves and in other illicit ways steal
and sell their neighbours to the Portuguese. Thus, we ourselves are responsible for all the sins committed by the
Negroes, besides those we commit in buying them. The
Emperor assigned the money paid for these licences to import
slaves and the duties collected on the slaves for the construction of the palaces in Madrid and Toledo; and both of them
have been built with that money. Formerly, before there
were any sugar mills, in Hispaniola, it was the consensus
of opinion that, if a Negro was not hanged, he would never
die, because we had never seen a Negro die of disease.
For it is a fact that the Negroes, like oranges, found this
land more natural to them than their native Guinea; but
once they were sent to the mills they died like flies from the
hard labour they were made to endure and the beverages they
drink made from the sugar cane. Thus large numbers of them
die daily. Therefore, in order to escape from their slavery,
whenever they can they run away in bands; they rise in
rebellion, kill the Spaniards and wreak cruelties on them.
As a result the small towns of Hispaniola are never very
safe, and this is yet another calamity which befell the island.

---

## No. 153 — THE INHUMANITY OF THE NEGRO SLAVE TRADE

*(Fray Tomas Mercado, Suma de Tratos y Contratos,
Seville, 1587)\**

It is public opinion and knowledge that no end of
deception is practised and a thousand acts of robbery and
violence are committed in the course of bartering and
carrying off Negroes from their country and bringing them
to the Indies and to Spain. Under the guise of just warfare,
wars that are all or for the most part unjust are waged,

*Cited in Saco, *Historia de la Esclavitud de la Raza Africana*, Tomo II,
pp. 80—82,

inasmuch as Negroes are uncivilised and are never moti-
vated by reason but only by passion. They neither examine
nor question the righteousness of their acts. Moreover, since
the Portuguese and Spaniards pay so much for a Negro,
they go out to hunt one another without the pretext of a
war, as if they were deer; even the very Ethiopians, who
are different, being induced to do so by the profit derived.
They make war on one another, their gain being the capture
of their own people, and they go after one another in the
forests where they usually hunt — the chase being a common
pastime among them—or cut wood for their huts. In this way
and contrary to all justice, a very great number of prisoners
is taken. And no one is horrified that these people are illtreating and selling one another, because they are considered uncivilised and savage. In addition to the pretext
of parents selling their children as a last resort, there is
the bestial practice of selling them without any necessity
to do so, and very often through anger or passion, for some
displeasure or disrespect they have shown them....The
wretched children are taken to the market place for sale,
and as the traffic in Negroes is so great, there are Portuguese, or even Negroes themselves, ready everywhere to buy
them. There are also among them traders in this bestial and
brutal business, who set boundaries in the interior for the
natives and carry them off for sale at a higher price on
the coasts or in the islands. I have seen many acquired in
this way. Apart from these acts of injustice and robberies
committed among themselves, there are thousands of other
forms of deception practised in those parts by the Spaniards
to trick and carry off the Negroes finally as newly imported
slaves, which they are in fact, to the ports, with a few
bonnets, gewgaws, beads and bits of paper which they give
them. They put them aboard the ships under false pretences, hoist anchor, set sail, and make off towards the high
seas with their booty....I know a man who recently sailed
to one of those Islands and, with less than four thousand
ducats for ransom, carried off four hundred Negroes without licence or registration....Delighted with the chase, he
has now returned and is there at the moment trying to
bring off a similar catch. There has been no small number
of similar cases. Further, those pretexts and false pretences
which I have recounted above, are growing and increasing
more than ever now, because of the great profit and the
money given to the Negroes themselves. Wherefore, it is
and has always been public opinion and knowledge that,
of every two persons who leave, one is duped, taken captive tyranically or forced to do so. They all treat them most
cruelly (though this is accidental) on the voyage, as regards
clothing, food and drink. They think that they are saving
by carrying them separated and by killing them of thirst

and hunger. They are certainly mistaken, because they are losing in the first place. They embark four and five hundred of them in a boat, which, sometimes, is not a cargo boat. The very stench is enough to kill most of them, and, indeed, very many die. The wonder is that twenty per cent of them are not lost. So that, no one may think that I am exaggerating: it is less than four months since traders took five hundred from Cape Verde to New Spain in one boat, and one hundred and twenty died in one night because they packed them like pigs or even worse, all below decks, where their very breath and excrement (which are sufficient to pollute any atmosphere and destroy them all) killed them. It was indeed a just punishment, from God that these brutal men who were responsible for carrying them also died. The sad affair did not end there, for before they reached Mexico, almost three hundred died. The tale of how those who survived were treated would never end.

## No. 154—THE INJUSTICE OF THE NEGRO SLAVE TRADE

*(Fray Alonso de Sandoval, De Instaurando Aetiopum Salute, Seville, 1627)* *

Apart, from these acts of injustice and robberies committed among themselves, a thousand other acts of treachery are performed by Spaniards who trick them and carry them off afterwards, as newly imported slaves and ignorant persons, to our harbours. This shows how uneasy the conscience of many of these slave traders is, yet they do not on this account mend their ways. One of them told me in all honesty that, he did not know how to quiet his conscience since he was very uneasy about the way in which he had brought over certain Negroes as it seemed to him that he had burdened it in Guinea by the method he had employed in obtaining them. Another who brought almost three hundred adult Negroes said almost the same thing to me and added that, in reality, half the number of wars reported among the Negroes would not be waged if they knew that the Spaniards were not coming to buy Negroes....On another occasion one of these slave traders who usually carried a few Negroes sent to call me while he was ill to settle a certain matter of conscience for him. This matter being resolved, I asked him what he thought of the manner of capturing the Negroes brought from Guinea. He answered me by saying that he thanked God that he had only carried a few and these, in his opinion, with a clear conscience. He could not, however, help feeling badly over what he had seen happening on some ships, namely, that sometimes

*Cited in Saco, *Historia de la Esclavitud de la Raza Africana*, Tomo II, pp. 109—110,

those who went aboard the ships free men left it as captives; and, on other occasions, the captain waited to be supplied with certain Negroes whom he bought at a lower price from other Negroes, at midnight and in a secret manner.

---

## No. 155 — THE ATTACK ON THE RATIONALISATION OF NEGRO SLAVERY

### (Bartolome de Albornoz, Arte de los Contratos, Valencia, 1573)*

When war is waged between public enemies, there is provision for making slaves in the law of dominion, but where no such war exists....how do I know that the slave that I buy was captured justly? For the supposition is always in favour of his freedom. In so far as natural law is concerned, I am forced to favour the one who suffers unfairly and not to make myself an accomplice of the delinquent, for, inasmuch as he has no right over the person whom he sells to me, I have so much less right in purchasing the latter. Therefore, what shall we say of children and women who cannot be guilty, and of those sold through hunger? I find no reason to make me hesitate in the matter, far less to prove my hesitation. There are those who say that it is better for the Negroes to be brought to these parts where they are taught the law of God and live rationally, although they are slaves, than to leave them in their country where, though free, they live like beasts. I hold the first view, and I would advise any Negro who sought my opinion in this matter that he should rather remain king in his country than come among us as a slave. For his welfare does not justify, but rather aggravates, the reason for holding him in servitude....It will only be justified where that Negro cannot be a Christian without being a slave. I do not believe that those persons will tell me that there is anything in Christ's law to the effect that freedom of the soul must be paid for by slavery of the body. Our saviour first cured the ills of the soul of all those whose bodily infirmities he healed. Saint Paul did not seek to deprive Philemon (although he was a Christian) of the service of his slave Onesimo; and now they wish those who become Christians to lose the freedom which God gave to man. Everyone looks after his own business, but very few look after the business of Jesus Christ. How great would be the reward in Heaven of the one who would go among those barbarous peoples to teach them the natural law and prepare them for Christ's law which is founded on the former! While these parts are won over to God, those places are starved of His doctrine. Great is the harvest, but the labourers are few. Because the country is hot and not as pleasant as Talavera or Madrid, no one wishes to take the role of Simon of Cyrene to assist in carrying the Cross, unless his hire is paid him in advance. If the Apostles had behaved thus and each one had taken shelter in Jerusalem, then, as far as preaching is concerned, the law of Jesus Christ would be today where it was ten years before His incarnation. It is His cause: let Him defend it.

## No. 156—DANGER OF SLAVE REVOLTS

### (Fray Alonso de' Sandoval, De Instauranda Aetiopum Salute, Seville, 1627)*

However flourishing kingdoms may be they ought not to consider themselves safe from servile wars while they have not succeeded in subjugating the slaves and are still at their mercy. Wherefore magistrates should fine any person who inspires the merchants' greed, which has been responsible for introducing into Europe no less than into the Indies, very prosperous businesses dealing in slaves, to such an extent that they are maintained and enriched by the bringing of slaves from their native land, now by deceit and now by force, even as people go out to hunt rabbits and partridges and bring them from some ports to others like linen or kersey. Two grave ills result from this business. The first is, that having made merchandise of men's liberty, many of the pretexts on which some of the slaves are captured and sold cannot be but unhealthy. The second is that the Republics are swelled with this supply at the risk of disturbances and revolts. Even as in a moderate degree captivity may be effected without these scruples and with notable benefit to slaves and masters, even so, when it is carried to excess it is very much endangered by any disturbance; not because of fear that the slaves may revolt against the state, for servile minds rarely beget noble thoughts, but because love of freedom is natural and, in exchange for obtaining it, they may unite and give their life for it.

*Cited in Saco, Historia de la Esclavitud de la Raza Africana, Tomo II, pp. 143—144,

## No. 157—THE VALUE AND BEAUTY OF FREEDOM

### (Fray Alonso de Sandoval, De Instauranda Aethiopum Salute, Seville, 1627)*

It is said that of all human possessions none is more valuable or more beautiful than freedom....All the gold in the world and all earthly possessions are not enough to purchase human liberty....God created man free, not only in respect of other men but also of God Himself, for He gave us full control of our free will to carry out our desires, following good or evil, vice or virtue....Finally, the value of freedom is nowhere better observed than in the evils and toils of slavery for, as the divine Plato said, captivity and slavery constitute one continuous death and, therefore, they should be shunned and avoided with greater care and diligence than death. With the latter, captivity and misery come to an end and it finalizes all evils. On the other hand, all ills and toils begin in slavery; it is one with continuous death since slaves live as dying men and die as living men. Philo Judaeus and Euripides stress the same point. For, if the civil laws classify exile as a form of civil death, with how much more reason may we call abject slavery death? For it involves not only exile but also subjugation, and hunger, gloom, nakedness, outrage, imprisonment, perpetual persecution, and is, finally, a combination of all evils.

---

*Cited in Saco, *Historia de la Esclavitud de la Raza Africana*, Tomo II, pp, 113—114,

# CHAPTER VI

# The Spanish Colonial System

## (i) THE SYSTEM OF MONOPOLY

### No. 158—THE ROYAL MONOPOLY OF GOLD
### (Christopher Columbus to Ferdinand and Isabella, King and Queen of Spain, 1493)*

Most High and Powerful Lords: In obedience to what your Highnesses command me, I shall state what occurs to me for the peopling and management of the Spanish Island and of all others, whether already discovered or hereafter to be discovered, submitting myself, however, to any better opinion....

....in order to secure the better and prompter settlement of the said island, that the privilege of getting gold be granted exclusively to those who actually settle and build dwelling-houses in the settlement where they may be, in order that all may live close to each other and in greater safety....

Likewise, that no settler be allowed to go and gather gold unless with a permit from the governor or mayor of the town in which he lives, to be given only upon his promising under oath to return to the place of his residence and faithfully report all the gold which he may have gathered, this to be done once a month, or once a week, as the time may be assigned to him, the said report to be entered on the proper registry by the clerk of the town in the presence of the mayor, and if so deemed advisable, in the presence of a friar or priest selected for the purpose.

Likewise, that all the gold so gathered be melted forthwith, and stamped with such a stamp as the town may have devised and selected, and that it be weighed and that the share of that gold which belongs to your Highnesses be given and delivered to the mayor of the town, the proper record thereof being made by the clerk and by the priest or friar, so that it may not pass through only one hand and may so render the concealing of the truth impossible.

Likewise, that all the gold which may be found without the mark or seal aforesaid in the possession of any one who had formerly reported once as aforesaid, be forfeited and divided into two halves, one for the informer and the other for your Highnesses.

*Cited in Bourne, The *Northmen, Columbus and Cabot,* pp, 273—277,

Likewise, that one per cent of all the gold gathered be set apart and appropriated for building churches, and providing for their proper furnishing and ornamentation, and to the support of the priests or friars having them in their charge, and, if so deemed advisable, for the payment of some compensation to the mayors and clerks of the respective towns, so as to cause them to fulfil their duties faithfully, and that the balance be delivered to the governor and treasurer sent there by your Highnesses.

Likewise, in regard to the division of the gold and of the share which belongs to your Highnesses, I am of the opinion that it should be entrusted to the said governor and treasurer, because the amount of the gold found may sometimes be large and sometimes small, and, if so deemed advisable, that the share of your Highnesses be established for one year to be one-half, the other half going to the gatherers, reserving for a future time to make some other and better provision, if necessary.

Likewise, that if the mayors and clerks commit any fraud or consent to it, the proper punishment be inflicted upon them, and that a penalty be likewise imposed upon those settlers who do not report in full the whole amount of the gold which is in their possession.

Likewise, that there be a treasurer in the said island, who shall receive all the gold belonging to your Highnesses, and shall have a clerk to make and keep the proper record of the receipts, and that the mayors and clerks of the respective towns be given the proper vouchers for everything which they may deliver to the said treasurer.

Likewise, that whereas the extreme anxiety of the colonists to gather gold may induce them to neglect all other business and occupations, it seems to me that they should be prohibited from engaging in the search of gold during some season of the year, so as to give all other business, profitable to the island, an opportunity to be established and carried on....

Likewise, in regard to the gold to be brought from the island to Castile, that the whole of it, whether belonging to your Highnesses or to some private individual, must be kept in a chest, with two keys, one to be kept by the master of the vessel and the other by some person chosen by the governor and the treasurer, and that an official record must be made of everything put in the said chest, in order that each one may have what is his, and that any other gold, much or little, found outside of the said chest in any manner be forfeited to the benefit of your Highnesses, so as to cause the transaction to be made faithfully....

Likewise, that in the presence of the Justice of the said city of Cadiz and of whomsoever may be deputed for the purpose by your Highnesses, the said chest shall be opened in which the gold is to be brought and that to each one be given what belongs to him.

---

### No. 159—THE ROYAL MONOPOLY OF TRADE

*(Ferdinand and Isabella, King and Queen of Spain, to Admiral Christopher Columbus and Councillor D. Juan de Fonseca, May 23, 1493)* \*

You well know or should know how, after the Islands and mainland....were discovered under our command, we....through our Decrees and provisions which were presented and. published, forbade, prohibited, and commanded that no person should dare to go to the said Islands and mainland of the Indies without our license and command, under certain penalties....And now we command that a certain armada be sent over there, to the places which have been discovered....as well as to discover other Islands and mainland; of which armada we name as Captain General you, our said Admiral of the Islands. Our pleasure and will is that in the said Armada....no vessel, or no person or persons, may go, except those whom we or the said Admiral and Archdeacon, to whom we entrust the responsibility of forming the said armada in our name, appoint to go with you....Likewise, that those who go there may not take and will not be allowed to take to the said Indies any sort of merchandise or things for exchange; and in order that an account be kept of everything which it is decided should be taken, everything will be kept and will be entered and is entered in our books, so that nothing more will go than what we have allowed. In order that in this matter there should not or might not interfere any sort of fraud, deceit, or collusion, we command this our Decree to be given for the said reason, through which we forbid, prohibit and command that no person of any state or condition, preeminence or dignity, dare to go, or may go to the said Islands and mainland in the said armada or. in any other, and that no masters or captains of any ship or ships dare to shelter them and take them.... to the said Indies in their vessels and lighters....except those whom we or you have appointed and will appoint in our name to go in this armada.... Those who do go will not take any merchandise without our permission and command; and in order that everything may be accounted for and listed, and that the vessels and persons who are going, what they take and what they bring, be known, we command that at the time of the armada's departure from

*Cited in Navarrete, *op. cit.*, Tomo II, Num. XXXV, pp. 68—70.

our Kingdoms it be written down when they embark, and that the ships and lighters on which they will go be laden before Juan de Soria, Secretary to Prince Don Juan, our very dear and beloved Son....Everything that is laden in them, persons as well as sailors, guns, and other persons, will be recorded in a book which will be kept by each Official of our Treasury who will go on each ship of the said armada. Upon arriving at the said Islands and main-land, everything will be presented to the other Lieutenant of our Treasury....before whom all persons will dis-embark, unload their effects, merchandise, arms, and other things....in order that he may keep account of every-thing, and no collusion, fraud, or deceit may take place. When they leave the Indies to come back to our Kingdoms, they will make a similar presentation before the said Lieutenant....which he will send with the Officials of our Treasury who come on the ships from there, who will give an account of everything to the said Juan de Soria....here, so that, as we have said before, there may be an account of everything, and no deceit done. So, we command that everything be done and obeyed as it has been commanded, and according to what has been stated in this Decree, under the penalty that whoever is found to have laden more than what he registered at the time of departure from our Kingdoms or to have unloaded in our Kingdoms at the time of his return more than what was laden at the time of depar-ture from the said Indies, will lose all of it, two-thirds of it going to our Chamber, and the remaining one-third being divided equally among the informer and the Judge who shall sentence him.

---

## No. 160—THE ROYAL MONOPOLY OF MINES

*(Ferdinand and Isabella, King and Queen of Spain, to the Governors and Royal Officials in the Indies, September 3, 1501)* \*

Be it known that we have been informed that, even though the mines of metal and other commodities which have been found and discovered up to now, and will be found and discovered hereafter in the islands and main-land of the Ocean sea, belong to us, some persons, without our licence and command, have on their own initiative discovered and found mines of certain metals called *"guanines"*\*\* in the islands of Paria, Caquebacoa and in other islands and parts of the mainland, and have brought and bring it for sale to the Indians of Hispaniola, and other places, which is to our detriment and prejudicial to our

\*Cited in Navarrete, *op. cit.*, Tomo II, Num. XIII, pp. 470—471.
\*\*Gold under legal standard.

revenues and the Royal Patrimony of our Kingdoms and Dominions; and since our will and pleasure is that this practice shall not be continued hereafter, we have decided to issue this Decree forbidding, ordering and commanding that no person or persons, our subjects and nationals, settlers and inhabitants of our Kingdoms and Dominions, and of the islands and mainland, or any other persons from foreign Kingdoms and Provinces, dare to seek, discover or sell to the Indians of Hispaniola, or to any other place, the said or other metals, or hides from the said Islands of Paria and Caquebacoa or from any other islands and mainland, without our licence and command.

---

### No. 161—THE EARLY MONOPOLY OF CADIZ

*(Decree of Ferdinand and Isabella, King and Queen of Spain, April 10, 1495)\**

....all the ships sailing to the said islands....will depart from the city of Cadiz, and from no other place; and before sailing they will present themselves before our Officials.... so that they may know who is going to the said Indies....

Item: That any of our subjects and natives may go from now on....if they wish to discover islands and mainland in the....Indies, both to the islands already discovered as well as to any others, and to trade in them, as long as it is not in the said Hispaniola; that they may buy from the Christians who are or may be there anything or any merchandise, provided that it is not gold; this they may do with whatever ships they wish, provided that at the time of departure from our kingdoms, they leave from the said city of Cadiz....and....that whatever the said persons may find in the said islands and mainland they may keep nine-tenths of it for themselves, and the remaining one-tenth will be for Us, which they will pay to us on their return to our Kingdoms in the said City of Cadiz, where they must first come to pay it....and at the time of departure from the city of Cadiz they must give security that they will comply with this.

---

### No. 162—MONOPOLY IN THE COLONIES

*(Ferdinand and Isabella, King and Queen of Spain, to Christopher Columbus, August 3, 1499)\*\**

Be it known that Pedro de Salcedo has advised us how the settlers and residents of Hispaniola were in lack and

---

*Cited in Navarrete, *op. cit.*, Tomo II, Num. LXXXVI, pp. 196—198.
\*\*Cited in Navarrete, *op. cit.*, Tomo II, Num. CXXXI, pp. 281—282.

much need of soap, because of the increase in population, and the distance from our Kingdoms of Castile. He would like us to give him the privilege of supplying the island with it; but without having to use his money on it, for after having supplied this necessity and any future one, it may be that other persons might enter the trade and he would suffer a great loss. In view of the fact that the said Pedro Salcedo has served us in the discovery of the Indies, and that harm would be done to him if he started and used his money in the said soap and, after he had opened this way and supplied and satisfied the settlers and residents of Hispaniola, others would come to take away and make him lose what he had started, which would all be against reason; seeing that if we do not give him the opportunity to provide and take soap to the Island, or to produce it in the Island, the settlers and residents would suffer from a great need of it, and would spend a long time without it, therefore, We.... as a reward for his service in the Indies and in their discovery, hereby give the said Pedro Salcedo the right to carry or arrange to carry soap to Hispaniola, in whatever quantity he may think necessary to furnish a supply and an abundance for the settlers and residents, and to sell it and have it sold for not more than its present price. We positively forbid any other person to take soap to Hispaniola for sale, or to manufacture it in the Island....

---

## No. 163 — THE MONOPOLY OF HISPANIOLA

*(Antonio de Herrera, Historia General de los Hechos de los Castellanos en las Islas y Tierra Firme del Mar Oceano, Madrid, 1601-1615)\**

On the occasion of the arrival of the English ships in the harbour of the city of Santo Domingo in Hispaniola, and of the French ships.... the Bishop of Santo Domingo, President of the Audiencia, summoned a council of persons of all ranks to consider what steps should be taken for the security of that island and all the others, mindful of the novelty of strangers roaming in those parts and the danger contained in the report that they captured the goods of the Indies and the gold, on which the King depended to keep up the war which he was fighting against other princes.... And having thoroughly discussed the matter, the council was of the opinion that the King should be informed of existing conditions and of the remedy deemed necessary. In their opinion, the islands of San Juan and Hispaniola were the principal ports of entry in those parts, where there was a large quantity of victuals and other provisions; the captains

*Op. cit., Decada Quarta, Libro Sexto, Cap. XIII, Tomo V, pp. 323—327.

and sailors who sailed in those regions had lost all fear of the law, and no other pirates were necessary. . . .

They recommended. . . . first, that incoming and outgoing ships should be restricted to a single port, whether it involved people, merchandise and provisions, gold, silver and other products of the Indies, so that a single place should be designated, the most appropriate, where the Fair should be held and the trade of the New World concentrated. Secondly, that in the place designated, there should also be the highest authority, and equipment of war, for their security and defence. Thirdly, that a Royal Audiencia should be established in that place, to endorse the King's decrees, and to supervise the execution of the Royal Ordinances. . . . They recommended also that orders should be given that all ships leaving Castile should go direct to the place designated and should there unload. . . . Once unloaded, they should return, without entering any other port, unless given a licence to do so, and should there pay the import, export and other duties. On the return voyage to Castile they should be registered, with the express licence and approval of the Royal Audiencia. . . . No captain should be allowed to sail from Castile to the Indies without giving sufficient security at the House of Trade. . . .

The Province which seemed most appropriate was Hispaniola, which combined all the qualities necessary for navigation, victualling, etc. and which was the point of departure for all the discoveries and pacifications of all parts of the Indies. This would result in the preservation of all the Indies and the increase of the royal revenues, for the following reasons. First, this being a powerful island, if the three recommendations above were implemented, it would unaided be able to defend itself against the armadas of other kingdoms, however large they might be, because the number of ships ordinarily in the island exceeded one hundred, large and small, so that the King would have to spend nothing from his revenues and could be relieved of expenses on that score. Secondly, an infinite number of ships would be constructed in Hispaniola, because of the large supply of wood and facilities for raising hemp, abundance of local bread, fish and meat, and these activities would contribute considerably to the settlement of the country; with the immigration of settlers a city would be built, like Palermo in Sicily, or London in England; and trade would increase in gold, silver, copper and other metals, sugar, cassia, wool, cotton and the many other commodities with which it abounds. If this island were fully populated, all the others would necessarily be subject and obedient to it. . . . there would be an end to the crimes which have been and are daily committed. . . . and the fear of the Negroes would be eliminated, and greater efforts would be made for the cultivation of sugar

and the rearing of livestock, which had been abandoned, in a desire to profit only by the hides, a great pity, and all because of the small population. If all the trade was restricted to Hispaniola, it would be easy to know from month to month what was happening in the Indies, and the Supreme Council could govern with less difficulty....
The view was expressed that the objection might be raised that these recommendations would be prejudicial to the new Audiencia of Mexico, to which the reply was given: "That nothing was being proposed which was contrary to the decisions reached with respect to the preeminence of that Audiencia.... And if the city of Seville should argue that it was being deprived of the liberty it enjoyed of sending its ships freely where it pleased, the reply was that what was being recommended was better, since nothing would be lost which came from the Indies, that nothing would be smuggled to other parts of Europe, but that everything would go in good faith to Seville, making allowance for the thefts of the captains and pirates and the perils of the sea; besides which, if the trade of the Indies were planned, there would be many underwriters and more shippers in Seville."

---

### No. 164 — THE MONOPOLY OF SPANIARDS FROM CASTILE, LEON AND ARAGON

*(J. Veitia de Linaje, Norte de la Contratacion, de las Indias Occidentales, Seville, 1672. English Translation by John Stevens, The Spanish Rule of Trade to the Indies, London, 1702)\**

1. No stranger is allowed to trade, or deal in the Indies, either going over himself, or remitting his effects, without express license and permission from His Majesty. Those who have such leave, in form as shall be shown hereafter, may trade with only their own stocks, upon pain of forfeiting them and their license. Persons naturalized, tho' they may ship their effects, and if considerable enough, go over to follow their own business, yet may they not be owners, nor masters of ships, nor enjoy any other employment, nor have any vote in the Court of Consulship, for the naturalization does not take off this prohibition.

2. ....D. John de Solorzano says, they are all positively to be looked upon as strangers or aliens, who are not born in the Kingdoms of Castile and Leon, and that the Navarrois are admitted, as being dispensed with and naturalized in the years 1553 and 1581. I was surprised he should say he found no such permission for the Aragonians, but rather looked upon them as aliens: and John de Hevia

Bolanos   plainly says that the natives of the kingdom   of
Aragon are strangers, but it seems he had not seen the
King's Order of the last of April, 1560, which directs the
expelling all Portugueses out of the Indies, and has these
words, *You shall expel them, and for the future not suffer
such as go over to remain there; the same shall ye do by all
other strangers, who have gone from other parts without
these Kingdoms of Castile and Aragon.* And it is not to be
doubted, but that the Aragonians were looked upon as
natives ever since the first discovery of the Indies, without
standing in need of such a dispensation as the Navarrois,
the difference between them being very great, because
Aragon and Castile were united when the Indies were discovered, which Navarre was not till 20 years after; and Their
Catholic Majesties, from the first discovery, provided, that
the Indies should not be peopled by any but natives of the
Kingdoms of Castile, Leon and Aragon, as was ordered in
the Year 1501....

5.   It was decreed in the Year 1562, that such strangers
as resided in Spain, or in the Indies, the term of ten years,
being settled housekeepers,   and married to Spanish   or
Indian women, should   be   accounted   natives;   but that
bachelors should not enjoy this privilege, tho' they had been
resident above ten years. This was afterwards repealed....

7.   There is a law that directs, there be a book in the
India House of such strangers as may trade to the Indies,
and such as may not, to show whether what is ordained in
that case be observed.   Another enjoins, that there be no
trade allowed strangers, in any port of the West Indies,
upon pain of death and forfeiture of goods. And in the
year 1557, it was ordained that, whosoever bought anything
of a foreigner should be sent, prisoner into Spain, and forfeit
half his goods.   Another law forbids all strangers residing
in the Indies, or going over thither, and directs such as are
there should be expelled, and if they went without leave to
lose all they have got there: and this, as has been observed
before, comprehends not only strangers, but natives going
over without, leave, who are supposed not to get anything
for themselves, or their heirs, but for the Exchequer.   There
are several orders against carrying any strangers as sailors,
or on any other pretence whatsoever, upon pain of forfeiting
of 100,000 maravedis to the master that shall carry any,
which in those days was no small sum.

8.   When any fleet sails for the Indies, inquiry is to be
made what strangers put any goods aboard, and they are to
be proceeded against.   All strangers and enemies to the
Crown of Castile, taken beyond the Canary Islands, either
coming or going to the West Indies, were to be executed
without acquainting His Majesty; how this was understood
formerly I know not, but at present none are punishable

for being in those seas, since other nations have islands there, and in case they be taken as pirates, all seas are alike to bring them to condign punishment.

9. Strangers residing at Seville and the adjacent ports, tho' forbid the trade of the Indies, are obliged to advance their quotas upon loans for fitting out of armadas and flotas, and all other contributions paid by natives....

## (ii) — THE ORGANISATION OF SPANISH TRADE IN THE COLONIES

### No. 165 — THE HOUSE OF TRADE IN SEVILLE

*(Decree of Ferdinand and Isabella, King and Queen of Spain, January 20, 1503)\**

First of all, we order and command that in the City of Seville there will be established a House of Trade where will be stored, for the time needed, all the merchandise and supplies and all other equipment needed to provide what is necessary for the trade of the Indies....and to send there everything that might be appropriate; where will be received all the merchandise and other commodities which will be sent from the Indies to these our Kingdoms, and where will be sold everything that is to be sold, or is to be sent for sale and trade to other places as necessary. We command that the said House be established so that there will be provision in it for all the aforesaid.

Moreover: we order and command that in the said House convenient apartments be prepared, as appropriate, in which the above-mentioned commodities will be stored: so that everything to be put there will be well kept, and in places where they will not spoil, and one commodity will be separated from the other, as the quality of the merchandise may require.

Besides: we order and command that within the said House there will be established and designated a separate place, where the Officials, who shall be appointed by Us to be and reside in the said House, will meet every day for the necessary hours, so that there as a group they will be responsible for providing all the goods which would be advantageous for the said business, and for the good shipping and dispatch of the merchandise which will be brought to the said House, and for trading, selling or sending it where necessary, and negotiating all the other matters pertinent for the administration of the said business.

Moreover: we order and command that in the said

*Cited in Navarrete, *op. cit.*, Tomo II, Num. CXLVIII, pp. 332—337.

House there will be and reside a Factor who is to be an able and diligent man, who will be in charge of the said business; and a Treasurer, who will receive and receives all the goods and merchandise, supplies, money and anything else stored in or consigned to the said House; and an Accountant or Scrivener, who are to be competent persons of good reputation, who will have their ledgers bound, in which they will write and enter all the goods which they receive from the said Treasurer, and those which it will be their responsibility to collect, merchandise as well as supplies, and money stored in or consigned to the said House, and likewise everything which the said Factor might ship and get in the said business, entering each item by itself under separate titles, first, entering what was received and collected, and what it will be his responsibility to collect, and then the data of the expenses, how and for what payment was made, to what persons and for what reasons. We command that the persons mentioned above will be the ones whom you will appoint, and commission, and the said persons will do all of the aforesaid inside the said House and as a group, so that there will be greater security; and in the said books we command that the said Factor, Treasurer and Scrivener will sign under each entry.

Besides: we order and command that all the merchandise which the said Treasurer of the said House might receive, he shall receive before the said Factor and the said Scrivener or Accountant, and will receive each merchandise of whatever sort it might be, declaring everything in detail, its price, and the quantity of each received; for some merchandise is worth more than others, and in this there cannot or must not be any fraud or deceit.

Moreover: we command that the said Factor and Treasurer of the said House take care to learn and inform themselves of all the merchandise and other goods which would be profitable and necessary for the said Trade, and at what time it will be necessary to send them and what ships will be needed to take them, and that at the appropriate time they shall have assembled and ready all the merchandise and supplies which would be necessary for said voyage of said Trade, in the ships which will be utilized, so that the said voyage will not be delayed or hindered by their fault or negligence, and everything will be done as convenient for the good conduct of the said Trade.

Besides: that the said Officials will be wise and careful with the merchandise, supplies and things which they may take on credit at good prices so that no great loss will result from them or from the prices paid for them; similarly with the merchandise and supplies which they may buy on the instalment plan, they will be careful as to the time when they buy it, so that it will be at the most profitable prices possible for the said Trade....

Likewise: we command that the said Officials will be careful to look for suitable and reliable persons as Captains of the ships which will make the said trips with the said merchandise, and likewise Scriveners who are to be good trustworthy persons in whose presence they will deliver and entrust to the Captains all the merchandise and supplies.... and the Captains will give and deliver it in the presence of the said Scriveners, to the persons who by our orders are to receive it in the Indies.... and will get signed documents from the persons to whom it was delivered and from the Scriveners in whose presence it was delivered, which they will give to the said Officials of the said House....

Likewise: we command that the said Officials will take great care to see and know the cost incurred by the said vessels on the said trips for the freight they carried, and consider whether, for the good of the said business and for reducing its cost, they should order some ships to be made for the said Trade, and what advantage there is in both procedures, and which is more appropriate for our service and the good of the said business, and to let us know so that we can command what should be done.

Moreover: we command that the said Officials, whenever they ship the said vessels for the said voyages, will give to each and every Captain of the said vessels and to the Scrivener who is to go in them, signed written instructions of everything they are to do, of the trip they will undertake, as well as of the order they will follow in giving and delivering the said merchandise to the persons who will receive it by our orders.... and what they are to do on their return with what they bring, so that they may not exceed their instructions....

Besides: we command the Officials of the said House to take great care to ascertain from the Officials who by our orders will be in the said Indies in charge of affairs over there, their needs of merchandise and supplies, so that.... they may provide the merchandise and supplies necessary according to the need existing there and the time when they are sent, and to advise these Officials of all the commodities which they have sent over there, and those they think should be sent from there to here, according to the need there may be here for them, so that the said Officials who reside in the Indies will send to these lands the commodities and merchandise which they have there and which are lacking here....

Moreover: we command the said Officials of the said House that all the gold which may come from the Indies is to be received by the said Treasurer in the way in which we have commanded them to receive the above-mentioned merchandise in the presence of the said Factor and Scrivener, and then as soon as it has arrived and been received they are to write to us and advise us of the quantity.... and its probable worth after being stamped, and they are to send us every year an account of everything in their charge and all data of the things which have been received and given, so that we will be kept informed. And likewise they shall send us a signed copy of all the debts of the said House, of all the orders for payment which we have given to whatever persons and that have been accepted by them, so that we may provide for everything as it fits our service, and order them what they are to pay and do after we have seen what has come in and what is owed; and in the meanwhile we command that the said Officials of the said House are not to spend, nor will spend any of the said gold which may come to the said House and into their hands from the Indies without our license and special command, and until we through our Decree and signed instructions direct them, how and in what things we wish the sum to which the gold will amount to be spent; telling them to take and spend so much for the expenses and debts of the said House, and with the remainder to do what we prescribe, because we wish that while they inform us of the aforesaid, the said Officials will have said gold stamped in the mint of the said City of Seville.

Moreover: we command the Captains and Scriveners of the ships in which the gold and other merchandise and things are brought from the Islands to the said House, to bring a certificate or a copy signed by the Officials of the Indies in charge, of the quantity of gold and other goods which they bring.

---

### No. 166—THE GREATEST HOUSE IN THE WORLD

*(J. Veitia de Linaje, Norte de la Contratacion de las Indias Occidentales, Seville, 1672. English Translation by John Stevens, The Spanish Rule of Trade to the Indies, London, 1702)\**

It will not....be improper....to observe the greatness of this Court, whose jurisdiction is so large, as its territory is boundless; whose authority is so extraordinary, that it has supplied the place of a Council, and acted as such, not only in reference to the Indies, but to the revenue and military affairs, when orders passed immediately from the King to it; whose wealth is such, that none in Europe can compare with it; whose credit is so high, that no private person could equal it; whose preeminences were such, that they had the appointing of all officers, even to the Admirals of fleets and Civil Magistrates; the giving passes to ships to all parts, and sending advice-boats with only their own orders. One of whose Judges or Commissioners, being want-

*Op. cit., pp. 10—11.

ing at the Board, the place has been supplied by an Assistant of Seville, being a Nobleman of Castile; the appointing of whose officers, the Emperor Charles V. reserved
to himself, together with Viceroys and Archbishops, when
he went into Flanders, leaving the disposal of all other
places to the Prince his Son, afterwards King Philip II,
tho' the poverty and vicissitude of times have of late
deprived it of the privilege of choosing officers, those
places being since sold. Notwithstanding the decay time
and several accidents have caused in the greatness of this
India-House, there is not in all the Spanish Monarchy a
nobler Court, next to the King's Councils; for the Commissioners of both the Chambers of Direction and Justice
enjoy all the same privileges and immunities with the
Judges in Chancery and other Courts, and may be termed
a Council inasmuch as their advice is asked upon several
occasions by His Majesty... the Licentiate, D. Francis de
Mosquera, had reason to say of this House, *that it is of the
greatest moment of any in the World.* And the Licentiate,
Alonso Morgado, *that the Treasure which has been in it
would suffice to pave the streets of Seville with tiles of silver
and gold.* Roderick Caro, *that it was part of the Palace and
Royal Apartment in it, and its authority so great, that no
ship can sail to the West Indies without its leave.* And
again, *that for this reason, authors justly call Seville
Queen of the Ocean.* D. John De Solorzano, with Antony de
Herrera, says, *it is a tribunal of great power, having to do
with all business concerning the commerce and trade of
the Indies, and arising from it; and no Magistrate can
intermeddle in what concerns it.*

---

## No. 167—ROYAL INSTRUCTIONS TO THE BUREAUCRACY

*(Ordinance of Ferdinand I, King of Spain, for the House of
Trade, June 15, 1510)\**

First: We order and command  that, in  accordance
with the charter of the said organisation, you officials will
meet in the House twice daily, on days which are not holidays, in the following way: from Michaelmas to the feast
of Saint Mary in March, from ten to eleven in the morning, and then from five to six in the afternoon; and from
the feast of Saint Mary in March to Michaelmas, from nine
to ten in the morning, and from five to six in the afternoon; and you will in a group, and in no other way, dispense
justice as well as despatch business, unless one of you

*Cited in Navarrete, *op. cit.*, Tomo II, Num. CLXX, pp. 391—399.

should be absent, from the City or ill, or busy attending to our affairs.

Item:   We command that all the transaction which are made in the Court for the Indies, will be registered in the House by you, entering the transfer in a book so that there will be a complete account of all that has been provided; and you will take good care to see if there is anything in it that is not in our interests, or which might be harmful to the business. in which event you will inform us of it so that we will provide for it a convenient....

Item: We order and command that henceforth all the goods for the trade loaded and unloaded in this House will be specially entered in ledger books which you have in the House, in accordance with the charter of the organisation, each commodity as it arrives, and the three of you will sign the books at the end of each chapter or chapters as each transaction is entered, under penalty of dismissal from office and of reimbursing us for any loss to our revenue.

Item: We command that after entering the goods, in accordance with the entries in said books, you' will give to the parties the order or orders of payment signed by you for the Treasurer of that House, for everything that should be given and paid for, so that he may pay for them; he will note what he pays to the parties on the back of the orders of payment, because henceforth he will make up his accounts from them. But as sometimes small sums will have to be paid, and it would be tedious to make out an order of payment for each, we command that for the payment of less than two hundred maravedis no order of payment will be given, but that it will be entered in a separate book; and finally, every fifteen days it will be transferred to the general book....

Item: We command that in the aforesaid   form you will charge to the Treasurer in another separate book or books, all the clothes, armour, artillery, parcels and any other goods which may be bought or consigned to the House, up to the smallest item; and when you give any of it to the armadas or to any individual, be it done with your order of payment, and taking note of the parties to whom it has been consigned on the back of said order of payment; and when the arms or any other item thus given are returned to the House, you will take great care that they are recovered, and you will charge them to the Treasurer, so that in everything there will be the necessary caution....

Item: We order and command that upon the arrival of any ship or ships from the Indies in the port, you will go to the said ship or ships accompanied only by your constable and ministers, and by no persons from outside, and with your customary diligence you will chase everybody off the ship and will take great care to ascertain if there is any stolen gold to be stamped or registered, and whatever you find stolen plus a fourth of the goods of the person importing it will be confiscated to our Chamber and the National Treasury; and our will is that whoever discovers it will have the third part of the gold, that you arrest the importer, and inform us of the case, so that we may have him punished as he deserves, and that you assign a person to guard the ships, who will be faithful and knows his job, and pay him a decent salary.

Item: If anyone buys gold not yet stamped or registered, we command that the same punishment will fall upon the buyer as upon the one who has stolen the gold, and the informer will have a third of it....

Item: We have commanded our Admiral and officials of the Indies not to allow henceforth any ship to leave for these Kingdoms without taking on enough supplies for eighty days, or for the time which they think convenient, so that they will not lack anything before they reach Seville....and so that they will not stop at any land on the pretext of taking on supplies....as they have done heretofore; we command you to ascertain when the ships arrive whether they have stopped in any foreign country or committed any fraud or deceit, or exceeded the tenor of their instructions....

Item: We command the said Admiral and officials henceforth to send to you an account of all the goods for the trade loaded and unloaded in particular, so that in that House there will be a record of everything; we command you to enter in a separate book the account and record which will be sent to you from there (Hispaniola), and similarly for the Island of San Juan and the other islands and lands which may hereafter be settled.

Item: We command that all judicial questions of importance be determined with the approval and opinion of your lawyer or lawyers, signing together with you the sentence or sentences; and when these are pronounced the lawyer is to be present, so that everything may be done legally....

Item: We order that when the captain of a merchant ship notifies you that he wishes to freight a ship for the Indies, all of you together will examine whether the ship is capable of making the trip and the freight which it can take, and the quantity which, in your opinion, it can carry; you will give him licence to obtain money for the victualling of the ship and its needs, and you are not to visit the ship until the lading has been completed, and the captain gives you the record of the clothes he is carrying....this done, you shall then visit him, and once you have visited him, you are not to allow him to take a larger cargo than what was determined by the visitors, so that due to the excess of cargo he will not be in danger during his trip. . . .

Item: We command that, should there be at any time a difference of opinion among you, if it is of importance and of such a nature that delay will not be hazardous, you will apprise us of the case and your votes thereon, so that we will provide for it; and in matters of lesser importance the majority vote will decide, provided you keep a book to enter in detail the vote of any dissentient.

Item: We command you to transfer in order to a separate book all the provisions and ordinances which have been made up to the present for this House and for the Indies since its foundation, and also the ordinances which may hereafter be made, so that you will have them all available, and this original one and all the others you will put in a chest where they may be locked up and safe.

---

### No. 168—COLLECTIVE RESPONSIBILITY OF THE BUREAUCRACY

*(Ordinance of Ferdinand I, King of Spain, for the Organisation of the House of Trade, May 18, 1511)*\*

In the first place: whereas in the ordinance made that the officials of the said House are to meet in it at certain hours, it is convenient to impose penalties on those who do not obey it. . . .I order and command: that, any official who does not come to the said House at the hours stated in the said ordinance, will pay for each offence half a real of silver for the upkeep of the House, unless he had a just reason for not coming, which he is required to send to the other officials, his colleagues, so that business will not be delayed by waiting for him; which penalty he will be forced to pay on the same day on which it is incurred, and he shall pay a similar fine for each day he postpones pay-ing it, and the Scrivener of the House is to be the depository, and to adopt measures for collecting the fines. . . .

Item: With regard to the cargo of clothes going to the Indies, I command that the pertinent ordinance of the House be obeyed; and besides, it is my will that anyone taking clothes to the Indies without first registering in the House whatever he carries, will lose them, and whoever discovers it will receive one-third of it, the remaining two-thirds being for the expenses of the House; and that in the Indies everything which has not been registered in the House of Seville is to be confiscated, the proceeds being distributed as prescribed.

Item: I command the Lawyer of the House of Seville

\*Cited in Navarrete, *op. cit.*, Tomo II, Num. CLXX, pp. 399—404.

to attend every Thursday, after lunch, at the hour appointed
for the officials to meet in the House....

Item: I declare and command that in all matters,
those pertaining to justice as well as to finance....the following method be followed: that in doubtful or important
matters no official will answer in public or in private, until
they have talked it over among the three of them, and
whatever seems best to all three of them shall be given as
the answer and taken as the conclusion; and if one holds
a different opinion from the other two, he will sign, according to the pertinent ordinance of the House, except in cases
of such importance that the third person thinks it proper
to consult us; in that case, the three of them, or those of
them together at that time, will explain the case in a letter
and will send it to me signed, so that I may tell them what
to do.

Item: I command that, when any trader comes to any
official privately, outside the hours prescribed for the
handling of business, the said official will refer him to the
House at the hours specified, without taking any action in
the matter; except in cases where, if all of them had been
together, the matter in question would have been assigned
to him alone so that he should give it special study....

Likewise: I command the said officials to keep a chest
with three keys, in which they will put the incoming bundles
and despatches, from the Court as well as from the Indies
and from any other place, where they will stay until they
are dealt with, and in which likewise will be kept incoming
letters for the officials from all places until they have been
answered. The three of them will handle the questions and
give their replies to the messengers and persons responsible for delivering them. These will be entered in a book
that will be kept in the said chest, where an account of
the despatches will be kept, with a certificate of the time
at which they are despatched....and once the replies have
been sent out the letters are to remain in possession of
the Accountant in order that he may give an account and
explanation of them when necessary, and the despatches
are to be sent with the seal of the House, which is to be
kept in the said chest.

Item: I command that, with respect to incoming orders
or messengers, the ordinance of the House of Seville is to
be followed, and that none of the officials is to open the
letter or despatch privately or until they are all together
in the House, and that whoever hears first of the messenger
and letters will advise his colleagues so that they may come
to the House, to take such action as may be appropriate.

Item: I order and command the officials....to keep
secret and deal faithfully with all matters involving the

business in general, and particularly those matters requiring secrecy, and I order them not to write individually to Me or to any other person, much less to publish or say anything concerning the business, directly or indirectly, until they are all agreed as to how and in what way they will do it, write it, publish it, or provide for it; and when they have agreed, together they will publish it and will not write it privately; and when they meet to transact business, they are to state and declare to one another clearly and openly their opinion on all matters pertaining to the business, in general as well as in particular....

Item: Because I have been informed that among the officials of the House there has been some difference of opinion as to who should sign first, I declare and command that henceforth, whenever an official is replaced due to a vacancy or for any other reason, the senior official shall have precedence both in voting and in signing....

---

### No. 169—THE ARMADA

*(Antonio de Herrera, Historia General de los Hechos de los Castellanos en las Islas y Tierra Firme del Mar Oceano, Madrid, 1601-1615)* *

Three ships arrived from the Indies, with many passengers, and the usual merchandise, cassia, sugar, and hides. As they had unloaded in Lepe and Palos, the captains were ordered to be punished for infringing thereby the ordinances of the House of Trade of Seville, although they were excused because they were obliged to do this by the weather and did not wish to detain the passengers. They brought the King, for his fifth, 136,874 pesos of gold, 983 marks of pearls of all sorts, and 382 large, fine, round pearls. They passed four French free-booters and one galleon, on the coast of Andalusia which were awaiting them....and as it was learned about the same time that eight other ships coming from the Indies had been detained in the Azores by the reports they had received of pirates....the King decreed, at the instance of the merchants trading to the Indies, that an Armada should be organised for the security of the ships coming and going, and that the cost of the Armada should be defrayed by a special tax, the *averia,* as had previously been done....

The seven ships which left Hispaniola....brought, besides large quantities of grain, cassia, sugar and hides, 51,082 pesos of gold for the King, as his fifth, 350 marks of ordinary pearls, 183 select pearls from Cubagua....and one very beautiful pearl, with which the King was vastly pleased,

*Op. cit., Decada Tercera, Libro Septimo, Cap. I, Tomo IV, pp. 343—344; Libro Decimo, Cap. XI, Tome V, pp. 111—112.

and he ordered the Members of the Audiencia of Hispaniola that, whenever anything valuable was discovered, whatever it might be, they should pay to the discoverer the share which belonged to him and take it for His Majesty....And as the French privateers still continued to prowl, the Members of the Audiencia of Hispaniola and all Ministers of the Indies were ordered to take steps that the ships sailing for Castile came well equipped with arms and all that was necessary for their defence, assembled in Hispaniola, and sailed thence together under convoy.

## No. 170—THE FLOTA

*(J. Veitia de Linaje, Norte de la Contratacion de las Indias Occidentales, Seville, 1672. English Translation by John Stevens, The Spanish Rule of Trade to the Indies, London, 1702)**

2. In the Year 1521 on account of the pirates that infested the coast of Andalusia and Algarve, lying in wait for the ships homeward bound from the Indies, it was ordered, that an Armada or convoy consisting of four or five ships should be fitted out; the charge to be defrayed out of the gold, silver, and merchandize brought to the ports of Andalusia from the Indies and Canary Islands, whether belonging to the King or private persons, at the rate of a shilling per pound, which was accordingly put in execution. The following year 1522 the seas being still infested with pirates, it was resolved another squadron should be fitted out, to be defrayed as the former, and to cruise not only on the coast, but as far as the Islands Azores, commonly called Terceras. This was the original not only of the Armada appointed to secure the navigation of the West Indies, but of the Haberia, or duty for convoys, and other things relating to it: the first imposition towards defraying this charge was one in the hundred, but that not answering, it came to five in the hundred.

3. One of the principal duties of the Committee of War, made out of the Council of the Indies, is to give the necessary orders for fitting out of Armadas and Flotas, and as the dangers increase, so to make the more effectual provisions against them. The Laws of Trade direct that, provided there be no special order to the contrary, two Flotas be set out, one for the Firm-land, the other for New Spain, and the Armada to convoy them; but this name of Armada was meant of the Admiral and vice-admiral only, which were fighting ships; and at first, there was one man–of–war to convoy the rest; her burthen 300 tun, and carrying eight

brass, and four iron guns, and till that time, the merchant ships carried 100 tun less than their burden, and 30 soldiers each, because they had no convoy of men-of-war. The times appointed for these Flotas to sail were, that of New Spain in May, and that of the Firm-land in August, both of them to go off with the first spring tides. The galleons were appointed to be out in January, that they might coast along the Firm-land, and come about mid April to Portobello, where the Fair would be over; they might take aboard the plate, and be at Havana with it, about mid June, where the New Spain Fleet would soon join them, and they might come together safer to Spain: To which effect the Viceroy of Peru was to take care the plate should be at Panama by the middle of March: the plate is 15 days carrying from Potosi to Arica; eight days generally from thence by sea to Callao, and 20 from Callao to Panama, taking in by the way the plate at Paita and Truzillo. To prevent the fleet being detained by contrary winds, as has happened, it was proposed to fit the galleons in the river of Seville in August and September, and then send away to Cadiz, where they might go out with any wind, and need not expect spring tides; and that to secure the ports, two Forts should be built upon the points of Puntal and Matagorda. The reasons why it was judged absolutely necessary that the Flota for the Firm-land should sail in September, were because that was a safe season to ship off the goods; they came to Portobello at a healthy season of the year; the merchandize were conveyed over to Panama at a cheaper rate, and with less danger of receiving damage; the merchants had leisure to sell their goods; the buyers had a fit season to travel to Peru with safety; and the Armadas and Flotas to return to Carthagena and Havana, to get clear of the Channel of Bahama, and to return to Spain in the best month for the sea. In fine it is agreed and found by experience that the month of September is the fittest for the fleets to sail, and tho' several accidents retard them till October or November, yet that season is fitter than March.

4, As to the number of ships whereof the Armada is composed, it is not fixed. In the year 1568 there were 20, which, as was mentioned before, were built galley fashion, and carried oars, being about 200 tun burden. Ever since that time there are some frigates that can make use of oars, whence the name of galleons is derived....afterwards the charge increasing, it was found necessary to lessen the number, so that in the Ordinances of the Haberia, or duty for convoys, it was established there should be twelve men-of-war, and five tenders fitted out every year, that is, for the Armada of Galleons, eight ships of 600 tun burden each, and three tenders, one of a 100 tun for the Island Magarita, and two of 80 each, to follow the Armada. For the New

Spain fleet, two ships of 600 tun each, and two tenders of 80 each, and for the Honduras fleet two ships of 500 tun each, and in case no Flota happened to sail any year, three galleons and a tender should be sent to New Spain for the plate.

---

## No. 171—THE PILOTS

*(J. Veitia de Linaje, Norte de la Contratacion de las Indias Occidentales, Seville, 1672. English Translation by John Stevens, The Spanish Rule of Trade to the Indies, London, 1702)\**

There are three several principal pilots belonging to the West-India voyage, viz. The Chief Pilot of the India House, instituted to examine and give their degrees to other pilots, and judges of the charts, and other instruments of navigation. The next is the Chief Pilot of the Armada, or Navy Royal to secure the Trade of the Indies, commonly called the Galleons. And the third the Chief Pilot of the New Spain Fleet....

2.  We are first to speak of the Chief Pilot of the India-house, because he takes place, and ought to be most know-ing, as being to choose the Pilots for the India ships, out of which are chosen those for the Galleons and Flotas, tho' as to seniority, there is no doubt but there were chief Pilots of Armadas before there was any of the India-house, because those discovering that New World made way for an India-house, and consequently for a chief Pilot of it, who ought to be universal in the theory, not only for the voyage to the Firm-land, New Spain, the coasts of those provinces, and the Windward Islands, but for the River of Plate, for which there was once a particular chief Pilot.

3.  The first Chief Pilot of the India house was Americus Vespucius, settled at Seville, to draw charts upon the discoveries of others, and the salary assigned him 50,000 maravedis; this was in the year 1507, and the reign of King Ferdinand. Not only the Chief, but all others whom the King received as his pilots, had salaries settled on them, and such as were as well skilled in warlike, as in sea affairs, were received as Sea Captains as was done with Ferdinand Magal-lanes, whom we call Magellan. who discovered the strait of his name and Ruy Fallero his companion, in 1518. Assign-ing each of them 40,000 maravedis salary, and in general, great encouragement was given to all that were skilled in this profession.

4.  The municipal laws of the Court of the India-House ordained that there be in the said House a Chief Pilot, to be preferred by Edict, which is thus. When the place is vacant, the King and his Council of the Indies are acquainted with it, and there are Edicts or Proclamations put up in

*op., cit., pp. 242—248.

Seville, the Universities of Salamanca, Valladolid, and Alcala, and also in those parts where sailing pilots are known to reside, as Cadiz, S. Lucar, Port S. Mary, and Ayamonte, for tho' it be rare to find among the practical pilots anyone so well skilled in the theory as to be fit to carry the place of Chief Pilot to the India-house yet they have sometimes been allowed as candidates, and the same may happen again. When the candidates have made their claims, the Court acquaints the King how the parties are qualified, both by their own acts, and the information the President and Commissioners have of them, declaring whom they judge most deserving, and what they think of the rest, that the Council may advise, and the King decree, as shall be most expedient. The Professor of Cosmography is made after the same manner, but as for the Cosmographer, who is to be instrument maker, his skills being of such sort as is not learnt at the Universities the Edicts are sent to Court and put up at the Council, and in Seville, at the India-house and Exchange, and the candidates are remitted by the Council, to make out their ability before the President and Commissioners of the India-house.

5. Tho' some of the practical pilots have been proposed as candidates, yet none of them has hitherto carried the employment; the Council wisely providing that he who fills this place be the most knowing that can be found, not only in the art of navigation, but in other parts of the mathematics, because his is not only to examine the pilots for the India Voyage, but to judge of the Professor of Cosmography, and the Cosmographer instrument maker, whom he is to examine and censure, as much as he does the mariners that have been his scholars, in order to take the degree of pilots. Vice-admirals have been proposed to fill this post. The design in instituting this Chief Pilot was only to examine and give their degree to the other pilots, forbidding him to teach navigation, or the use of any instruments, upon the penalty assigned, and he that learns of him to be incapable of being examined in two years, which was done to the end that affection for his own scholars might not cause him to wink at their ignorance. For the same reason he is forbid making any sea charts or instruments to sell, because it being his business to judge of them used in the voyage to the Indies, he could never see any faults in his own, for no master will speak ill of his own work. For these reasons the two employments of Chief Pilot and Cosmographer were never but once conferred upon the same person, and many inconveniences appearing in it then, they were ever since accounted incompatible.

6. When any are to be examined in order to be declared pilots, it is to be done in the India-house, and no

other place. The Cosmographers and Pilots that are then in Seville are to be present to the number of six at least, being men well skilled in sea affairs, the candidates are to be strictly examined, all the examiners taking an oath to do it fully, and give their votes according to the best of their judgment, and the person so approved is to be declared a Pilot, and not otherwise, upon forfeiture of 10,000 maravedis. . . .

8. There are two Cosmographers, as has been said before: the one is Professor of Cosmography, instituted by King Philip II, in the Year 1552, to teach the art of navigation and cosmography, with order that none should be admitted Pilot or Master who had not learnt under him a year or thereabouts. This time was afterwards shortened to three months, and at last to two, in order to fit them for examination; and as for reading and writing it was thought enough if they could read the sailing orders, and write their own names; what was ordered to be taught was as follows. The Treatise of the Sphere, or at least the first and second book of it. The Treatise that teaches how to take the sun's altitude, and the elevation of the pole, with all the rest taught in it. The use of the sea chart, and how to find out the point where the ship is. The use of instruments, and manner of making them, to discover whether they are faulty, that is, the compass, astrolabe, quadrant, and Jacob's staff, and how to observe the needles, to discover whether they vary East or West, which is a matter of great moment, to keep an exact account when they sail. The use of a general dial for day or night, and the pilots must know either by memory, or by writing, what the age of the moon is any day in the year, that they may know how the tides fall out to enter any rivers, or bars, and other matters in continual use. A lesson upon these subjects is to be read every day, at the hours appointed by the President and Commissioners of the India-House, that may be most convenient for the learners. There is a great room in the Exchange appointed for this use.

9. The other Cosmographer is Instrument-Maker, the use of which the Professor teaches, but the first of these is the ancientest employ. Both the Cosmographers are to sit with the chief pilot upon examining of pilots, and to put questions to them and the Law appoints that if the Cosmographer of the India-House informs the Commissioners that the examination is not duly made, the said Commissioners shall take care to see right done. It is also the duty of the chief Pilot and Cosmographers to approve of and mark the sea charts and other instruments; and they are to have marks for that purpose, which are to be kept in the India-House in a chest under two keys, whereof the chief

Pilot is to keep one, and the younger Cosmographer the other, that no instruments may be sold or approved without the consent of all three, to which purpose they meet every Monday, and no instrument to be sold without the mark, under the forfeiture of 30 ducats. Two practical Pilots were to be appointed by the Commissioners of the India-House, to examine instruments, together with the Chief Pilot and Cosmographers; but if the instrument were made by the Cosmographer himself, then he was to have no vote in the approbation. If an astrolabe be faulty, it is to be broken and cast again; and a chart that cannot be mended must be cut and left in the Treasury Chamber, that it may not be put together again. When the Pilot and Cosmographers meet, if there are any to be examined for Pilots, that is the first thing to be done; what time remained after marking instruments, was to be employed in examining the general map, and adding what they think necessary, but all these things are now out of use, there being no further discovery made, and the instruments and sea charts generally used, being those made by the Cosmographer of the India-house, of which he makes some profit, but nothing considerable, nor is he to take any fee for touching the needles to the loadstone.

---

### (iii)—THE GOVERNMENT OF THE COLONIES
#### No. 172 — THE ABSOLUTE MONARCHY

*(Ferdinand II, King of Spain, to Diego Columbus, Governor of the Indies, May 3, 1509)\**

First of all you will give very careful attention to the service of God our Lord; I have sent a petition to our very Holy Father regarding the Prelates who are to be provided for in said Hispaniola, and while this goes into effect, I would like the Churches of said Island to be as well served and provided for as possible. You will take with you Miguel de Pasamonte, our general Treasurer, to whom I am writing about this, and you shall get information from the Major Prefect of Alcantara, who until now has been our Governor in said Indies, about the Clergymen and Sacristans there are in each of the said churches of the said island, and how and in what way they have served and serve, and what has been given and is given to each one of them annually, and said Miguel de Pasamonte will pay them from the tithes what they should have according to what they have been paid until now.

Item: You shall try to make all those who reside in the said Island live as honestly and without offending Our Lord as they can, for which purpose you must see that the

\*Cited in Navarrete, *op. cit.*, Tomo II, Num. CLXIX, pp. 370—390.

laws and royal ordinances that I and the Queen Dona Isabella, my wife, of glorious memory, have commanded, especially those regarding swearing and gambling, are obeyed....

Item: Because I have been informed that most people who go from here fall ill upon arriving in the said island, and if there were not adequate facilities in the hospitals of Buenaventura and Concepcion, which are now finished, many persons would be in danger of death; you must take special care that said two hospitals are well provided with the necessary things; and as I sent alms of two hundred dollars of gold to each one of said hospitals, you should ascertain the way in which it is spent; and if it is not spent as it should be, you will give orders as to how it should be well spent; and likewise you should ascertain if it is necessary that some additional hospitals be built, and, in the event that they are needed, give orders as to how they should be built....

Moreover: My principal desire has always been and is in these affairs of the Indies that the Indians be converted to our Holy Catholic Faith so that their souls will not be lost, for which it is necessary that they be informed of the things of our Holy Catholic Faith; you will take care that, without treating them with any violence, both the religious persons as well as those to whom they have been given in our name in *encomienda* instruct them in and teach them the things of our Holy Catholic Faith with much love, so that those who have already been converted to our Holy Faith will persevere in it and will serve God as good Christians, and those who have not yet been converted may be as soon as possible; and you must give orders that in each town there be one Ecclesiastical person.... so that he will take care to see that they be well treated as we have commanded, and will likewise take special care to teach them the things of Faith; and you will have a house built for this person near the church, where you will command all the children of the town to meet, so that there this person may teach them the things of our Holy Faith, and you are to command that this person be given what you think appropriate, but more than the other Clergymen, in return for the work he has to do with respect to the aforesaid....

Item: You will say in my name to the Cacique and other principal Indians of said Island, that my will is that they and their Indians be well treated as our good subjects and nationals, and if hereafter anyone should do them harm or evil they are to advise you of it, because you carry our orders to punish such cases very severely.

Moreover: You will see that the Indians are well treated, and that no one does them violence, or steals anything from them or ill-treats them by word or otherwise, and that they and their wives walk safely the length and breadth of the land, assigning for the aforesaid the penalties you deem necessary, and inflicting them on those who incur them; and as for the women, take special care of them, because I have been informed that if much caution were not taken, there would be much dissoluteness, which would be a great disservice to me.

Item: Tell the said Caciques in my name that our will is that they shall treat their Indians well likewise.

Item: You must command that the Indians will not have the festivals and ceremonies which they used to have, if by chance they have them, but instead they are to follow the pattern of life of the other people in our Kingdoms, and you must endeavour to achieve this gradually and with much tact, without scandalizing or illtreating them.

Likewise: Because we had commanded said Major Prefect to take great care that the Indians of said Hispaniola live together in towns as our natives live in these Kingdoms, and that each one should have in a separate house his women, children, and property; ascertain what has been done about this, and if there is something still to be done, try to get it done as soon as possible, ordering the towns to be built where you think it best for the good of its inhabitants.

Item: Inasmuch as the Indians roam like vagabonds and do not want to work for a just wage, a Decree was given by the Queen Dona Isabella, my wife, of glorious memory, with common consent from the Council....so that paying each the usual daily wage as was their just due, they may be compelled to work; and you must see that it is obeyed according to the said provision....with the greatest contentment on the part of the Indians and their Caciques.

Item: Because we have commanded that the Indians to whom we thus gave said property should not sell it or exchange it at a low price as they used to, you will command the people in the said towns that they do not allow them to sell or exchange said property, and if necessity obliges the Indians to sell it, that they will try to sell it at a just price; likewise the aforesaid person will endeavour to make the Indians dress and walk like rational men.

Item: So that among the Christians and the Indians there may be peace, friendship and union, and no disputes or scandals, you will forbid all of them to give or sell, exchange or pawn or lend, offensive or defensive weapons to the Indians, assigning for it the penalties which you deem appropriate; and if you should find some in possession of the Indians, you are to take them away, and have them surrendered to our Treasurer so that he may do with them what he has been told.

Item: I have sent Miguel de Pasamonte....that he,

together with said Major Prefect of Alcantara, will be responsible for mining the gold from the rich mines for Us, and it is fitting to our service that this be done with diligence and caution. For this reason when you arrive in said Hispaniola ascertain what has been provided for said mines, and together with said Pasamonte provide for everything which may be needed; so that all the gold possible will be taken out, for Us from said mines, and let us know constantly the supply there is of it.

Item: Since as in the collection and melting of gold much fraud and deceit can be committed, you will order the miners to go in brigades, as they go now in groups of ten, or whatever number you may think best, and to each brigade you will assign a trustworthy person who is to be present when the gold is collected, and who will accompany it as it is taken to the smeltery. . . .

Item: Once you have arrived at said Hispaniola you will ascertain the number of Indians there are in it, and the persons who have them; and as I sent Gil Gonzalez Davila to bring some information of said Indians, if he has not gathered it, you should help him acquire it; so that you will bring us a true report, and in the distribution of Indians made by the Major Prefect you shall not interfere, until you have seen from the account I ordered sent to you what you have to do about it. . . .

Moreover: You will see to it that all who live in the said island work each one in his occupation, so that nobody will be lazy, because from laziness always follow many difficulties like gambling as well as swearing and offending God Our Lord in many other ways; in this connection, you are to see to it that all the royal ordinances concerning gambling and swearing are obeyed. . . .

Moreover: It is my will that the Christians who reside now and hereafter in said Indies do not live scattered; you will forbid anyone to live outside of the towns there are in said island, or those which will be founded hereafter. . . .

Item: Since we have a suspicion that in the Island of Cuba there is gold, you should try, as soon as possible, to know the truth, and if you find out anything in relation to it you are to let us know. . . .

Likewise said Major Prefect of Alcantara. . . .has reported to me that some of the men married to native women believe that their wives and children own and inherit the lands which belonged to their fathers and mothers, and notwithstanding occasional reprimands, the thoughts they have about it have not changed. To remedy this he said that he takes away from these married men the Indians which they were given with the Caciques who are relatives of their wives, and in their place they are given some others. Those he found living on the lands of their fathers-in-law or relatives were taken somewhere else where they might forget their purpose. And as I wish that all cause he removed so that said persons should not have the thought they have about this, therefore, in order to get them out of worse danger, you are to be very careful and diligent in continuing the aforesaid. . . . and you are to urge the religious men who confess said persons to take away their thoughts and desires from this, telling them how wrong they are in wishing the aforesaid.

Item: Because some of the persons who are there, or of those who would go to live there hereafter, are said to go with no other intention and purpose than to reside there for two or three years, or, at best, until they have acquired a considerable sum of gold, and in their cupidity to come with it to these Kingdoms, and anxious to come soon, they seek gold in every way and do much fraud and sell things under cost price until they have it; for that reason you are to be very careful not to allow any such person to come here, unless he has a special licence from me or has just cause, such as illness, or has resided at least — years.

Likewise, because I have been informed that, due to the fact that Indians have been given to the Priests who have charge of the administration of some churches, they do not administer in them the Sacraments or celebrate the Divine Worship as it should be celebrated, by reason of their supervision of and relations with said Indians, which is a disservice to God, our Lord, you are therefore not to give or allow any Indians to be given to those Priests, so that they may be more disposed and have more time to administer the Sacraments, as they are obliged to by virtue of the salary they receive as Priests. . . .

---

### No. 173 — SPANISH COLONIALISM

*(Gil de Lemos, Viceroy of New Spain, to a Deputation from the Collegians of Lima, n.d.)* [*]

Learn to read, write, and say your prayers, for this is as much as any American ought to know.

---

### No. 174 — TOWN PLANNING BY THE METROPOLITAN GOVERNMENT

*(Ordinance of the King of Spain, July 3, 1573)* [**]

110. . . . After having made the discovery and selected the province, district and land to be peopled and the sites where new settlements are to be founded, those who intend to settle are to proceed in the following manner:

---

*Cited in H. **Merivale**, *Lectures on Colonization and Colonies, delivered before the University of Oxford in 1839, 1840, and 1841*, Oxford, 1928 edition, p. 14.
** Cited in *Contribuciones a la Historia Municipal de America* pp. 18—34.

On arriving at the locality where the new settlement is to be founded (which according to our will and ordinance must be one which is vacant and can be occupied without doing harm to the Indians and natives or with their free consent), the plan of the place, with its squares, streets and building lots, is to be outlined by means of measuring by cord and ruler, beginning with the main square from which streets are to run to the gates and principal roads and leaving sufficient open space so that even if the town grows it can always spread in a symmetrical manner. Having thus laid out the chosen site the settlement is to be founded in the following form :

111.   The chosen site shall be on an elevation; healthful; with means of fortification; fertile and with plenty of land for farming and pasturage; fuel and timber; fresh water, a native population, commodiousness; resources and of convenient access and egress. It shall be open to the north wind. If on the coast, care is to be taken that the sea does not lie to the south or west of the harbour. If possible, the port is not to be near lagoons or marshes in which poisonous animals and corruption of air and water breed.

112.   In the case of a sea-coast town, the main plaza, which is to be the starting point for the building of the town, is to be situated near the landing place of the port. In inland towns the main plaza should be in the centre of the town and of an oblong shape, its length being equal to at least one and a half times its width, as this porportion is the best for festivals in which horses are used and any other celebrations which have to be held.

113.   The size of the plaza shall be in proportion to the number of residents, heed being given to the fact that towns of Indians, being new, are bound to grow, and it is intended that they shall do so.   Therefore, the plaza is to be planned with reference to the possible growth of the town.   It shall not be smaller than two hundred feet wide and three hundred feet long nor larger than eight hundred feet long and three hundred feet wide.   A well proportioned medium size plaza is one six hundred feet long and four hundred feet wide.

114.   From the plaza the four principal streets are to diverge, one from the middle of each of its sides, and two streets are to meet at each of its corners.   The four corners of the plaza are to face the four points of the compass, because thus the streets diverging from the plaza will not be exposed to the four principal winds, which would cause much inconvenience.

115.   The whole plaza and the four main streets diverging from it shall have arcades, for these are a great convenience for those who resort thither for trade. The eight streets which run into the plaza at its four corners are to

do so freely without being obstructed by the arcades of the plaza. These arcades are to end at the corners in such a way that the sidewalks of the streets can evenly join those of the plaza.

116. In cold climates the streets shall be wide; in hot climates narrow; however, for purposes of defence, and where horses are kept, the streets had better be wide.

117. The other streets laid out consecutively around the plaza are to be so planned that, even if the town should increase considerably in size, it would meet with no obstruction which might disfigure what had already been built or be a detriment to the defence or convenience of the town.

118. At certain distances in the smaller town, well proportioned plazas are to be laid out on which the main church, the parish church or monastery shall be built so that the teaching of religious doctrine may be evenly distributed.

119. If the town lies on the coast, its main church shall be so situated that it may be visible from the landing place, and so built that its structure may serve as means of defence for the port itself.

120. After the plaza and streets have been laid out, building lots are to be designated, in the first place, for the erection of the main church, the parish church or monastery, and these are to occupy respectively an entire block, so that no other structure can be built next to them excepting such as contribute to their commodiousness or beauty.

121. Immediately afterwards, the place and site are to be assigned for the Royal and Town Council House, the Custom House and Arsenal, which is to be close to the church and port, so that in case of necessity one can protect the other. The hospital for the poor and sick of noncontagious diseases shall be built next to the church, forming its cloister.

122. The lots and sites for slaughter houses, fisheries, tanneries, and such like productive of garbage shall be so situated that the latter can be easily disposed of.

123. It would be of great advantage if inland towns, at a distance from ports, were built on the banks of a navigable river, in which case an endeavour should be made to build on the northern river bank, all occupations producing garbage being relegated to the river bank or sea situated below the town.

124. In inland towns the church is not to be on the plaza but at a distance from it, in a situation where it can stand by itself, separate from other buildings, so that it can be seen from all sides. It can thus be made more beautiful and it will inspire more respect. It should be built on high ground, so that in order to reach its entrance people will have to ascend a flight of steps. Nearby and between

it and the main plaza, the Royal Council and Town House and the Custom House are to be erected in order to increase its impressiveness but without obstructing it in any way. The hospital of the poor who are ill with non-contagious diseases shall be built facing the north, and so planned that it will enjoy a southern exposure.

125. The same plan shall be carried out in any inland settlements where there are no rivers, much care being taken that they enjoy other conveniences requisite and necessary.

126. No building lots surrounding the main plaza are to be given to private individuals, for these are to be reserved for the church, Royal and Town House, also shops and dwellings for the merchants, which are to be first erected. For the erection of the public buildings the settlers shall contribute, and for this purpose a moderate tax shall be imposed on all merchandise.

127. The remaining building lots shall be distributed by lottery to those of the settlers who are entitled to build around the main plaza. Those left over are to be held for us to grant to settlers who may come later or to dispose of at our pleasure. In order that entries of these assignments be better made, a plan of the town is always to be made in advance.

128. After the plan of the town and the distribution of the lots have been made, each settler is to set up his tent on his lot if he has one, for which purpose the captains shall persuade them to carry tents with them. Those who own none are to build huts of such materials as are available, wherever they can be collected. All settlers, with greatest possible haste, are to erect jointly some kind of palisado or dig a ditch around the main plaza so that the Indians cannot do them harm.

129. A common shall be assigned to each town, of adequate size, so that even though it should grow greatly, there would always be sufficient space for its inhabitants to find recreation and for cattle to pasture without encroaching upon private property.

130. Adjoining the common there shall be assigned pastures for team oxen, for horses, for cattle destined for slaughter and for the regular number of cattle which, according to law, the settlers are obliged to have, so that they can be employed for public purposes by the Council. The remainder of land is to be subdivided into as many plots for cultivation as there are town lots, and the settlers are to draw lots for these. Should there be any land which can be irrigated, it is distributed to the first settlers in the same proportion and drawn for by lottery. What remains over is to be reserved for us so that we can make grants to those who may settle later.

131.  As soon as the plots for cultivation have been
distributed, the settlers shall immediately plant all the seeds
that they have brought or are obtainable, for which reason
it is advisable that all go well provided. All cattle
transported thither by settlers, or collected, are to be taken
to the pasture lands so that they can begin at once to breed
and multiply.

132.  Having sown their seeds and provided accommodation for their cattle in such quantities and with such
diligence that they can reasonably hope for an abundance
of food, the settlers, with great care and activity, are to
erect their houses, with solid foundations and walls, for
which purpose they shall go provided with moulds or planks
for making adobes and all other tools for building quickly
and at little cost.

133.  The building lots and the structures erected
thereon are to be so situated that in the living rooms one
can enjoy air from the south and from the north, which are
the best. All town houses are to be so planned that they can
serve as a defence or fortress against those who might
attempt to create disturbances or occupy the town. Each
house is to be so constructed that horses and household
animals can be kept therein, the courtyards and stockyards
being as large as possible to insure health and cleanliness.

134.  Settlers are to endeavour, as far as possible, to
make all structures uniform, for the sake of the beauty of
the town. . . .

---

## No. 175—THE COLONIAL MUNICIPALITY

*(Ordenanzas para el cabildo y regimiento de la villa de la
Habana y las demas villas y lugares de ésta isla que hizo
y ordeno el ilustre Sr. Dr. Alonso de Caceres, oidor de la
dicha Audiencia real de la cuidad Santo Domingo, visitador
y juez de residencia de esta Isla, January 14, 1574)\**

1.  We order and command both the judges and the
administrators of this island to meet every Friday at 8.00
o'clock, to discuss and make provision for the good government of this city and for the public welfare. These meetings should be held in the houses of the Municipal Council
which have been established for that purpose and in no
other place. For these Friday meetings it will not be necessary to inform the aldermen, governor or mayors, because

*Cited in Instituto Panamerica de Geografia y Historia, *Contribuciones a la
Historia Municipal de America*, Mexico, D.F., 1951, pp. 89—93, 97.

the time and day of the week have been set in advance; thus they should be there at the appointed time. If Friday is a holiday. the meeting should be held on Thursday.

2. The governor or anyone of the mayors of this town without the others. and not less than three aldermen (resident in this town) constitute a quorum.

3. When important matters are to be discussed, the governor and all the aldermen and mayors should be present, even if they are away on their plantations as these are not very far away. This applies to the election of mayors and other office holders. They must be compelled to come under penalties imposed by the judges.

4. In the election of mayors and other office holders, the governor must allow the aldermen to vote freely, and neither he nor his deputy should vote because they are present in a judicial capacity and must be judges of whatever may be done.

5. If there is any need to convene an extraordinary meeting on other days besides Friday, the governor or any of the mayors....may convene the meeting at any time provided that the governor, the mayors and aldermen are given due notice by the messenger who is to certify it to the Council's notary.

6. That ordinary meetings be held every Friday, even though there may be nothing to do, and that they should last at least one hour, discussing and conferring as to what can be done for the welfare and development of this town.

7. That the aldermen sit and vote according to age, the oldest voting first and the youngest last; that when one of them is voting, and expressing his views, none is to interrupt or contradict him; when his turn comes he can express his own views. The judges are to take great care in this respect and see to it that there is neither clamour nor obstinacy but that the discussions and deliberations are conducted temperately and modestly.

8. That in the election of mayors and other office holders and in all other matters dealt with at the meetings, the decision of the majority will prevail and that the governor or mayors see to its execution without delay, because appeal to the Supreme Court is very difficult....if there is any controversy between the governor and mayors over the orders to be executed and enforced, the vote of two out of the three of them will prevail.

9. That every time a meeting is held, the book containing these ordinances should be available so that they may read the Law on the subject under discussion....

10. That in this town the number of aldermen is not to exceed six, because this number is in proportion to its population.

11. That nobody may enter the meeting or city hall

armed, under the penalty that if anyone enters wearing a sword, it is to be confiscated for the Council's chest; and if he carries a dagger, since it can be hidden and is a more dangerous weapon, he shall be suspended from the Council for two months.

12. That the ordinary mayors shall be elected annually by the Council on January 1, as aldermen are now elected. The one who receives the majority of votes is to be mayor; in case of a tie, another vote will be taken to see if there is agreement as to who is to be elected; but if there is a tie for a second time, they shall draw lots between them and the one to come out first shall be elected.

13. That a mayor cannot be re-elected for a second term until three years have elapsed after his term has ended.

14. That the mayors are to visit in due course the entire municipal area, and if on their visits to the plantations, ranches and pig farms they find any confusion, they are to inform the Council, punish those who are guilty and remedy matters.

15. Because some mayors go off to their plantations and do not live in this town, we order them to live in town and to give audiences every afternoon at a fixed time and place so that their working hours may be known....They may not leave town without the permission of the Council, so that the business they have to attend to may not be neglected, to the detriment of the parties concerned.

16. Because the aldermen frequently are absent from meetings and these meetings are deferred for many days, any alderman who, residing in town and not being sick, is absent from the Friday meetings is to pay four reales for the day he is absent, and if he absents himself contumaciously for a longer period, the judge will increase the punishment.

17. That there should be, in this town no more than one Chief Constable and his deputy, and another deputy to handle rural matters; the latter is to have no authority in the town unless he comes from the country with a prisoner....

————

### (iv) THE COLONIALS AND THE METROPOLITAN MONOPOLY

*No. 176 — THE COLONIAL OPPOSITION TO MONOPOLY*

*(The Colonists of Cubagua to Count Luis Lampunano\*, 1527)\*\**

The Emperor, too liberal of what was not his own, had

*Given a monopoly of pearl fishing.

\*\*Cited in Southey, *op. cit.*, Vol. I, p. 159.

not the right to dispose of the oysters which live at the bottom of the sea.

---

## No. 177—THE SHORTAGE OF ESSENTIAL COMMODITIES

*(Dean and Council of Hispaniola to Charles V, Emperor of the Hapsburg Empire, May 27, 1555)* *

We are dying of hunger through lack of Negroes and labourers to till the soil. As a result of the fact that ships come only in fleets, provisions arrive from Spain at intervals of years, and we are without bread, wine, soap, oil, cloth, linens. When they arrive, the prices are exorbitant, and if we attempt to have them valued, the merchandise is hidden.

---

## No. 178—HIGH PRICES OF IMPORTS

*(Dr. Fray Diego Sarmiento, Bishop of Cuba, April, 20, 1566)* **

So many calamities and so much misery have befallen this island in recent times that it seems to be gradually approaching ruin. The sacrifice of the Mass has not been offered many a time for lack of wine. Today, when extreme poverty exists here, the fleet arrives and a yard of canvas costs a castellan, a sheet of paper a real; everything from Spain, even what the soil produces, is very expensive. Everyone is anxious to leave the country, and if the few Spaniards who are still here are not leaving, it is because no customer can be found to buy their property, even though they would be willing to sell for three what is worth ten.

---

## No. 179—THE SCARCITY OF SHIPS

*(Pedro de Beltranilla to President of the Council of the Indies, Trinidad, January 8, 1613)* ***

The Licenciado Pedro de Beltranilla, a vecino of the Town of San Joseph de Oruna in the Island of Trinidad, as Procurator General of the said Town, reports that some 18 years ago, at the order of Your Highness, he went to the

*Cited in Saco, *Historia de la Esclavitud de la Raza Africana*, Tomo II, p. 39.
** Cited in Saco, *Historia de la Esclavitud de la Raza Africana*, Tomo II, pp. 40—41.
***Cited in The Trinidad Historical Society, Publication No. 150.

conquest and settlement of this Island and to reduce the Indians to our Holy Catholic Faith.

During all this time he has never seen at this Island a single Spanish ship with which to trade. On the contrary there have been many enemy ships, the trade with which has led to many troubles and much difficulty as is well known to Your Highness.

The only remedy for this is to make the Spaniards afraid to trade with the enemy and of dealing with them in the produce of these lands. Any who would thus trade should not be allowed into this Island which has cost our people so much blood and which is so much wanted by the enemies of our faith in view of the great advantages which would result and of the raids which they could effect along the Main as also from reducing the Indians to their wicked beliefs.

I humbly beg Your Highness to arrange that a royal order be sent to the President and Officers of the Casa de la Contratacion* to send to this Island each year two ships of small size, about two hundred tons, to bring to this Island food and other necessary things, and to take back in return the produce of the Island.

Further that these vessels may be sent without carrying a certificated master pilot. Also that of the two vessels, one may be convoyed by the fleet to New Spain and the other by the fleet to Tierra Firme, just as is done with vessels going to the Islands of Santo Domingo, Puerto Rico, Margarita and Venezuela and others to the windward.

This would be of great advantage to the Island of Trinidad and its people.

———

## No. 180—THE SPANISH FLEETS FOR THE NEW WORLD

*(Thomas Gage, A New Survey of the West Indies, 1648)***

To Puerto Rico went that year (1625) two ships; to Santo Domingo three; to Jamaica two; to Margarita one; to the Havana two; to Cartagena three; to Campeche two; to Honduras and Truxillo two; and to St. John Dilua, or Vera Cruz, sixteen; all laden with wines, figs, raisins, olives, oil, cloth, carsies, linen, iron, and quicksilver for the mines.

*House of Trade at Seville.
**Op. cit., 1946 edition, London, p. 14.

## No. 181—COMMERCIAL CONCESSIONS TO TRINIDAD

*(Council of the Indies to Philip IV, King of Spain,
November, 22, 1630)\**

By the Cedula of the 21st November of the year 1625,
Your Majesty was pleased to extend for six years to the
vecinos of the Island of Trinidad and of Guayana, the time
during which the tobacco taken to the City of Seville should
be exempt from the dues of Almoxarifago and Alcabala
belonging to Your Majesty and also from the dues of Diezmo
and Chancelleria.

Now on behalf of the vecinos of this said Island of
Trinidad and of Guayana, it has been represented that this
time expires shortly and that these vecinos are in greater
distress now than when this exemption was extended, that
the enemy have settled these coasts and sacked the town
of Guayana in the month of December in the year 1629,
and that this land is new and has no other produce by
which the vecinos can maintain themselves and extend and
increase the settlement.

The vecinos now therefore beseech Your Majesty to
be pleased to extend this privilege for eight years more.
After carefully considering the circumstances and reasons
for this application, it appears to the Council that it would
be advisable to extend these privileges for three years more.

May Your Majesty direct as may be your pleasure.

## No. 182 — THE BANKRUPTCY OF THE SPANISH COLONIAL SYSTEM

*(Council of the Indies to Philip IV, King of Spain,
October 24, 1653)\*\**

On behalf of the Island of Trinidad and Town of St.
Thome de la Guayana, it has been represented that it is
20 years since an authorised ship went to these parts and
consequently they are suffering great want of clothing and
other things and their crops are worthless as they have no
market for them, and that in one of the covenants made
with the Govenor, Don Martin de Mendoca, permission was
given to the vecinos of that Island and Town to send their
produce to these Kingdoms for ten years free of duties and
that they have neither had ships nor means to make use
of this favour.

\*Cited in The Trinidad Historical Society, Publication No. 243.
\*\*Cited in The Trinidad Historical Society, Publication No. 47.

They beg Your Majesty to grant them in perpetuity or for ten years two authorised ships, one for Trinidad and the other for Guayana

This has been considered in the Council together with the report from the Casa de Contratacion thereon of the 16th September last; it appears advisable if it please Your Majesty, that one authorised ship may be granted them for four years allowing one voyage each year to Trinidad and Guayana, and that produce of that country which may be registered for Spain be free of duty so that thereby they may be encouraged to cultivate their land and to trade and may have clothing to wear, wherefrom profit will accrue to the Royal Treasury and advantage to those subjects; upon condition that the products they bring to Spain are to pay the customary entrance dues of the Custom Houses thereof.

Your Majesty will order what may be your good pleasure.

# CHAPTER VII

# The International Struggle for the Caribbean

## (i) THE DIPLOMATIC AND INTELLECTUAL ATTACK ON THE SPANISH MONOPOLY

### No. 183—THE PAPAL DONATION OF THE NEW WORLD TO SPAIN

*(Bull of Pope Alexander VI, Inter Caetera, May 4, 1493)* *

We of our own motion, and not, at your solicitation, do give, concede, and assign forever to you and your successors, all the islands, and mainlands, discovered; and which may hereafter be discovered towards the west and south; whether they be situated towards India, or towards any other part, whatsoever, and give you absolute power in them; drawing, however, and affixing a line from the Arctic pole, viz., from the North, to the Antarctic pole, viz., to the south; which line must, be distant from anyone of the islands whatsoever, vulgarly called the Azores and Cape de Verde Islands, a hundred leagues towards the west and south; upon condition that no other Christian king, or prince, has actual possession of any of the islands and mainlands found....Let no person, therefore, presume to infringe, or, with rash boldness, to contravene this page of our commendation, exhortation, requisition, donation, concession, assignation, constitution, deputation, decree, mandate, inhibition and will. For if any person does, he will incur the indignation of Almighty God, and the blessed apostles Peter and Paul.

---

### No. 184 — THE PORTUGUESE REFUSE TO ACCEPT THE DONATION

*(Ferdinand and Isabella, King and Queen of Spain, to Christopher Colombus, August 16, 1494)* **

....With respect to the disputes with Portugal, a convention has been entered into here with their ambassadors, which appeared to us less subject to inconveniences; and in

*Cited in Southey, *op. cit.*, Vol. I, p. 22.
**Cited in Southey, *op. cit.*, Vol. I, p. 38. The original document is cited in Navarrete, *op. cit.*, Tomo II, Num. LXXIX, pp. 185—186.

order that you may be fully and distinctly informed of it, we send you a copy of the articles agreed upon: so that it is not necessary for us to dilate here upon the said subject, except to order and charge you to observe them fully, and cause them to be observed by every one, according to the tenor of the said convention.

With respect to the boundary which is to be determined, it appearing to us a very difficult thing, and an affair which requires much knowledge and confidence, we would wish, if it were possible, that you were present there, to assist in its determination, along with the commissioners on the part of the king of Portugal. And if your going upon this affair should be attended with difficulty, or your absence be productive of inconvenience, see whether your brother, or any other of the persons about you, be fit for the trust; give them the fullest information in writing, and verbally, and by picture, and every other means proper to instruct them; and send them immediately to us, by the first caravel that sails, in order that we may send other persons from hence with them, within the period of time agreed upon. And whether you are to go yourself upon this affair or not, write to us fully respecting all you know of it, and which may appear to you proper to be done, for our information, and that our interests may be in all points attended to; and take care that your letters, and the persons whom you have to send, may arrive soon, that they may proceed to the place where the line is to be determined, before the time agreed upon with the king of Portugal be elapsed, as you will see by the capitulation.

---

## No. 185—THE PARTITION OF THE WORLD BETWEEN SPAIN AND PORTUGAL

### (Treaty of Tordesillas, June 7, 1494)*

Whereas a certain controversy exists between the said lords, their constituents, as to what lands, of all those discovered in the ocean sea up to the present day, the date of this treaty, pertain to each one of the said parts respectively; therefore, for the sake of peace and concord, and for the preservation of the relationship and love of the said King of Portugal for the said King and Queen of Castile, Aragon, etc., it being the pleasure of their Highnesses, they, their said representatives, acting in their name and by virtue of their powers herein described, covenanted and agreed that a boundary or straight line be determined and

*Cited in F. Davenport, European Treaties bearing on the History of the United States and its Dependencies 1648, Carnegie Institution of Washington D.C., Publication No. 254, 1917—1937, Vol. I, p. 84.

drawn north and south, from pole to pole, on the said ocean sea, from the Arctic to the Antarctic pole. This boundary or line shall be drawn straight, as aforesaid, at a distance of three hundred and seventy leagues west of the Cape Verde Islands, being calculated by degrees, or by any other manner as may be considered the best and readiest, provided the distance shall be no greater than aforesaid. And all lands, both islands and mainlands found and discovered already, or to be found and discovered hereafter, by the said King of Portugal and by his vessels on this side of the line and bound determined as above, toward the east, in either north or south latitude, on the eastern side of the said bound, provided the said bound is not crossed, shall belong to, and remain in the possession of, and pertain forever to the said King of Portugal and his successors. And all other lands, both islands and mainlands, found or to be found hereafter, discovered or to be discovered hereafter, which have been discovered or shall be discovered by the said King and Queen of Castile, Aragon, etc., and by their vessels on the western side of the said bound, determined as above, after having passed the said bound toward the west, in either its north or south latitude, shall belong to, and remain in the possession of, and pertain forever to, the said King and Queen of Castile, Leon, etc., and to their successors.

---

## No. 186—SPAIN'S WARNING TO ENGLAND

*(Ferdinand and Isabella, King and Queen of Spain, to Dr. de Puebla, Spanish Ambassador in England March 28, 1496)* *

You write that a person like Columbus has come to England for the purpose of persuading the King to enter into an undertaking similar to that of the Indies, without prejudice to Spain and Portugal. He is quite at liberty. But we believe that this undertaking was thrown in the way of the King of England by the King of France, with the premeditated intention of distracting him from his other business. Take care that the King of England be not deceived in this or in any other matter. The French will try as hard as they can to lead him into such undertakings, but they are very uncertain enterprises, and must not be gone into at present. Besides they cannot be executed without prejudice to us and to the King of Portugal. ,

*Cited in *Calendar of State Papers, Spanish Series*, Vol. I, 1485-1509, London, 1862, pp. 88-89.

## No. 187—ENGLAND REFUSES TO HEED THE WARNING

### (Letters Patent of Henry VII, King of England, to Sebastian Cabot, 1497)*

Be it known that we have given and granted, and by these presents do give and grant for us and our heirs, to our well beloved John Cabot citizen of Venice, to Lewis, Sebastian, and Santius, sons of the said John, and to the heirs of them and every of them, and their deputies, full and free authority, leave, and power to sail to all parts, countries, and seas of the East, of the West, and of the North, under our banners and ensigns, with five ships of what burthen or quantity soever they be, and as many mariners or men as they will have with them in the said ships, upon their own proper costs and charges, to seek out, discover, and find whatsoever isles, countries, regions or provinces of the heathen and infidels whatsoever they be, and in what part of the world soever they be, which before this time have been unknown to all Christians....

---

## No. 188—THE IMPENDING ANGLO-SPANISH CONFLICT

### (Don Pedro de Ayala, Spanish Ambassador in England, to Ferdinand and Isabella, King and Queen of Spain, July 25, 1498)**

I think Your Majesties have already heard that the King of England has equipped a fleet in order to discover certain islands and continents which he was informed some people from Bristol, who manned a few ships for the same purpose last year, had found. I have seen the map which the discoverer has made, who is another Genoese like Columbus, and who has been in Seville and in Lisbon, asking assistance for his discoveries. The people of Bristol have, for the last seven years, sent out every year two, three, or four light ships, in search of the island of Brazil and the seven cities, according to the fancy of this Genoese....I have seen, on a chart, the direction which they took, and the distance they sailed; and I think that what they have found, or what they are in search of, is what Your Highnesses already possess....I write this because the King of England has often spoken to me on this subject, and he thinks that Your Highnesses will take great interest in it....I told him that, in my opinion, the land was already in the possession of Your Majesties; but though I gave him my reasons, he did

*Cited in Richard Hakluyt, *The Principal Navigations, Voyages, Traffiques and Discoveries of the English* Nation, London, 1599; 1927 edition, London, Vol. V., p. 83.

**Cited in *Calendar of State Papers, Spanish Series,* Vol. I, pp. 168–179.

not like them. I believe that your Highnesses are already informed of this matter; and I do not now send the chart, or mapa mundi which that man has made, and which, according to my opinion, is false, since it makes it appear as if the land in question was not the said islands.

---

## No. 189—THE IMPENDING FRANCO-SPANISH CONFLICT

*(Statement of Francis I, King of France, 1526)* *

The sun shines on me as well as on others. I should be very happy to see the clause in Adam's will which excluded me from my share when the world was being divided.

---

## No. 190—"GOD HAD NOT CREATED THOSE LANDS FOR SPANIARDS ONLY"

*(Antonio de Herrera, Historia General de los Hechos de los Castellanos en las Islas y Tierra Firme del Mar Oceano, Madrid, 1601-1615)* * *

Influenced by the persuasions of some of his vassals and by jealousy of the Emperor Charles V. . . . and to further his interests, by chance excited by the signs of the wealth of the Indies which the freebooters brought to his court, Francis I, King of France, decided to send a captain, Juan Verrazano, a Florentine, to make discoveries, saying "That God had not created those lands for Spaniards only".

---

## No. 191—ENGLAND'S OPPOSITION TO THE PAPAL DONATION

*(Sir William Cecil to the Spanish Ambassador in England, 1562)* * * *

The Pope had no right to partition the world and to give and take kingdoms to whomsoever he pleased.

---

*The statement is a well known one and is frequently cited. The present phraseology is taken from Hanke, *The Spanish Struggle for Justice*, p. 148.
**Op. cit., Decada Tercera, Libro Sexto, Cap. IX, Tomo IV, p. 316.
***Cited in J. A. Williamson, *The Age of Drake*, London, 1946, p. 33.

## No. 192 — ENGLAND'S INSISTENCE ON THE FREEDOM OF THE SEAS

*(William Camden, Annales Rerum Anglicarum et Hibernicarum regnante Elizabetha, London, 1615, Edition)* *

Bernardinus Mendoza, Ambassador for Spain in England, made an angry and vehement demand for satisfaction from the Queen, complaining that the Indian Ocean was navigated by the English. The reply that he received was as follows:— That the Spaniards by their unfairness towards the English, whom they had prohibited from commerce, contrary to the right of nations, had brought these troubles upon themselves; that Drake would be ready to answer in due form of law if he were convicted by sufficient evidence and proof of having done anything contrary to law; that the wealth referred to had been put aside with the design of satisfying the Spaniards, although the Queen had freely expended a greater amount of money than Drake had brought against the rebels whom the Spaniards had stirred up in Ireland and England. Besides, Her Majesty does not understand why her subjects and those of other Princes are prohibited from the Indies, which she could not persuade herself are the rightful property of Spain by donation of the Pope of Rome, in whom she acknowledged no prerogative in matters of this kind, much less authority to bind Princes who owe him no obedience, or to make that new world as it were a fief for the Spaniard and clothe him with possession: and that only on the ground that Spaniards have touched here and there, have erected shelters, have given names to a river or promontory; acts which cannot confer property. So that this donation of alien property (which by essence of law is void) and this imaginary proprietorship, ought not to hinder other princes from carrying on commerce in these regions, and from establishing Colonies where Spaniards are not residing, without the least violation of the law of nations, since prescription without possession is of no avail; nor yet from freely navigating that vast ocean, since the use of the sea and the air is common to all men; further that no right to the ocean can inure to any people or individual since neither nature or any principle of public user admits occupancy of the ocean.

*Cited in *British Guiana Boundary, Arbitration with the United States of Venezuela, Appendix to the Counter Case on behalf of the Government of Her Britannic Majesty,* London, 1898, p. 317.

## No. 193—QUEEN ELIZABETH'S "WESTERN DESIGN"

*(Letters Patent of Elizabeth, Queen of England, to Sir Humphrey Gilbert, 1584)* *

Know ye that of our especial grace, certain science and mere motion, we have given and granted, and by these presents for us, our heirs and successors, do give and grant to our trusty and well-beloved servant Sir Humphrey Gilbert of Compton, in our County of Devonshire knight, and to his heirs and assigns forever, free liberty and licence from time to time and at all times for ever here-after, to discover, find, search out, and view such remote, heathen and barbarous lands, countries and territories not actually possessed of any Christian prince or people, as to him, his heirs & assigns, and to every or any of them, shall seem good....

---

## No. 194—THE ASS IN THE LION'S SKIN

*(Richard Hakluyt, A particular discourse concerning the great necessity and manifold commodities that are like to grow to this Realm of England by the Western discoveries lately attempted, 1584)* * *

....The planting of two or three strong forts upon some good havens....between Florida and Cape Breton would be a matter in short space of greater damage as well to his fleet as to his western Indies; for we should not only often times endanger his fleet in the return thereof, but also in few years put him in hazards in losing some part of Nova Hispania....

....And entering into the consideration of the way how this Philip may be abased, I mean first to begin with the West Indies, as there to lay a chief foundation for his over-throw....

....If these enter into the due consideration of wise men, and if platforms of these things be set down and executed duly and with speed and effect, no doubt but the Spanish Empire falls to the ground, and the Spanish king shall be left bare as Aesop's proud crow, the peacock, the parrot, the pye, and the popingay and every other bird having taken home from him his gorgeous feathers, he will in short space become a laughing stock for all the world, with such a maim to the Pope and to that side, as never happened to the See of Rome....If you touch him in the Indies, you touch the apple of his eye; for take away his treasure which

* Cited in Hakluyt, *op. cit.*, Vol. V, pp. 349—350.
* *Cited in *The Original Writings and Correspondence of the Two Richard Hakluyts* Vol. II, Works issued by the Hakluyt Society, Second Series, No. LXXVII, London, 1935. Document 46, pp. 240, 246, 249, 252, 256, 290, 293, 298, 300, 303, 305, 307, 309—311, 315.

is *nervus belli,* and which he hath almost, out of his West
Indies, his old bands of soldiers will  soon be dissolved,
his purpose defeated, his power and strength diminished,,
his pride abated, and his tyranny utterly suppressed....
....For he being in those parts exceeding weak hath
nothing such numbers of people there as is given out:
neither do his dominions stretch so far as by the ignorant
is imagined....So when we shall have looked and
narrowly pried into the Spanish forces in America, we
shall be doubtless ashamed of ourselves, that we have all
this while been afraid of those dissembling and feeble scare-
crows....I may therefore conclude this matter with com-
paring the Spaniards unto a drone, or an empty vessel,
which when it is smitten upon yieldeth a great and terrible
sound and that afar off, but come near and look into them,
there is nothing in them, or rather like unto the ass which
wrapped himself in a lion's skin and marched far off to
strike terror into the hearts of the other beasts, but when
the fox drew near he perceived his long ears and made
him a jest unto all the beasts of the forest. In like manner
we  (upon peril of my life) shall make the Spaniard
ridiculous to all Europe, if with piercing eyes we see into
his contemptible weakness in the West Indies, and with true
style paint him out *ad vivum* unto the world in his faint
colours....
To confute the general claim and unlawful title of the
insatiable Spaniards to all the West Indies, and to prove
the justness of Her Majesty's title and of her noble
progenitors if not to all, yet at least to that part of America
which is from Florida beyond the Circle Arctic....are we
to answer in general and particularly to the most injurious
and unreasonable donation granted by Pope Alexander the
Sixth, a Spaniard born of all the West Indies to the Kings
of Spain and their Successors, to the great prejudice of all
other Christian princes but especially to the damage of the
Kings of England....
But leaving this abuse offered to the King of England
either by Christopher Columbus or the Kings of Spain in
taking that enterprise out of his hands which was first sent
to him and never refused by him, and to put the case that
Columbus first discovered part of the Islands of Hispaniola
and Cuba, yet we will prove most plainly, that a very great
and large part as well of the continent, as of the Islands
was first discovered for the King of England by Sebastian
Cabot an Englishman born in Bristol, the son of John Cabot
a Venetian, in the year of our Lord 1496....
....No Pope had any lawful authority to give any such
donation at all....our Saviour Christ confessed openly to
Pilate that his kingdom was not of this world. Why then
doth the Pope that would be Christ's servant take upon him

the division of so many kingdoms of the world? If he had but remembered that which he hath inserted in the end of his own Bull, to wit that God is the disposer and distributor of kingdoms and empires, he would never have taken upon him the dividing of them with his line of partition from one end of the heavens to the other. . . . none of the Prophets made Bulls or donations in their palaces under their hands and seals and dates, to bestow many kingdoms which they never saw nor knew, nor what nor how large they were, or to say the truth whether they were extant *in rerum natura,* as the Pope hath done in giving all the West Indies to the Kings of Spain. . . .

The inducements that moved His Holiness to  grant those unequal donations unto Spain were, first, (as he saith) his singular desire and care to have the Christian Religion and Catholic faith exalted, and to be enlarged and spread abroad throughout the world especially in his days, and that the salvation of souls should be procured of everyone, and that the barbarous nations should be subdued and reduced to the faith, &c.

To this I answer that if he had meant as indeed he saith he should not have restrained this so great and general a work belonging to the duty of all other Christian princes unto the Kings of Spain only, as though God had no servants but in Spain. Or as though other Christian kings then living had not as great zeal and means to advance God's glory as they. Or how meant he that everyone should put their helping hand to this work, when he defended all other Christian Princes, in pain of his heavy curse and excommunication to meddle in this action, or to employ their subjects though it were to the conversion of the inhabitants in those parts. . . . it was no marvel that His Holiness being a Spaniard born set apart all other respects of justice and equity and of his mere motion and frank liberality was ready to raise and advance his own nation with doing secret wrong and injury as much as in him lay and more unto all other Princes of Christendom. . . .

God never gave unto the Popes any such authority. . . . But that either Peter or any of the Apostles did teach or affirm that they had authority to give away kingdoms of heathen Princes to those that were so far from having any interest in them, that they knew not whether there were any such countries in the world or no, I never read nor heard, nor any man else as I verily believe. . . . the Kings of Spain have sent such hellhounds and wolves thither as have not converted but almost quite subverted them, and have rooted out above fifteen millions of reasonable creatures as Bartholomew de Casas. . . . doth write. . . .

Those things being thus, who seeth not that the Pope is frustrated of the end which he intended in his donation, and so the same ought not to take effect? . . . .

And whatsoever Pope should excommunicate or curse any Chrisstian prince for seeking to reduce to the knowledge of God and to civil manners those infinite multitudes of Infidels and heathen people of the West Indies, which the Spaniards in all this time have not so much as discovered much less subdued or converted, his curse would light upon his own head, and to those which he cursed undeservedly would be turned to a blessing....

....How easy a matter may it be to this Realm swarming at this day with valiant youths rusting and hurtful by lack of employment, and having good makers of cable and of all sorts of cordage, and the best and most cunning shipwrights of the world to be lords of all those seas, and to spoil Phillip's Indian navy, and to deprive him of yearly passage of his treasure into Europe, and consequently to abate the pride of Spain and of the supporter of the great Antichrist of Rome, and to pull him down in equality to his neighbour princes, and consequently to cut off the common mischiefs that come to all Europe by the peculiar abundance of his Indian Treasure, and this without difficulty....

---

## No. 195 — ENGLAND'S PLACE IN THE SUN

*(Richard Hakluyt, Preface to the Second Edition of The Principal Navigations, Voyages, Traffiques and Discoveries of the English Nation, London, 1598)* *

For....will it not in all posterity be as great a renown unto our English nation, to have been the first discoverers of a Sea beyond the North Cape (never certainly known before) and of a convenient passage into the huge Empire of Russia....as for the Portugales to have found a Sea beyond the Cape of Buona Esperanza, and so consequently a passage by Sea into the East Indies; or for the Italians and Spaniards to have discovered unknown lands so many leagues Westward and Southwestward of the Straits of Gibraltar, & of the pillars of Hercules? Be it granted that the renowned Portugale Vasques de Gama traversed the main Ocean Southward of Africa: Did not Richard Chanceler and his mates perform the like Northward of Europe? Suppose that Columbus that noble and highspirited Genoese escried unknown lands to the Westward of Europe and Africa: Did not the valiant English knight Sir Hugh Willoughby; did not the famous Pilots Stephen Burrough, Arthur Pet, and Charles Jackman accoast Nova Zembla, Colgoieve, and Vaigatz to the North of Europe and Asia? Howbeit you will say perhaps, not with the like golden success, not with such deductions of Colonies, nor attaining of conquests. True it is, that our success hath not been corres-
*Cited in *The Two Richard Hakluyts*, Vol II, Document 76, pp. 434—437.

pondent unto theirs; yet in this our attempt the uncertainty of finding was far greater, and the difficulty and danger of searching was not whit less....Since therefore these two worthy Nations had those bright lamps of learning (I mean the most ancient and best Philosophers, Historiographers and Geographers) to show them light; and the loadstar of experience (to wit those great exploits and voyages laid up in store and recorded) whereby to shape their course: what great attempt might they not presume to undertake? But alas our English nation, at the first setting forth for their Northeastern discovery, were either altogether destitute of such clear lights and inducements or if they had any inkling at all, it was as misty as they found the Northern seas, and so obscure and ambiguous, that it was rather meet to deter them, than to give them encouragement....

And here by the way I cannot but highly commend the great industry and magnanimity of the Hollanders....yet with this proviso; that our English nation led them the dance, broke the ice before them, and gave them good leave to light their candle at our torch. But now it is high time for us to weigh our anchor, to hoist up our sails, to get clear of these boisterous, frosty, and misty seas, and with all speed to direct our course for the mild, lightsome, temperate, and warm Atlantic Ocean, over which the Spaniards and Portugales have made so many pleasant prosperous and golden voyages. And albeit I cannot deny, that both of them in their East and West Indian Navigations have endured many tempests, dangers and shipwrecks: yet this dare I boldly affirm; first that a great number of them have satisfied their fame-thirsty and gold-thirsty minds with that reputation and wealth, which made all perils and misadventures seem tolerable unto them; and secondly that their first attempts (which in this comparison I do only stand upon) were no whit more difficult and dangerous, than ours to the Northeast. For admit that the way was much longer, yet was it never barred with ice, mist, or darkness, but was at all seasons of the year open and navigable; yea and that for the most part with fortunate and fit gales of wind. Moreover they had no foreign prince to intercept or molest them, but their own. Towns, Islands, and mainlands to succour them. The Spaniards had the Canary Isles: and so had the Portugales the Isles of the Azores, of Porto Santo, of Madeira, of Cape Verde, the castle of Mina, the fruitful and profitable Isle of S. Thomas, being all of them conveniently situated, and well fraught with commodities. And had they not continual and yearly trade in some one part or other of Africa, for getting of slaves, for sugar, for elephant's teeth, grains,

silver, gold, and other precious wares which served as
allurements to draw them on by little and litle, and as props
to stay them from giving over their attempts?

---

### No. 196 — ENGLAND'S OPPORTUNITY

*(Richard Hakluyt, "The Epistle Dedicatorie" to Sir Robert
Cecil in the Second Volume of The Principal Navigations,
Voyages, Traffiques and Discoveries of the English Nation,
London, 1599 edition)* *

And here by the way if any man shall think, that an
universal peace with our Christian neighbours will cut off
the employment of the courageous increasing youth of this
realm, he is much deceived. For there are other most convenient employments for all the superfluity of every profession in this realm. For, not to meddle with the state of
Ireland, nor that of Guiana, there is under our noses the
great & ample country of Virginia; the In-land whereof is
found of late to be so sweet and wholesome a climate, so
rich and abundant in silver mines, so apt and capable of
all commodities, which Italy, Spain, and France can afford,
that the Spaniards themselves in their own writings printed
in Madrid 1586, and within few months afterward reprinted
by me in Paris....acknowledge the In-land to be a better
and richer country than Mexico and Nueva Spania itself....
if upon a good & godly peace obtained, it shall please the
Almighty to stir up her Majesty's heart to continue with
her favourable countenance....with transporting of one or
two thousand of her people, and such others as upon mine
own knowledge will most willingly at their own charges
become Adventurers in good numbers with their bodies and
goods; she shall by God's assistance, in short space, work
many great and unlooked for effects, increase her dominions,
enrich her coffers, and reduce many Pagans to the faith
of Christ....No sooner should we set footing in that pleasant and good land, and erect one or two convenient Forts
in the Continent, or in some Island near the main, but every
step we tread would yield us new occasion of action, which
I wish the Gentry of our nation rather to regard, than to
follow those soft unprofitable pleasures wherein they now
too much consume their time and patrimony, and hereafter will do much more, when as our neighbour wars being
appeased, they are like to have less employment than
now they have, unless they be occupied in this or some
other the like expedition.

*Cited in *The Two Richard Hakluyts*, Vol. II, Document 74, pp. 455—457.

## No. 197—THE DRAGON OF THE GOLDEN FLEECE

*(Sir Francis Bacon, Speech in the House of Commons, June 17, 1607)\**

The policy of Spain doth keep that treasury of theirs under such lock and key, as both confederates, yea and subjects, are excluded of trade into those countries; insomuch as the French king, who hath reason to stand upon equal terms with Spain, yet nevertheless is by express capitulation debarred. The subjects of Portugal, whom the state of Spain hath studied by all means to content, are likewise debarred; such a vigilant dragon is there that keepeth this golden fleece. Yet nevertheless such was His Majesty's magnanimity in the debate and conclusion of the last, treaty, as he would never condescend to any article, importing the exclusion of his subjects from that· trade: as a prince that would not acknowledge that any such right could grow to the Crown of Spain by the donative of the pope whose authority he disclaimeth; or by the title of a dispersed and punctual occupation of certain territories in the name of the rest; but stood firm to reserve that point in full question to further times and occasions.

---

### (ii)—THE COMMERCIAL ATTACK ON THE SPANISH MONOPOLY

### No. 198—THE FIRST VIOLATION OF THE MONOPOLY

*(Charles V, Emperor of the Hapsburg Empire, to the Judges, of the Audiencia of Hispaniola, March 27, 1528)\*\**

With respect to what you say of the English ship which anchored in the harbour of the city of Santo Domingo in that island, I would have been much pleased had you taken and detained it, and had there not been such carelessness in this matter; for, as you will have learned we are at war with the King of England, and even were we not, it would have been well had you learned what voyage the ship was making and what she carried, and had not let the master and men of said ship go (as go they did), and after they had landed and visited the city, and seen how it lies, and its harbour, inasmuch as they were from a foreign kingdom, and this was a thing not heretofore experienced in those parts. Nor can you exonerate yourselves in the matter, for there was great carelessness and negligence.

*Cited in L. F. Stock (ed.), *Proceedings and Debates of the British Parliaments respecting North America*, Vol. I, 1542—1688, Carnegie Institution of Washington, 1924, p. 17.
**Cited in Irene A. Wright, *Spanish Documents concerning English Voyages to the Caribbean*, 1527—1568, Works of the Hakluyt Society, Second Series, No. LXII, London, 1928, Document No. 2, p. 57.

*No. 199—HAWKINS AND THE BEGINNINGS OF THE
ENGLISH SLAVE TRADE*

(Richard Hakluyt, The Principal Navigations, Voyages,
Traffiques and Discoveries of the English Nation, London,
1597)*

Master John Hawkins having made divers voyages to the
Isles of the Canaries, and there by his good and upright dealing being grown in love and favour with the people, informed
himself amongst them by diligent inquisition of the state
of the West India, whereof he had received some knowledge by the instructions of his father, but increased the
same by the advertisements and reports of that people. And
being amongst other particulars assured, that Negroes were
very good merchandise in Hispaniola, and that store of
Negroes might easily be had upon the coast of Guinea,
resolved with himself to make trial thereof, and com-
municated that device with his worshipfull friends of
London: namely with Sir Lionell Ducket, Sir Thomas Lodge,
M. Gunson his father–in–law, Sir William Winter, M. Brom-
field, and others. All which persons liked so well of his
intention, that they became liberal contributors and
adventurers in the action. For which purpose there were
three good ships immediately provided: The one called the
*Salomon* of the burthen of 120 tons, wherein M. Hawkins
himself went as General: The second the *Swallow* of 100
tons, wherein went for Captain M. Thomas Hampton: and
the third the *Jonas* a bark of 40 tons, wherein the Master
supplied the Captain's room: in which small fleet M. Hawkins
took with him not above 100 men for fear of sickness and
other inconveniences, whereunto men in long voyages are
commonly subject.

With this company he put off and departed from the
coast of England in the month of October 1562, and in his
course touched first at Teneriffe, where he received friendly
entertainment. From thence he passed to Sierra Leona,
upon the coast of Guinea, which place by the people of the
country is called Tagarin, where he stayed some good time,
and got into his possession, partly by the sword, and
partly by other means, to the number of 300 Negroes at
the least, besides other merchandises which that country
yieldeth. With this prey he sailed over the Ocean sea unto
the Island of Hispaniola, and arrived first at the port of
Isabella; and there he had reasonable utterance of his
English commodities, as also of some part of his Negroes,
trusting the Spaniards no further, than that by his own
strength he was able still to master them. From the port
of Isabella he went to Puerto de Plata, where he made like

*Cited in Donnan, op. cit., Vol. I, pp. 45—47.

sales, standing always upon his guard: from thence also he sailed to Monte Christi another port on the North side of Hispaniola, and the last place of his touching, where he had peaceable traffic, and made vent, of the whole number of his Negroes: for which he received in those 3 places by way of exchange such quantity of merchandise, that he did not only lade his own 3 ships with hides, ginger, sugars, and some quantities of pearls, but he freighted also two other hulks with hides and the like commodities, which he sent into Spain. And thus leaving the Island, he returned and disemboqued, passing out by the Islands of the Cacos, without further entering into the bay of Mexico, in this his first voyage to the West India. And so with prosperous success and much gain to himself and the aforesaid adventurers, he came home, and arrived in the month of September 1563.

## No. 200 — THE COLONIALS CONNIVE AT CONTRABAND TRADE

*(Licentiate of Hispaniola to King of Spain, May 20, 1563)* *

A Lutheran Englishman with a large ship and a shallop, both well supplied with artillery, and a caravel and a large bark, both handsome vessels, which they had taken from merchants as they left, the Portuguese islands, arrived off the town of Puerto de Plata in this island. As soon as the captain and *alcaldes* of this town saw them, fearing lest they march inland to pillage the country, they entered into negotiations with them to the end of procuring their departure and inquired of them what they wanted. The English said they would go if they were shown a port where they could careen a caravel and shallop. In order to get rid of them they sent them to the port of La Isabela, which is twelve leagues from there.

The *alcalde* at once advised me of what was happening and immediately I sent a certain Licentiate Bernaldez, lawyer of this *Audiencia*, who is a diligent man and knows the country thoroughly. He was instructed to use all possible means to endeavour to arrest those Lutherans and seize their goods and not allow a man to trade an article.

He went and in the adjacent settlements raised as many as seventy horsemen, who proceeded to a hut to which the English were accustomed to come. Advancing by night and endeavouring to discover and encounter them, they came upon three Englishmen, very well armed with arquebuses, who were spies and sentinels for the English, whom they seized. When the English became aware of their presence

*Cited in Wright, op. cit., Document No. 5, pp. 61—63.

they retired and put to sea, believing this was a larger body of men than it was in fact, and sent to demand the prisoners of the said licentiate adding that they would conduct themselves courteously and give what might be desired. Seeing how small a force he had compared with the Englishman's, the licentiate replied that he was agreeable. They then came up and the Englishman said that he would give one hundred and four head of slaves. In fine, they reached an agreement, but when it came to delivery the Englishman hung back a little in handing them over, demanding that the licentiate first give his written authorization to dispose by barter of thirty other pieces he had. The licentiate answered that he could not do this since his commission read quite to the contrary—that he could do no such thing. Nevertheless the Englishman again insisted that he give him this authorization as best he could, since it was nothing to him; wherefore, in order to get possession of his Negroes, the licentiate gave it to him in so far as he was legally empowered to do so and no further. He obtained the slaves and turned them over to the treasurer of that town. Having consulted Your Majesty's royal officials, the *Audiencia* sent order to sell these slaves to the burghers of those places, who had had to do with the matter, because of their need of slaves.

They wrote me from that town that the English had another hundred slaves hidden and were trading them to the settlers there and elsewhere. Instantly Licentiate Villoria, Your Majesty's counsel's assistant, was despatched with a receiver of the *Audiencia* to investigate the whole matter aforesaid and arrest the culprits and sequester their goods and sell the said pieces in that town in the presence of Your Majesty's officials.

I have reported this matter to Your Majesty at such length because I am aware that many persons intend to write to Your Majesty concerning it, and are writing, in sense quite contrary to this (which is the truth of the business) with intent to fix blame on certain persons without cause or reason except their own ends which they must have in view, themselves being, perhaps, the most guilty in the affair. I will advise Your Majesty of what action they may take.

I entreat Your Majesty to deign to employ me in some other post where I may serve Your Majesty better. These people oppose justice here and bear a not friendly attitude toward me because ever since I arrived I have endeavoured to enforce Your Majesty's commands and royal *cedulas*, particularly with respect to vessels which enter this port without manifests and are seized....

## No. 201—THE BASIS OF CONTRABAND TRADE

*(Antonio de Berrio to Licentiate Bernaldez of Hispaniola, April 4, 1565)* *

The situation is that yesterday....there appeared off this town seven sails, one of which vessels is very powerful. The fleet is English and so rich in slaves and merchandise that they affirm it to be worth more than 100,000 *pesos*. The commander is an Englishman who time past came to Santo Domingo. He advertises, that he is a great servitor of His Majesty. His intention is to sell with authorization and unless this license is given him he threatens with great oaths to do what harm and damage he may be able.

Your honour is already aware of the necessity existing in all the province and of the serious illnesses all the province is suffering because of its penury. I entreat your honour to deign to come to apply the remedy, for the best good of all. All the settlements will ask and formally demand it and even furnish depositions as to the general need and hardship and epidemics due to this situation, in which matter neither God, Our Lord, nor His Majesty is well served. The royal revenues would be augmented and the country benefited, for this captain promises to please everybody. He brings more than four hundred Negroes.

If by chance your honour does not come to apply the remedy, as we all desire and entreat your honour to do, having taken the measures above said, of having all the people ask it and furnish depositions, I beg your honour to deign to extend the license and open the way, for in addition to the benefit and relief this would mean to all, and increase of the royal revenue, to do so will obviate the great damage and hardship we anticipate.

The captain has agreed to wait ten days, to be reckoned from tomorrow....and so it behoves your honour to hurry or at least send some messenger to advise of your honour's arrival, for which we confidently hope, since it would be an act of great charity and relief to all.

---

## No. 202 — HAWKINS REFUSES TO OBSERVE THE MONOPOLY

*(John Hawkins to Licentiate Bernaldez of Hispaniola, April 16, 1565)* * *

I, John Hawkins, captain general of my fleet, in the person of Cristobal de Llerena, my procurator, appear before

*Cited in Wright, *op. cit.*, Document No. 9, pp. 76—77.
**Cited in Wright, *op. cit.*, Document No. 11, pp. 82—88.

your honour in the manner most advantageous to my
interests, and state that:
    Whereas by order of Elizabeth, Queen of England, my
mistress, whose fleet this is, I cleared on a certain voyage,
and was by contrary weather driven to these coasts where,
since I have found a convenient harbour, it behoves me to
repair and refurnish my ships to continue said voyage;
    And whereas to do this I have need to sell the slaves
and merchandise I carry;
    And whereas I am a great servitor of the majesty of
King Philip, whom I served when he was King of England;
    I therefore petition your honour to grant me license
to sell my cargo. I stand ready to pay His Majesty the
duties usual in this land and to sell the said merchandise
at acceptable prices;
    And whereas in addition to repairing and refurnishing
my fleet, I am obliged to pay my ships and men in each
port entered;
    And whereas I do not desire to offend or occasion diffi-
culties, petitioning, as I petition, your honour to grant me
the license requested under which to sell to the Spanish
in order that I may purchase of them;
    If this petition be not granted, I shall seek my own
solution, for I cannot leave this port, nor will I leave, without supplying my said necessities for even were I willing
to do so, yet am I unable, for I cannot prevail with my
people;
    Therefore, since between Spain and England there is
no enmity nor war, and this fleet belongs to the Queen,
my mistress, of which and of all else herein stated I am
ready to furnish depositions, let your honour not anger me
nor move me to aught that I should not do, as will be inevitable if your honour refuse me the license I ask. I protest
that if from its refusal harm and damage follow, the
fault and responsibility will be your honour's.

-----

*No. 203—QUEEN ELIZABETH SUPPORTS HAWKINS*

*(Guzman de Silva, Spanish Ambassador in England, to
Philip II, King of Spain, July 12, 1567)* *

    I hear that the ships that Hawkins is going to take
out are being got ready rapidly, and I am now told that there
are to be nine of them, four of the Queen's and five which
Hawkins has in Plymouth, where they say the others are
to join them. The four belonging to the Queen are off
Rochester. They are fine vessels. the principal of them being

* Cited in Donnan, *op. cit.*, Vol. I, pp. 63—64.

called the *Jesus de Lobic* of 800 tons, and another of 300, the other two being somewhat smaller. They are armed with fine bronze cannon. The five ships which are to join them consist of one of 130 tons, another of 100 tons and another of 80 tons, the rest being smaller, but all very well fitted. They have brought out from the Tower of London lately the artillery, corslets, cuirasses, pikes, bows and arrows, spears, and other necessary things for the expedition. They say that 800 picked men are to go, and the sailors to work the ships are engaged by order and permission of the Queen, paid at the same rate as for her service. All this looks as if the object was different from that which they say, namely, to go to the Cape de Verde Islands and Guinea to capture Negroes, and thence to go and sell them for gold, silver, pearls, hides, and other merchandise in Your Majesty's Indies. They are taking linens, cloths, merceries, and other things of small value to barter for the Negroes. The admiral went yesterday with his officers to Rochester where the Queen's ships are being fitted out; they say that they will sail in ten days, and many sailors have come from the West Country to man them.

The Queen, as I have written, assures me that they will not go to places prohibited by Your Majesty, and the secretary has done the same. I returned to the subject again yesterday, and had Cecil informed on my behalf that the ships would certainly go to Your Majesty's Indies, whereupon he sent word to me that I might believe his assurance that they would not. I have nevertheless asked for an audience of the Queen to warn her again.

---

## No. 204—THE ROYAL OFFICIALS CONNIVE AT CONTRABAND TRADE

*(Accountant of Venezuela to Philip II, King of Spain, April, 21, 1586)* *

These corsairs come fully supplied with all lines of merchandise, oils and wines and everything else which is lacking in the country. The colonists' needs are great and neither penalties nor punishments suffice to prevent them from buying secretly what they want. As a matter of fact, they make their purchases, but nothing can be learned of them, for they buy at night and cover each other, and no measures suffice to prevent it. Truly we, Your Majesty's officials, feel conscientious scruples about putting them on oath, when investigating; all we accomplish, as we think, is to make them perjure themselves. This jurisdiction would

* Cited in Wright, *op. cit.*, Document No. 21, pp. 114—115.

not, suffer as it does for lack of necessary articles if Your Majesty would deign to order that when the fleet passes to Tierra Firme a ship should call here, to supply the colony. The colonists then could no longer justly complain nor would they dare, because of their necessities, to buy of the French as they now do. This could easily be done, for from here the vessel can go to Cabo de la Vela and Santa Marta and Cartagena.

## No. 205—THE ONLY WAY

*(Bernardino de Mendoza, Spanish Ambassador in England, to Philip II, King of Spain, 1580)\**

....no foreign ship should be spared in either the Spanish or Portuguese Indies, but....everyone should be sent to the bottom....This will be the only way to prevent the English and French from going to those parts to plunder; for at present there is hardly an Englishman who is not talking of undertaking the voyage, so encouraged are they by Drake's return.

### (iii)—THE CORSAIRS

## No. 206—NO PEACE BEYOND THE LINE

*(Treaty of Cateau Cambresis, 1559)\*\**

West of the prime meridian and south of the Tropic of Cancer....violence done by either party to the other side shall not be regarded as in contravention of the treaties.

## No. 207—LORDS OF THE SEA

*(Lazaro de Vallejo Aldrate and Hernando Costilla to Phillip II, King of Spain, September 26, 1568)\* \*\**

We entreat Your Majesty to remedy the grievous condi-

* Cited in *The Cambridge History of the British Empire*, Vol. I, The Old Empire, from the Beginnings to 1783, Cambridge University Press, 1929, p. 116.
\*\*Cited in *The New Cambridge Modern History*, Vol. I, The Renaissance, 1493—1520, Cambridge University Press, 1961, p. 467.
\*\*\* Cited in Wright, *op. cit.*, Document No. 22, pp. 118—119.

tions prevailing today in the Indies. For every two ships that come hither from Spain, twenty corsairs appear. For this reason not a town on all this coast is safe, for whenever they please to do so they take and plunder these settlements. They go so far as to boast that they are lords of the sea and of the land, and as a matter of fact daily we see them seize ships, both those of the Indies trade and also some that come here from Spain itself. They capture towns, and this so commonly that we see it happen every year. Unless Your Majesty deign to favour all this coast by remedying the situation, all these settlements must necessarily be abandoned, from which will result grave detriment to Your Majesty's royal patrimony and an end will be put to inter-Indies traffic, trade with the Canaries will suffer, as will also those ships which come out of Spain between fleets.

---

## No. 208—THE LUST FOR GOLD

*(The City of Panama to Philip II, King of Spain, May, 25, 1571)* *

The cause of much of the trouble has been the certain and widespread knowledge that this country has great wealth, and that to this city is sent all the gold, silver and pearls of Potosi, Chile and the rest of Peru, for shipment to Spain, and that from this city it is all sent to the city of Nombre de Dios by the Chagre River, from the House at Cruces, which is five leagues from this city by land. This knowledge has given courage to many French and English corsairs, many of them Lutherans, enemies of the holy Catholic faith, to come to sack the city of Nombre de Dios and plunder the barks in which the gold and silver goes down the Chagre River from this city to Nombre de Dios; in which barks also the major portion of all the merchandise brought from Spain is conveyed from Nombre de Dios to the House at Cruces.

---

## No. 209 — EL DRAQUE

*(Philip Nicholls, Sir Francis Drake Revised; calling upon this dull or effeminate age to follow his noble steps for gold and silver: by this Memorable Relation of the Rare Occurrences (never yet declared to the world) in a Third Voyage made by him into the West Indies, in the years (15) 72 and (15) 73, London, 1626)* **

He had brought them to the mouth of the Treasure of

* Cited in Wright, op. cit., Document No. 13, p. 31.
**Op. cit., p. 144.

the World,* if they would want it, they might henceforth blame nobody but themselves!

. . . . He advised the Governor "to hold open his eyes, for before he departed, if GOD lent him life and leave, he meant to reap some of their harvest, which they get out of the earth, and send into Spain to trouble all the earth!"

They** presently came forth upon the sand, and sent a youth, as with a message from the Governor, to know, "What our intent was, to stay upon the coast?"

Our Captain answered: "He meant to traffic with them; for he had tin, pewter, cloth, and other merchandise that they needed".

The youth swam back again with this answer, and was presently returned, with another message: that, "The King had forbidden to traffic with any foreign nation for any commodities, except powder and shot; of which, if he had any store, they would be his merchants".

He answered that "He was come from his country, to exchange his commodities for gold and silver, and is not purposed to return without his errand. They are like, in his opinion, to have little rest, if that, by fair means, they would not traffic with him".

---

### 210—THE FEAR OF DRAKE

#### (Venetian Ambassador in Spain, 1580)***

Should the *flota* (from the Indies) fall into Drake's hands, that would mean the ruin of half Spain, as indeed will happen if the fleet does not arrive this year; for they say that a mere delay will cause the failure of many merchants in Seville.

---

### No. 211—THE ENGLISH CAPTURE OF SANTO DOMINGO

#### (The Audiencia of Santo Domingo, to Philip II, King of Spain, February 24, 1586)****

On January 10 of the present year, at about ten o'clock in the morning, warning reached this city and eleven sail were sighted which seemed to be steering for this port. At this news a person was immediately sent to endeavour to identify them and to determine their intention and course. So also for this purpose Don Diego Osorio, captain of Your

*Nombre de Dios.
**Before Cartagena.
***Cited in *Cambridge History of the British Empire*, Vol. I, p. 120.
****Cited in Irene-Wright (ed.) *Further English Voyages to Spanish America, 1583—1594*, Works of the Hakluyt Society, Second Series, XCIX, London, 1951, Document No. 19, pp. 32—37.

Majesty's galleys, went out in person. Meanwhile, with the diligence and efficacy possible, given the scanty means we possessed, everybody was busied in preparing this city for whatever the event might prove to be. For not only was the powder in the fort and city scarce and of poor quality, but also the galley was dismantled, for it was being careened.

Nevertheless, with great activity, what men could be mustered were assembled, both foot and horse. After we had consulted with those residents who seemed best informed, in order to reach a determination as to what should be done, and been by them assured that there was no fear whosoever that from the landward the enemy, if this were an enemy, could do us damage or disembark, unless it were at a certain inlet the sea forms at a place called Guibia, we sent thither troops who stood guard all night, to send warning and to defend that place. Meanwhile, all our effort was addressed to strengthening this harbour and its defences.

At nine o'clock that night Don Diego Osorio, captain of the galley, came in with the report that he had seen seventeen vessels which he believed to be English, owing to the cut of their sails and rigging. Whereupon preparations to defend the harbour and protect the city were redoubled; and the spirits of many of its residents commenced to weaken, who forthwith began to flee. Proclamations which were issued and other measures taken to the end of preventing this, proved unavailing.

The morning of the following Saturday (which was the 11th) seventeen vessels appeared off this port, and seemed to intend to attempt to force an entrance. They tacked back and forth, without firing upon the fort, nor did the fort fire upon them, both because we were not sure that they were enemies (on the contrary, many asserted that they were Your Majesty's galleons) and also because the powder we had was of such wretched quality. In order not to lose reputation we delayed firing until it could no longer be avoided, which was very soon.

A shot was fired when the ships came up and stood off the streets ending on the waterfront, toward which these vessels turned their bows. A man we had sent to reconnoitre brought assurance that they were enemies. Since this shot did not reach them by a long stretch they determined to ignore our defence, as we learned afterwards.

We strengthened the harbour's defences and those at its entrance. We hastened to sink three ships along the bar, that theirs might not enter. Although with great diffi-culty, Don Diego also brought out his galley and laid it across at a point where with the artillery (and great effort which he put forth) he could do serious damage if the

enemy entered the haven. Certain pieces of artillery which
we planted in works and suitable positions would do no
less.

But all this and the great endeavour made to encourage
the people and to detain those who were leaving was of
no effect, for about midday we received news that over land,
half a league from the city, nine standards of very select
infantry were advancing rapidly upon the place. This, when
at the river's mouth for its defence we were not 200 men.
All the rest, to a total of more than 400, had fled and
abandoned their posts without our being able to prevent it.

Nevertheless, we brought out what cavalry there was—
about 40 horse, harquebusiers mounted behind the riders, in
order to do what we could. The rest were left to protect
the river. Half a league out they encountered the enemy,
who gave them a sprinkling of musket-shot in such fashion
that the few who had arrived within range turned back on
the run, to spread the certainty that we were entirely
unequal to defending ourselves against such numbers.

As a last effort and trial of fortune we brought out
what horse and foot remained, who in all were not 120
men, with the determination to attack and die rather than
witness such damage and loss as has befallen us. But upon
taking the field the men, especially the foot, began to
exhibit such poor spirit (recognizing the enemy's strength)
that many shamelessly abandoned their arms and took to
the bush, fleeing; and it was impossible to get the rest
into military formation or to attempt to fight, nor had the
men equipment or suitable weapons to meet even equal
numbers, much less as many as well armed and disciplined
foes as were advancing.

Ten or twelve of us who were mounted advanced within
musketshot, to oblige the rest to do the same, in order to
attack. Although we were in great danger from the many
shots they fired at us, we were unable to make the rest
move from where they stood. Therefore, on the advice of
certain experienced men who were present, we changed our
plan, or were forced to change it, because of the aforesaid
situation and because, in addition to the musketry fire to
which they subjected us from the land, their ships turned
their bows toward the field, against us, and swept it with
their artillery in such a manner that they left not a tree
standing. Therefore in good order we returned to the city
gate, where we had planted three pieces of artillery, which
we fired. This artillery fire killed only two or three of their
men, among them an ensign. In fine, they entered the city.

No other resistance was offered, because it was all open,
without gates or denfensive works. We fled from it as best
we could, for we found ourselves deserted. They took the
city and occupied it and the fortress, which has no defences

upon the side toward the city nor had its warden means or men to hold it.

Amidst so much evil God granted that the honour of no woman should be jeopardized, for they had all fled with their children. Very few men were killed, by shots which from the sea their ships fired into the streets. Presently we got some people together and removed subsistence from round about the city. A troop of horse under Don Diego Osorio has hung persistently on its outskirts and upon what occasions have offered has killed some of the enemy. We remained masters of the countryside although we never had the means to attack, lacking arms, and because the enemy, who entered by land and sea, was numerous.

According to the most reliable reckoning those who came up by land were as many as 1400, the third part musketeers and the others harquebusiers and cuirassiers. The rest raised the total to five or six thousand in all, very well armed and equipped, and so well disciplined that within a few hours they had so fortified themselves that a great force would have been required to retake the city.

In possession of it, they began to commit a thousand abominations, principally in the temples and with the images. They broke these all to pieces, heaping ignominy and vituperation upon our religion, profaning everything without distinction or consideration. Not content with this, they opened the sepulchres of the dead and into them threw filth and offal of cattle they slaughtered within the churches, which they converted into slaughter-pens. They made even viler use of these edifices.

They looted the private property of the residents. Very little was saved. There is no man but has suffered notable loss. Especially have we, for the enemy took everything we had and carried it off. We removed nothing opportunely in order not to afford the people occasion to do the same and so leave the city empty and defenceless while we considered defence possible. So have we all come to extreme poverty, being in want of everything both to eat and to wear, of money and of all sorts of clothing and means to sustain life.

So also they burned all the vessels which were in the harbour aboard which might have been shipped certain ginger which was left; this would in part have relieved our situation, but loss of the ships prevented this, too.

Seeing how unable we were to retake the city by arms, we entered into negotiations with them to recover it in exchange for money. The price they set upon it was excessive, for they asked a million at first, and, finally, a hundred thousand ducats, which we were as unable to raise as the million. Since they would not reduce that figure and we could not meet it, they began to burn the city and its temples, so that in a very short time they burned the greater part. Because the best portion still remained, through Garcia Fernandez de Torrequemada, Your Majesty's factor, we renewed negotiations with them to redeem it. He came to an agreement with them and arranged the matter at 25,000 ducats, which such sum was with great difficulty raised among all the citizens, the archbishop and the church.

At this price, after they had been in the city five weeks, they left it on February 9, taking with them all our wealth, even to the bells of the churches, artillery from the fort, and ships, and other smaller things of every sort. They carried off the copper coin which circulates in this city. Much of it they melted up and wasted.

They took with them the galley-slaves from the galley, whose irons had been removed that they might help us. Later they rose against us and did more looting than the English. Many Negroes belonging to private persons (who are the labourers of this country) went with them of their own free will.

The commanding officer of these people is Francis Drake —he who entered the Pacific by way of the Straits of Magellan. He is a cautious commander, equal to any undertaking. He brings with him veteran captains and soldiers from among the richest and most honoured in England.

The number of ships with which he arrived here was 30 or 31, including the seventeen with which he made the feint we have described, of intending to force the harbour entrance. The others came down at night, unobserved, to land troops at Hayna, which is a certain inlet, where we never anticipated a landing because, in addition to the heavy sea which runs there and reefs which obstruct the entrance of ships, the native residents of this island guaranteed it against everything. But the English brought with them people so well acquainted with the vicinity that they showed them safely in.

Their ships have the best possible armament and equipment, munitions and choicest powder in superabundance. There are ships of over 700 tons, armament some 70 heavy guns, most of them bronze, not counting those they took from us.

Their course is for Cartagena, according to what we understood. We have taken care to send warning, as Your Majesty will see by the evidence enclosed herewith. Similarly, we warned Havana and other places, in good season.

And if similar warning had been sent from Cape Verde or the Canaries to us, this city would not have suffered the damage it has received, or it would have cost the enemy dearer. We cannot comprehend why no warning was sent to us. We received none from any quarter. The ship which usually comes has not arrived, from which we infer that the fleet got in safely.

We have reported in such detail to Your Majesty lest advices which Licentiates Juan Fernandez de Mercado and Baltazar de Villafane, Your Majesty's judges, sent by way of La Yaguana and Puerto Plata may not have arrived.

At first it was supposed that the commander of these people was Don Antonio, prior of Crato, but later it was learned that this was not true, that he remains in England at the house of this Captain Francis, by whose hand so much damage has been inflicted.

To remedy which we humbly entreat Your Majesty to have pity on this sad city and its inhabitants, promptly providing as necessary for its restoration and taking measures such that it may hereafter protect itself and not be left so incapable to defence. We have neither artillery nor powder, neither harquebuses nor men experienced in war, which is what is most needed. Unless provided, these people are so terrorized, poor and defenceless that they will abandon the country, nor have we been able to prevent some from beginning to do so, seeing that the city's reputation of being impregnable by land (which alone sustained it) is lost, as well as its means of defence by sea, so that it has no recourse for its recovery except Your Majesty's clemency, which will not permit this country's ruin. Had it no other merit than that it was the first discovered in this New World, that it belongs to Your Majesty would suffice to assure its restoration, for Your Majesty is wont to relieve even the distress of others, how much more Your Majesty's own.

What else remains to be said of this matter we reserve until a person goes by whom Your Majesty may be fully informed of the condition in which we are left and of what is required for the protection and relief of this land, which lies at the mercy of a thousand ships, both English and French, which clutter the sea. A pair of galleys would be of very great service now; although they could not resist a royal armada, they would suffice against the attacks of petty marauders, which this port greatly fears.

For the love of Our Lord, may Your Majesty order measures to be opportunely taken while yet it is possible to remedy the dangers which impend, for we have understood both from these evil people and also from others that this and other fleets which cleared from England will meet at Cape Canaveral, where they have made a settlement. We have heard also that the French have settled on Dominica and there are many indications that it is all true.

God help and preserve the Catholic royal person of Your Majesty with increase of greater kingdoms and happy achievements, as Christianity has need.

## No. 212 — DRAKE THE "CRUSADER"
### (Dean and Chapter of the Cathedral of Santo Domingo to Philip II, King of Spain, February 19, 1586)*

God, Our Lord, permitted an English fleet which the people of this city of Santo Domingo sighted on Friday, the 10th of January of this present year, to land men immediately, on the following Saturday. That day they entered into the city and sacked and destroyed it. We understand that it was Heaven's punishment on this people's manifold sins.

Although the inhabitants were so inexperienced and untrained in military affairs, there was such lack of powder and munitions it has long been understood that this city lay, a prize and a spoil, at the mercy of any enemy who might care to attempt it.

The English remained here 36 days, during which they treated this city as an enemy of their religion, of their queen and of themselves. They carried away everything they wanted and could transport; everything else they burned and destroyed. Notably, they burned two-thirds of the residences and edifices of this city and all its churches and monasteries and nunneries, its hospitals and hermitages, excepting the cathedral.

I should say excepting only the shell of the cathedral; for its altars, retables, crucifixes, images, choir, screens, organs, bells and all other objects usual in such churches, they broke up, overthrew, burned and destroyed. When they threw the bells down these fell upon the dome and demolished part of the sacristy.

Further, they burned many buildings belonging to the foundation of this church and to its chaplaincies, as well as eight other houses which were the property of the church hospital and constituted its principal income and capital.

They made a jail of two chapels in this church wherein they confined many residents whom they arrested; and, confined therein, these persons used the chapels as prisoners must any place in which they are long detained.

This church was the enemy's centre for business, where they dealt in and negotiated their evil affairs. It was their warehouse and dispensary, and served them for even viler purposes. In fine, within its premises they committed other abominations worse than the conflagration itself and more horrible.

* Cited in Wright, *Further English Voyages to Spanish America*, Document No. 17, pp. 27–29.

The body of this church, then, and one hospital called Saint Nicholas's, and the third of the dwellings they left standing, because this much was ransomed with a certain sum of money. Nearly all the silver service of this church and all of the archbishop's (which he freely proffered although he had no house to be redeemed) went toward making up this sum.

By accounts of the matter which are being sent by the royal *Audiencia* and the municipal council Your Majesty will be more fully informed of other damage done in this city. Therefore we do not go into details.... We confine ourselves to consideration of what this church and its hospital have suffered, these being particularly our charge.

The church stands, then, sacked, defaced, in ruins. We are helpless. Before Your Majesty we lay the situation with entreaty made as humbly and earnestly as we are able that with that royal spirit of religious piety with which Your Majesty is wont to raise new and sumptuous churches, temples and edifices to the honour of God — with that same spirit Your Majesty will now come to the support of this church which still stands, by His grace....

*No. 213 — DRAKE'S GOSPEL OF RANSOM*

*(Pedro Fernandez de Busto to Philip II, King of Spain, Cartagena, May 25, 1586)\**

After we had set forth the poverty of this land and explained that there was no money here, he answered that he knew quite well that this was one of the principal cities in the Indies and very rich. In reply he was reminded that Santo Domingo, a very much larger place than this is, had been ransomed for little money, and we said that for Cartagena we would give him 25,000 ducats. He answered that in Santo Domingo he had obtained pillage, for the people there had saved only themselves and there had been no bloodshed, whereas in Cartagena there had been no booty and there had been bloodshed, for all of which he must be compensated with money, and that he must have 400,000 ducats as ransom. In view of this demand, nothing further was said in the matter and we returned. Therefore Francis began to burn the town, beginning with the least valuable portion; and he burned about 100 houses, the most worthless in the place.

In view of the damage he was doing, a person was sent to urge him not to burn, for the ransom would be negotiated. And so they went to offer him 30,000 ducats. He retorted that he would not accept less than he had demand-

* Cited in Wright, *Further English Voyages to Spanish America*, Document No. 29, pp. 142—146.

ed; unless he got, it he would destroy everything. The messenger returned with this answer and meanwhile the enemy burned another 100 houses of a better sort, tiled and of masonry.

Seeing the damage he was doing the people assembled and appealed to the prelate and to me, pleading that if I had no authority to negotiate the ransom, I should empower them to ransom each man his own house before the enemy should completely raze the city. Having consulted the bishop, who gave his opinion in writing signed with his name, to effect that the ransom could be effected without burdening of conscience, I gave them leave to ransom each his own house.

They sent in Diego Daca, lieutenant governor, and Tristan de Orive, with their authority to treat of the ransom. These persons went and with every visit increased their offer of ransom from the 30,000 which they had proffered to 80,000, and the bishop recommended that they make it as much as 100,000. On this recommendation and with the consent of the interested persons this sum was offered. And the enemy refused it.

At this juncture one morning showed that three arches of the cathedral had fallen in. It was completed, lacking only the tiling of the fourth part. Captain Francis had ordered it to be demolished by a culverin shot which he caused to be fired at it an hour before dawn. A ball struck a main support of one arch and this dragged down two more and all the woodwork with them. The damage he did here amounted to more than 10,000 ducats.

In view of this damage, which must have been more than he intended, although in my opinion because it was the church he would have preferred to do it very much more, he said that he would accept 107,000 ducats, and to this they agreed, and they paid it to him.

It would not have been possible to meet, his demands had not 79,000 ducats out of Your Majesty's treasury been lent to the citizens, each pledging himself, his person, goods and house, to repay his portion of it by Christmas Day. They assumed this obligation. Had this not been done the enemy would have razed the whole city, leaving not even the memory of it. To do so he had already brought ashore fireworks to blow up the large edifices and he meant to demolish all the rest. He said that when he had finished the utter des-truction of this place he would go and do the same to Nombre de Dios.

Four or five considerations moved me to make this loan and undue use of Your Majesty's revenues. First, because were this city and Nombre de Dios to be razed, when the fleet (which is expected soon) should arrive on this coast, it would find no place to discharge its cargoes and the vessels would be compelled to return laden to Spain. This would have meant a loss to Your Majesty of more than 300,000 ducats in duties and to this city a similar loss of 100,000. What is more, all that is owing to Your Majesty in this province would have been lost, because each creditor would have betaken himself elsewhere on his own account, and no collection could have been made. Second, 40,000 ducats in debts which are owing from Panama and Lima and Cartagena would also have been totally lost because the people would have been scattered, each going his own way. This would have meant a heavy loss to Your Majesty, arising out of the cessation of trade. Third, all the business of Seville with this city, Nombre de Dios, Peru and the New Kingdom of Granada would have come to a stop for some years, which also would have entailed very heavy loss on Your Majesty. Fourth, it would have meant the death of more than 4,000 persons, children and adults, which is the population which went out from this city. They were scattered in the bush and in the hills where they must have suffered hunger, there being no means of relief while the enemy held the sea, as he held it. Fifth, divine worship must have ceased in this city and province and three monasteries and one cathedral would have been lost. I considered that it was not for the good of Your Majesty's armadas and fleets for me to do otherwise than I did.

All these reasons moved me to take the course I took, believing that in so doing I was serving Your Majesty and avoiding all the losses above mentioned, without entailing that of a single *real* of the royal revenues. Nothing will be lost, because the parties will fulfil their obligations by Christmas, and the amounts taken from Your Majesty's royal treasury will be forwarded to Your Majesty by the fleet which must winter here.

The person who most importuned and persuaded me to make this use of Your Majesty's revenues and to ransom the city was the bishop of this province. Not that he wished to do the city a service but that he fancied that, in this manner he could do me grave harm, and that it would fare ill with me. Similarly he encourages every matter that bodes evil for me, because he is my enemy. I have deemed it advisable to write this to Your Majesty that Your Majesty may understand that insofar as they refer to me any relations he may make are prejudiced, and the reason of it is that I have defended the royal prerogative against him and have procured provisions from the royal *Audiencia* of the New Kingdom of Granada to prevent his encroachments upon it. Similarly, the royal officials in charge of Your Majesty's revenues urged me to effect the ransom and to

authorize negotiations and to make use for the purpose of
Your Majesty's money which was in their custody. I assert
this because they took certain steps to make it appear that
I did it against their will.

The persons interested paid the ransom of 107,000
ducats to the Englishman, as I have said, mostly out of Your
Majesty's revenues, some out of certain deposits, and other
persons paid with their own cash. The Englishman gave a
receipt for everything and left the city to its inhabitants.
On board his ships, he remained in the harbour until April
10, and on the 11th with his fleet cleared from the port on
a course for Jamaica where he expected to obtain meat and
water which he did not have when he left here.

He sailed four days and on the 14th returned to this
harbour because Coro's ship which he had seized at Santo
Domingo sprung a leak. It was laden with all the booty
he obtained in that city and the artillery he had seized. He
unloaded all this and distributed it among the other vessels
of his fleet.

He held a council of all his people, to whom he made
an address, informing them that Your Majesty's armada was
on its way to these parts and would soon arrive, that he
meant to await it for, if they would do their duty, he was
confident he could take it. All the principal persons and
officers of his fleet answered that without exception they
would all die or capture Your Majesty's armada. With this
intention the enemy remained in the port until the 24th of
the said month of April, when he left with his fleet, consisting as he left, of 22 large vessels and six pinnaces and
brigantines. The six galleons of this fleet were 600 tons
burden and upward, very well supplied with artillery and
thoroughly equipped. The flagship carried 60 pieces of
heavy brass artillery in tiers. The other vessels were 100 to
200 tons.

When the enemy entered the port of this city he
brought in 3,000 men. The muster he held when he left
showed that he had only 2,500. The night the city was lost
his casualties were about 150 and the rest died of sickness
during the time he was here.

He sailed on a course for Havana with the intention of
attacking that city and its fortress and, if they were successful, of awaiting the New Spain fleet there. I am quite certain
that he will not attack Havana because there was great dissen-
sion among them and they could agree on nothing. Three
days before they left there was much argument and dispute.
Therefore I am sure that he was going to Matanzas to take
on water and meat and continue his voyage to England.

Nevertheless Francis said publicly that he intended to
go to the island of Madeira and endeavour to take it, and

send word to England that they might furnish him food supplies and more ships in order that there he might await the fleets coming out of these parts, to take them. For the principal purpose of this corsair is to prevent Your Majesty and private persons from receiving revenues from these parts. I informed the realm of Tierra Firme that the enemy had left this harbour for Havana, in order to put an end to the expense they were incurring.

The damage this corsair did this city amounts to more than 400,000 ducats, including the artillery which he carried off. He burned and demolished 248 houses, two–thirds of them masonry and tile, and one–third of them palmboard and thatch. The principal buildings were left, which were appraised at 450,000 ducats in order to determine what amount each one must pay toward the ransom. This business will all be finished and done by the end of the present month in order that the royal officials may collect from the parties concerned by Christmas.

*No. 214 — "I WILL RETURN !"¹*
*(Alonso Suarez de Toledo to Philip II, King of Spain, Havana, June 27, 1586)\**

If the corsair has disembogued, as is understood to be certain, he has left very rich with booty obtained at Santo Domingo and in the many years during which he has suffered no loss. He will return again and in much greater strength. He has advised us to expect another call from him. May God provide the remedy in time and may Your Majesty be ready to apply it, that it may not be carried into effect as slowly and as tardily as the arrival of the galleons which are expected now that the enemy has gone. God grant the enemy encounter Your Majesty's armada out yonder, that this corsair's design may be frustrated....

*No. 215 — THE WRITING ON THE WALL*
*(Sir Francis Walsingham to Earl of Leicester, 1586)\*\**

The enterprise of Sir Francis Drake layeth open the present weakness of the King of Spain....

*No. 216 — THE WORLD SUFFICETH NOT*
*(Captain Walter Biggs, A Summary and True Discourse of Sir Francis Drake's West Indian Voyage, begun in the year 1585, London, ca. 1586)\*\*\**

Amongst other things which happened and were found

\*Cited in Wright, *Further English Voyages to Spanish America*, Document No. 38, pp. 172—173.
\*\*Cited in A. E. W. Mason, *The Life of Francis Drake*, London, 1950, p. 254.
\*\*\**Op. cit.*, p. 251.

at St. Domingo, I may not omit to let the world know one very notable mark and token of the unsatiable ambition of the Spanish king and his nation, which was found in the king's house, wherein the chief governor of that city and country is appointed always to lodge, which was this. In the coming to the hall or other rooms of this house, you must first ascend up by a fair large pair of stairs, at the head of which stairs is a handsome spacious place to walk in, somewhat like unto a gallery. Wherein, upon one of the walls, right over against you as you enter into the said place, so as your eye cannot escape the sight of it, there is described and painted in a very large scutcheon the arms of the King of Spain; and in the lower part of the said scutcheon there is likewise described a globe, containing in it the whole circuit of the sea and the earth, whereupon is a horse standing on his hinder part with the globe, and the other forepart without the globe, lifted up as it were to leap, with a scroll painted in his mouth, wherein was written these words in Latin, NON SUFFICIT ORBIS, which is as much to say, as, *The world sufficeth not.* Whereof the meaning was required to be known of some of those of the better sort that came in commission to treat upon the ransom of the town; who would shake their heads and turn aside their countenance, in some smiling sort, without answering anything, as greatly ashamed thereof. For by some of our company it was told them, that if the Queen of England would resolutely prosecute the wars against the King of Spain, he should be forced to lay aside that proud and unreasonable reaching vein of his; for he should find more than enough to do to keep that which he had already, as by the present example of their lost town they might for a beginning perceive well enough.

---

## No. 217 — THE COLOSSUS WITH FEET OF CLAY

*(Garcia Fernandez de Torrequemada, His Majesty's Factor for Hispaniola, to Philip II, King of Spain, February 1, 1587)\**

On February 23 and April 14 of last year I wrote to Your Majesty concerning the hardship which came upon this city with the arrival of the English fleet. I outlined the situation in the large, only, and dealt with the most urgent matters and the general state of everything and the great danger in which all this colony will be, invariably, if reliance is placed in force, arms, defensive measures, and the military prowess of this people, for among them there is not a

*Cited in Wright, *Further English Voyages to Spanish America*, Document No. 56, pp. 220—223.

soldier, nor a captain, who knows what war is, or strategy, or has seen, or perhaps even heard of such. That I may at no time fail to advise Your Majesty of the country's needs, in case Your Majesty be pleased to hear of them and order necessary provision made, it has seemed to me to be my duty to go into details in this despatch (as I did not in the other) concerning the matter which gave rise to the event.

Your Majesty is doubtless fully aware of the few precautions and little discipline usually observed by an untrained and untried population as against veteran and experienced soldiery; and also it is notorious that the inhabitants of this city are persons assembled to do business in trade and to attend to suits at law, and, further, that only one or another of them understands these matters although very few desire to know anything else. While musters are held as a matter of course and various sorts of persons figure in them, some are litigants and others are merchants, some are haggling shopkeepers and others those who find their profit and support in rural parts. These reviews usually bring out 500 men, but withal it is to be borne in mind that among them not a hundred nor even 60 can be called harquebusiers nor would dare to lift such a weapon to their shoulders because to do so is not their proper calling nor pertinent thereto, nor is it the purpose which brought them thither or the means of their support here.

Similarly, as to the horse, although 300 mounted men be assembled by summoning to such a muster those persons who live six and eight and ten leagues round the city, engaged in growing food crops and raising cattle, it is not easy to get them together in less than ten days, and the animals on which they appear will eat nothing but grass and are not accustomed to be shod. They are good only for field work and for nothing else and their riders are unarmed except for a sort of lance of little worth and a poorly cinched wooden saddle. Actually, to assemble in this city a couple of dozen horses for a tourney is impossible and explains why a mount in a proper stable represents a cost of 200 ducats a year. Few persons can afford it, and therefore on the day the Englishman appeared there were 36 horse, a number which diminished to sixteen; and it must be added that of these not more than ten or twelve were suitable mounts.

Both foot and horse were without defensive weapons except lances and shields (for the horse) and harquebuses (for the foot) — mostly without munitions — and mouldy pikes and rusty swords. The climate here is such that every harquebus, sword and halberd needs a man with no other occupation, to keep it clean, I speak of this from such experience that I assure Your Majesty that the sword I carry

in my belt is cleaned every time I return home and nevertheless it rusts. This happens to the most careful person,
and the same is true of all other weapons. Your Majesty
will realize what occurs, then, in the case of the merchant or
shop-keeper or litigant who comes and remains here only
to earn his living and get back to Castile, or, if he be a
resident of the colony, seeks only to feed his wife and
family, inasmuch as the misery and poverty of this land
yields no further profit, and even this only at the price of
much sweat and exertion and sickness.

As for powder, the little there is in my house is refined
in the sun nearly every day and nevertheless it deteriorates.
Further, it must be remembered that all the powder is imported into the island and usually it is not to be purchased,
nor are there any armourers who know their business, or
artisans acquainted with any sort of weapon, to repair it.
To put into condition 30 muskets which the officials at Seville sent as relief — they arrived four months after the
Englishman left — has required another four months time.

These muskets came with another 28 harquebuses
(mostly in bad condition) and ten hundredweight of powder,
arriving in the month of June following upon the catas-
trophe of the preceding January. This, as against a royal
armada of 32 sails, carrying five or six thousand men, provided with musketproof corselets as became the veterans
which most of them were, and the third part of their shot,
musketeers! Given, too, the whole course of the event, our
lack of warning, arms, preparation and of competent military officers of any experience whatsoever, from the first in
command down. This thing must have had Divine sanction,
as a punishment for the people's sins.

Although it is true that men become ministers and masters, it is understood that they usually pass through an apprenticeship and learn from a beginning, through means, in
training under experienced teachers. If this be not so, un-
desired results follow; and I humbly entreat Your Majesty
to deign to permit me to say that in makng appointments to
office consideration should always be had to each candidate's
qualifications, his aptitudes, condition, experience and talent.

I have written at length in order to give Your Majesty
a full account and, in fine, I will conclude by saying that if
the impetus and force which Francis Drake brought to bear
here had suddenly appeared at the gates of Seville it would
have put that city to flight, had it found the place as defenceless, without arms or soldiers, as was this city, and
without any previous warning. I speak as an eye-witness
who saw whereof I write, and measured the enemy's strength
and organization and know how many veteran troops he had

and what very experienced military officers, and I appreciate also the weakness of this city.

A third of the Englishman's foot were musketeers and he marched in good order with pikes in his van — and in his rearguard. He divided his forces into two columns with troops of shot, in which formations I know (from conversation with the enemy himself) that he had 2,500 men whom he landed three leagues from this city.

The place was only half, or little more, enclosed by a very weak wall, without gates or artillery. Only the fort had ordnance with which to offend any enemy entering by the river, and for this there were few munitions and powder so poor in quality that the necessary range could hardly be obtained or any real effect produced.

The fort itself is merely a strong site suitable for the construction of a fortification for the defence of the harbour only. Against an enemy advancing by land it is of no use whatsoever. If Your Majesty were pleased to remedy this situation it would be very necessary for engineers to make an inspection and plan other forts in the harbour itself and on the heights of the city, where the Franciscan monastery is, or the parish church of Santa Barbola, which shall be better adapted to the defence and protection of the city than this fort. is. As I wrote to Your Majesty on May 17, 1578, and on June 8 and 15 of 1580, and in other letters, it has many defects, and so I again do assure Your Majesty.

---

(iv) — **THE COLLAPSE OF THE SPANISH MONOPOLY**

*No. 218—THE DEFEAT OF THE SPANISH ARMADA*

*(Richard Hakluyt, The Principal Navigations, Voyages Traffiques and Discoveries of the English Nation, London, 1599)\**

The Spanish King having with small fruit and commodity, for about twenty years together, waged war against the Netherlanders, after deliberation with his counsellors thereabout, thought it most convenient to assault them once again by sea, which had been attempted sundry times heretofore, but not with forces sufficient. Unto the which expedition it stood him now in hand to join great puissance, as having the English people his professed enemies; whose Island is so situate, that it may either greatly help or hinder all such as sail into those parts. For which cause he thought good first of all to invade England, being persuaded by his Secretary Escovedo, and by divers other well experienced Spaniards and Dutchmen, and by many English fugitives, that the conquest of that Island was less difficult than the conquest of Holland and Zeeland. Moreover the Spaniards

*Op. cit.,* 1927 edition, London, Vol. II, pp. 370, 399—401.

were of opinion, that it would be far more behoveful  for
their King to conquer England and the Low Countries all at
once, than to be constrained continually to maintain a warlike Navy to defend his East and West India Fleets,  from
the English Drake, and from such like valiant enemies....
    For the perpetual memory of this matter, the Zeeland-
ers caused new coin of silver and brass to be stamped: which
on the one side contained the  arms of Zeeland,  with this
inscription :  GLORY TO GOD ONLY :  and on the other
side, the pictures of certain great ships, with these words :
THE SPANISH FLEET :  and in the circumference about the
ships :  IT CAME, WENT, AND WAS. Anno 1588.  That
is to say, the Spanish fleet came, went, and was vanquished
this year; for which, glory be given to God only.
    Likewise they coined another kind of money; upon the
one side whereof was represented a ship fleeing, and a ship
sinking: on the other side four men making prayers  and
giving thanks unto God upon their knees; with this sentence: Man purposeth; God disposeth.  1588.  Also, for the
lasting memory of the same matter, they have stamped in
Holland divers such like coins, according to the custom of
the ancient Romans.
    While this wonderful and puissant navy was sailing along
the English coasts, and all men did now plainly see and hear
that which before they would not be persuaded of, all people throughout England prostrated themselves with humble
prayers and supplications unto God: but especially the outlandish  Churches (who  had greatest  cause to fear, and
against whom by name the Spaniards had threatened  most
grievous torments) enjoined to their people continual fast-
ings and supplications, that they might turn away God's
wrath and fury now imminent upon them for their sins :
knowing right well, that prayer was the only refuge against
all enemies, calamities, and necessities, and that it was the
only solace and relief for mankind, being visited with afflic-
tion and misery. Likewise such solemn days of supplica-
tion were observed throughout the United Provinces.
    Also a while after the Spanish Fleet was departed, there
was in England, by the commandment of Her Majesty, and
in the United Provinces, by the direction of the States,  a
solemn festival day publicly appointed, wherein all persons
were enjoined to resort unto the Church, and there to render
thanks and praises unto God: and the preachers were commanded  to exhort  the people  thereunto.  The foresaid
solemnity was observed upon the 29 of November;  which
day was wholly spent in fasting,  prayer,  and  giving  of
thanks.
    Likewise, the Queen's Majesty herself, imitating  the
ancient Romans, rode into London in triumph, in regard of

her own and her subjects' glorious deliverance. For being attended upon very solemnly by all the principal estates and officers of her Realm, she was carried through her said City of London in a triumphant chariot, and in robes of triumph, from her Palace unto the Cathedral Church of Saint Paul, out of which the ensigns and colours of the vanquished Spaniards hung displayed. And all the Citizens of London in their liveries stood on either side of the street, by their several Companies, with their ensigns and banners: and the streets were hanged on both sides with blue cloth, which, together with the foresaid banners, yielded a very stately and gallant prospect. Her Majesty being entered into the Church, together with her Clergy and Nobles gave thanks unto God, and caused a public sermon to be preached before her at Paul's cross; wherein none other argument was handled, but that praise, honour, and glory might be rendered unto God, and that God's name might be extolled by thanksgiving. And with her own princely voice she most Christianly exhorted the people to do the same: whereupon the people with a loud acclamation wished her a most long and happy life, to the confusion of her foes.

Thus the magnificent, huge, and mighty fleet of the Spaniards (which themselves termed in all places invincible) such as sailed not upon the Ocean sea many hundred years before, in the year 1588 vanished into smoke; to the great confusion and discouragement of the authors thereof.

---

### No. 219 — THE CORSAIRS ATTACK WITH UTTER IMPUNITY

*(Juan de Texeda to Philip II. King of Spain, Havana, August 24, 1590)\**

This coast has been so overrun with corsairs, sailing in pairs and in quartets, that not a vessel left this port that it was not immediately captured. In view of this situation the generals of the fleets and armada which Your Majesty has here, and I also, agreed to make ready four ships which were lying here using up provisions to no profit, and to send them out to clean the coast. They went and fond nothing because the season is far advanced and the enemy had disembogued....

The galleys on patrol duty here have had little effect, yet they are as good as the best Your Majesty has today in Italy, which to me seems a pity and I have desired many times to take them in hand to see whether I might have

*Cited in Wright, *Further English Voyages to Spanish America*, Document No. 76, pp. 260—261.

better luck in meeting the enemy than they have had on
occasions when they have gone out....

The reason the galleys have accomplished nothing this
year, so many enemy ships having meanwhile sailed by the
entrance to this port, is because they are so restricted by the
order Your Majesty has issued to me that they must await
the passing of the fleets at Cape San Antonio. The enemy is
perfectly aware of this order and so with utter  impunity
frequents this coast, merely avoiding Cape San Antonio,
which they know is the place where the galleys are usually
lying.   Therefore I entreat Your Majesty to leave it to my
discretion to send the galleys wherever they can do most
damage to the enemy, even though it be only to try   out
their worth and report whether they should be maintained
here or not.   I would prefer to see four frigates of the armada detailed to protect this coast. They would cost less
and could go out in any weather....

## No. 220—POUR ENCOURAGER LES AUTRES

*(Antonio Navarro, Captain General of the New Spain*
*Fleet, to the House of Trade, October 12, 1591)\**

At the end of that time Agustin de Paz and Ygararan
and many other persons came into Havana in a boat with
the news that the corsairs had taken them and seven other
ships of the Santo Domingo fleet and had steered for England, having given them that boat in which to come to
Havana.

Forthwith I arrested Juan Gayon, pilot,  for having
steered off his course simply because he chose to do so.
I prosecuted him and, by a judge from Mexico called Dr.
Farfan and by the lieutenant governor of Havana,  he was
sentenced to public disgrace and ten years on the rowers'
bench in the galleys, loss of goods and privation of office.
I assure your lordship that if they had not taken the case out
of my jurisdiction I'd have hanged him.   I granted his appeal
that your lordship may do so, for if these things are tolerated,
as they have been hitherto, the great damage arising there-
from will much increase hence forward.

## No. 221 — SPAIN'S MANPOWER SHORTAGE

*(Antonio de Berrio to Philip II, King of Spain, July 27,*
*1592)\*\**

God alone knows how urgent it is to settle these large
provinces, may He help me to serve Your Majesty; the men

\*\*Cited in Wright, *Further English Voyages to Spanish America*, Document
No. 86, pp. 274—275.
\*\*Cited in The Trinidad Historical Society, Publication No. 14, p. 1.

who I have in the Island of Trinidad have prevented four English ships from trading with the Indians and from taking water and other supplies and making lanchas as they are accustomed to do then going along and raiding Tierra Firme; my people made an ambush, killing two and taking one alive from whom was taken a deposition which with the report of this affair is sent so that Your Majesty may understand how urgent it is that the Island should be settled.

---

## No. 222 — CARIBS WITHIN, CORSAIRS WITHOUT

### (Antonio de Berrio to Philip II, King of Spain, November 24, 1593)*

This Island of Trinidad is one of the best and largest in this district with circumference of more than 120 leagues and many Indians, a very fruitful land not more than four leagues from the mouth of the Orinoco; and the distance along the south coast and through the bocas which is where the ships pass, both of friends and enemies, is more than 40 leagues and quite smooth sea in all the places where vessels anchor and here there are usually found English ships which I have attacked always doing damage to them, killing men and taking prisoners and after four months there I found two English ships trading for tobacco with the Indians against which I at once went forth and took a Captain and five other prisoners for whom as a ransom I got a quantity of powder and lead, muskets and arquebuses of which there was great need because all the Governors nearby have been annoyed at my discovery of these provinces and none of them have allowed me to buy anything in their territories.

Besides these Englishmen whom I loathe and always injure, I am surrounded by Caribs who have tried to destroy this Island and have eaten a great number of Indians and since I have been here we have lost eleven Spaniards killed in two attacks and more than 100 Indians who with the few men we have, were sent with Domingo de Vera to attack them in their own lands where they found four pirogues on the point of starting, these Caribs were all killed and none escaped; but they are so many and so wide spread and I have so few people and so little help that I cannot do what I want.

It would be easy for Your Majesty to deal with these Caribs if your ministers wished without buying or sending anything at your cost or disturbing the mind of Your Majes-

*Cited in The Trinidad Historical Society, Publication No. 18, pp. 2—3.

ty; in Puerto Rico, Your Majesty keeps 400 paid soldiers and round about it are La Dominica, La Granada, Santa Lucia and many other settlements of Caribs who each year go forth with their fleets for their cannibal feast; and these soldiers have no orders from Your Majesty save only to guard the fort and draw their pay.

I have only 70 men, yet in this Island are more than 6,000 war Indians, the major part of them by no means peaceable; the greater part of the time my men are patrolling the sea for the security of our coast and to see what is happening; and none of the Governors nearby will allow me to recruit men in their district and this Island must be settled before settling the large provinces which I have discovered and for this I lack the remedy unless Your Majesty sends me from Seville some men and an express and precise cedula ordering the Governor of Puerto Rico to send me from the 400 men kept idle there, a hundred so that with those and the men which I have, I hope to patrol the coast and protect this Island and go to conquer and settle that which has cost me already so much.

Furthermore I beseech Your Majesty for the love of God be pleased to order them in Puerto Rico to give me 20 quintals of powder and an equal weight of lead and six culverins of those now unused in the fort each a quintal and a half and fifty muskets so that I may pursue the settlement of this Island of such importance to Your Majesty and to obstruct the Corsairs and the Caribs and prevent them doing harm to the human race and this is necessary for the conquest with which Your Majesty has charged me so much so that in truth without settling this Island it is not possible to settle the provinces which I have discovered.

---

## No. 223 — THE ENGLISH CAPTURE OF PUERTO RICO

*(Francesco Soranzo, Venetian Ambassador in France, October 24, 1598)*\*

The Earl of Cumberland has reached Spanish Isle in the West Indies, and has made a rich booty. He captured, by force of arms, St. John of Porto Rico, though at a heavy loss in men. This was a plan designed by Drake, but interrupted by his death. In England they are manning many ships to send them in that direction. If this be true it cannot fail to greatly injure the King of Spain. The Count of Freyra has put out from Portugal with a view to fighting the Earl of Cumberland.

*Cited in A. Morales Carrion, *Puerto Rico and the Non-Hispanic Caribbean: A Study in the Decline of Spanish Exclusivism*, University of Puerto Rico Press, 1952, p. 28, footnote.

## No. 224 — THE INFLUENCE OF SEA POWER ON WEST INDIAN HISTORY

*(Don Juan Malaonado Barnuevo to King of Spain, November 12, 1604)\**

....I should not be fulfilling the duty which I owe to your Majesty.... if I did not state in very plain truths the dangerous condition in which the affairs of the Indies now are....and the urgent necessity there is of coming to the help thereof. And, therefore, beginning the matter further back, I declare, Sire, that although the saying that whoever becomes master of the sea will also be master of the land, a very ancient proverb confirmed by all the great Councillors of State of our times, may be a general one and may refer to all the Kings and Potentates of the world it can only now, it seems, be said to refer to Your Majesty. Because leaving aside the Mediterranean Sea, which, though the same argument applies to it, does not at present concern our subject, and coming to the ocean, which is that of which we have more particularly to treat, if we run over the kingdoms and provinces which extend along its coasts, we shall find that of the Kings of France and England, and those of Denmark and Sweden, the Islands of Holland and Zealand, and the other free cities on the north, the one that has the most coast–line to guard has little more than 100 leagues, and in all cases the Provinces are so inaccessible, owing to the many shoals, sandbanks, and currents that they require no other defence. Your Majesty is the only one to whom God has been pleased to grant so many and such great kingdoms and lordships, and therein so many thousands of leagues of coasts to guard, that all your power and greatness is required for their defence. And considering that in the extremity of the east Your Majesty possesses the East Indies, and in the West the West Indies of Castille (for to be in the Philippines amounts to being very near the East Indies and almost completes the circuit of the world): on the north the defence and protection of the States of Flanders is to be provided for, and on the south all that extends beyond the Equator both in the North Sea and in the South Sea as far as the Straits of Magellan or very near them, besides an infinity of islands which Your Majesty possesses in all these seas, which, although they may be considered an accessory as compared with the mainland, would nevertheless make other Kings rich and powerful, and which as an appendage of your Crown and estate Your Majesty has under your protection: it is hardly possible to effect this union of so many kingdoms and their mutual support for preservation

*\*Cited in British Guiana Boundary. Arbitration with the United States of Venezuela. Appendix to the Counter Case on behalf of the Government of Her Britannic Majesty, London, 1898, pp. 1—6.*

and defence on account of their being so many thousands
of leagues apart, unless the seas are bridged by a great and
powerful fleet, which by being mistress of the seas, may
secure the coasts and free passage for all your Majesty's
subjects who sail from one Province to another in pursuit
of their trade and commerce.

This it was necessary for your Majesty to hold ready
and maintain when all the world was in profound peace and
tranquillity, without there being in England, France, or the
whole of the North, one ship of war....

Now, Sire, the times are different, and all is so changed,
and the enemies of your Majesty have continued making
themselves so powerful, and acquiring so much strength,
that it has now become very imperative that as there was
formerly a fleet, but not a large one, there should now be
a great one, and that it should be constantly increased and
strengthened in proportion to the enemies, so that in any
event your Majesty must be superior and master of the sea
....while in the time of the Emperor Charles V, grandfather
of your Majesty, of glorious memory, the most bitter wars
between Spain and France were in Lombardy and the State
of Milan, from this time forward they will be those which
your Majesty may have with the whole of the north by sea,
and this is to be our field of battle.   The reason of this
is the greatness of the Indies and the great quantity of gold
and silver, pearls and emeralds, and numerous products
which come from them every year.   This being what enriches
these kingdoms, and the source from which your Majesty
derives a large portion of your greatness, and the quantity
of money by which your armies are maintained, from the
moment of their discovery, and when they began to be conquered, the Indies have been envied and coveted by the
enemies of your Majesty.   But as there has not been anyone
who has had strength or means to attack them up to now, it
has all been limited to robbers and corsairs, who, at one time,
in different ports of the sea, lying in wait for the ships that
come separately, apart from fleets and "Armadas," and at
another trading and raiding on the same coasts, have become
rich at the expense of your Majesty and your subjects.   And
if so far they have been satisfied therewith because their
power was not equal to more, from now forward, on finding
themselves with greater forces, they will attempt more, not
only against the fleets which bring and carry the produce,
but even against the galleons of the "Armada" which bring
the gold and silver. And if they should succeed in this,
even in the case of a single galleon, they will not stop until
they attack the country itself, and try to make themselves
masters of it.

....I say, Sire, that up to now this vineyard has been

preserved solely through fear, because the reputation and greatness of your Majesty, and the belief of the world that kingdoms so important, and belonging to a King so powerful, must naturally be well defended, together with the fact that the distance is so great that immense difficulties would be encountered in sending great fleets thither, has been the cause why nobody has undertaken this expedition with the object of setting foot in the country, or preserving whatever he might acquire. But now things are quite altered, and are being changed to a very different state, since the enemies are taking a different course, for as the Dutch are now deprived of the trade in salt, which they had in Castile and Portugal, a class of merchandize without which they cannot live, and of that of the spices which they had in Portugal, they have been necessarily obliged to seek a remedy in other parts. Consequently they have betaken themselves to India in search of the spices; and have gone for the salt to the Indies of Castile to Point Araya where there is an immense quantity of it, and they take what they require for themselves and for sale in Germany.

From this beginning and first enterprise, which unless stopped, might well cause much loss, it has resulted that they are extending themselves along the coast of Terra Firma, where, in Margarita and in Cumana, and the coast of Venezuela, Rio de la Hacha and Santa Marta, they have been trading and exchanging their merchandise for pearls and other products of the country, and in like manner on the north side of Santo Domingo, and on the south side of Cuba, where they have found very great profit. This is increasing to such an extent that, as your Majesty will have learned from the reports of the Governors and other Ministers of your Majesty in those provinces, the number of ships and pilot boats which are generally there exceeds 100, and they are spread over different parts of those provinces, where they are better received by the inhabitants than they should be. Even now there is a report that there are some Dutch settling in the bay of Caros on the coast of Florida, which, were it the worst port of the Indies, would be highly inconvenient; so it is clearly evident that they must have surveyed the land and the sea, the ports and their entrances and outlets, so that it may be feared that they are marking with soap, as tailors do, so that they may cut and guide the scissors when furnished with power and means to undertake it.

....I therefore say, Sire, that taking the entry to the Indies from the first settlement thereby going from Spain along the coast of Terra Firma, namely the Island of Trinidad, passing by Margarita along the coast of Venezuela to Carthagena, and from there along that of Veragua, Hon—

duras, and Compeachy to the coast of new Spain, and afterwards that of Florida to the Martyrs Head and Channel of
the Bahamas drawing up in the port of Saint Augustjne,
which is the last settlement nearest to Spain on the north
side, Your Majesty will find that all this territory has a
coast line of more than 1,200 leagues; then the four principal
Windward Islands, namely Puerto Rico, Santo Domingo, Cuba
and Jamaica, have more than 600, in all making more than
1,800 leagues of coast, which Your Majesty possesses and
must protect, for there are many who covet them. In all
these Your Majesty possesses six fortresses, namely Carthagena, Puerto Rico, Portobelo, San Juan de Ulloa, Havana,
and Florida. Each of these only guards its own territory and
jurisdiction, without being able to help another, nor in any
case can men be drawn from them for any other parts, consequently the whole of the rest of the line, which covers
nearly the number of leagues I have stated, remains without
a fortress or a strong house, or even a soldier to guard it;
nor is there any other defence than the strength, or more
correctly the weakness of its residents, who, on seeing a ship-
of-war, fly with their clothes or effects to the woods, for
the sea coast defence is so abandoned that there is not, in all
the Indies, an armed cutter to guard them. Nor can the
galleons be reckoned on, as they go direct to load their
silver, and, when they are bringing it, even should they
encounter the enemies right before them, they must not
fight, nor is it right that they should do so.

So much for the weakness of that land and its being
in such a defenceless state, as has been set forth in this
account. As regards the advantage the enemies would have,
should they attempt to plant themselves therein, there is the
fact of their having so many coasts and ports in which they
may enter without finding anyone to hinder them. And
as, wherever they enter, the Spaniards will be very few, and
the Negroes, half-breeds, and mulattoes very numerous, it
will be the easiest thing for them to bring all those people
into their service, as they are all men without reflection and
lovers of novelty. The Negroes and Mulattoes long for
liberty, and they grant them that. The Indians and half-
breeds are all abandoned people, and as to their being
Christians and frequenting the churches and sacraments, —
most of them do so more from force than from duty, being
compelled by those who govern them, and by the clergy who
go to instruct them. Therefore upon anyone entering among
them and granting and preaching liberty of life and freedom
of conscience to whoever does not possess them, it is easy
to believe that they will accommodate themelves more
readily to live with them than with us.

To this must be added profit which, among these people,

and even among others more advanced in civilisation, has great influence. And as the Dutch go among them giving three yards of Rouen print and other cotton stuffs, where the Spanish merchant only gives them one, and buying the products of the land, and all the merchandise they have for sale, at double the price paid or current in the country, they will prefer their trade and traffic to that of Spain as we see they now do with the English, French and Flemish. For, although Your Majesty has commanded judges to go from these kingdoms, solely to punish with the greatest rigour, and prevent the bartering, and ordered your Audiencias and Governors to take extraordinary measures, it has not only been impossible to prevent it, but it has rather daily gone on increasing by the people trading with the foreigners and admitting them in the most familiar way into their houses and cattle farms, where they deliver the hides to them. And it may very well be feared that they will do this better and with more pleasure if they have them in their houses, and still more when they see them with so much force, and so powerful that they may not fear any punishment, but may expect a reward. To all these advantages is to be added the force of ships and mariners existing today in Holland and Zealand, for there are more than 2,000 ships of the mercantile marine in those provinces at a low estimate; and all manned with a sufficient number of sailors, for they are always engaged in navigation, as in this class of people these islands are most abundant. And although it be true that these are ships of the mercantile marine, it is a very easy thing to convert them in such a way that they may form a fleet of warships, for by unloading their cargoes and lading them with powder and ball it is done. For we well know that there is no want of artillery and all kinds of munitions among them.    ,

If, then, it be true that in these islands, which are today in rebellion against Your Majesty, and are enemies of your Crown, there is such a force and number of ships and mariners, and war material, and that where it is a question of the conquest of the Indies, so much desired by them, there would be no peace with either France or England which would suffice to restrain those Kings from assisting now secretly and now openly, each striving to get his share, and as the advantages that both would have in the Indies for the attainment of their ends are those which I have pointed out, it will be right, that Your Majesty should endeavour to foresee events, and so arrange the matter that the designs, thoughts and wishes of your enemies may be frustrated on seeing Your Majesty master of the sea, and with so great a force and power therein, that you are able to go with your "Armadas" not only to the defence of any part of your kingdoms they might desire to attack, but even to enter those of your enemies, whenever it shall please you, then each must then look to the defence of his own house and remain within the limits of his kingdom without troubling those of your Majesty....one absolute necessity is wanting which requires special attention, namely, rapid execution, and taking in hand whatever be agreed upon with the greatest despatch, for the enemies are not asleep, nor are they wont to give a long time for consideration, but rather the contrary — very few hours. And these last years there have been, and even today there are more than 100 Dutch ships in the Indies, and if a little force be added, they might, far quicker than imagined, be able to effect some great undertaking. That which could now, with little cost, be stopped, might afterwards need a great deal; and as maritime affairs such as levies of mariners and building and fitting out of fleets are naturally vast and lengthy, and even if these kingdoms contained abundance of everything necessary it could only be done with great difficulty, and with very long delays, it is necessary now to take it in hand vigorously, employing extraordinary means and measures, so that this end may be attained with the quickest despatch.

## No. 225 — THE WEAKNESS OF SPAIN

*(Sir Thomas Roe to Earl of Salisbury, Lord High Treasurer of England, Trinidad, February 28, 1611)\**

The Spaniards here are equally proud, insolent yet needy and weak; their force is reputation and their safety opinion....

## No. 226 — THE CONTRABAND TOBACCO TRADE OF TRINIDAD

*(Council of the Indies to Philip III, King of Spain, May 15, 1611)\*\**

Don Alonzo de Velasco, Ambassador in England, reports on the trade that the English carry on with Trinidad.

Quite lately three ships have arrived in England with tobacco from Trinidad and the least was valued at five hundred thousand ducats.

At the time there were preparing in London four ships for the trade at Trinidad. The Governor of that Island should be punished.

*Cited in The Trinidad Historical Society, Publication No. 98, p. 2.
**Cited in The Trinidad Historical Society, Publication No. 115.

## No. 227 — PROPOSAL TO BAN TOBACCO CULTIVATION IN TRINIDAD

(Bernardo de Vargas Machuca, Governor of Margarita, to King of Spain, August 16, 1612)*

He reports that while it is true that the ports of the Island of Trinidad and the Province of Guayana are closed yet the English and Dutch ships persist in going and trading there. Since the galleons had visited, about ten or eleven ships had visited.

He recommends that the sowing of tobacco be prohibited in the Island of Trinidad so that the enemy will find nothing to obtain and give up this trade and so no longer go there. In consequence the pearl fisheries of Margarita would be relieved from these raiders.

## No. 228 — THE DESTITUTION OF THE COLONIES

(Juan, Bishop of Puerto Rico, to Philip IV, King of Spain, February 23, 1634)**

I found its inhabitants who do not now exceed forty, poor and destitute through loss of their trade in tobacco and produce by which they were supported, and through no register ship having come to them from Spain for more than two years. Considering your Majesty's service, I find, among others, two very powerful reasons for which your Majesty may be pleased to favour this settlement: first on account of the attention and care which the Dutch pay to it, who are now settled close to this great river Orinoco in three rivers adjoining it, namely the river Berbice, Corentine and Essequibo, and if, the few residents could not protect the ascent up the river against the enemy the Provinces of Peru would not be safe; for 300 leagues up the river one reaches the New Kingdom of Granada. The other reason is that in the old town a very great quantity of quicksilver is found, and descending the river the residents succeed in collecting it, for it comes down to the shore from a great cliff. Being such a useful thing for working the mines, it might be discovered at very slight cost by a person acquainted with this subject; and I have seen with my own eyes a certain quantity among the residents. Likewise in the visitation I am making of this Island of Trinidad I find that it is very fertile and better ground for some produce than that of Puerto Rico, but twenty-six residents are keeping in subjection 4,000 warlike Indians who are in this island; and

* Cited in The Trinidad Historical Society, Publication No. 149.
**Cited in British Guiana Boundary. Arbitration with the United States of Venezuela. Appendix to the Counter Case on behalf of the Government of Her Britannic Majesty, London, 1898, p. 10.

if your Majesty be pleased to grant leave for twenty-five families of married people to come and settle it, the profit and improvement thereof will be quickly shown; likewise, at twelve leagues distance lies the island of Tobago peopled with many Dutch.

## No. 229 — THE KING OF SPAIN LOSES HIS TEMPER

### (Memorandum of Philip IV, King of Spain, on a Report from the House of Trade, January 23, 1638)*

You make reproaches about the money I have used as though I had taken yours or some private person's without compensation or as if I had ordered it to be taken for the purpose of making presents to certain people or as though if I had not taken it, a great portion of the State of Milan and of Flanders with the whole of Burgundy would not now have been lost, so you may see with what slight reason you advise repeatedly on this matter.

If the trade would voluntarily pay one per cent. or two or had been made to pay for the public cause on any of the many occasions on which I have so ordered, there would have been a totally different result and what has happened and is feared, would never have occurred, nor would so tardy a remedy as a visit by the ships of the Brazil route be proposed for they can only be a very small fleet and cannot arrive for four months nor can they alone effect anything of importance against those who may have taken possession over there.

What might be done is to send direct at once to the Island of Trinidad, in tenders and caravels or light vessels, 200 men with munitions and clothing and some provisions for the people there and a couple of good soldiers as leaders to ensure success and when this assistance has been despatched as I have resolved, this matter can be discussed to some purpose and on a firm basis.

## (v)—THE ESTABLISHMENT OF NON-SPANISH COLONIES IN THE CARIBBEAN

### No. 230 — EL DORADO

### (Sir Walter Raleigh, The Discovery of the large, rich, and beautiful Empire of Guiana, 1595)**

The country hath more quantity of gold, by manifold, than the best parts of the Indies, or Peru. All the most of the kings of the borders are already become Her Majesty's vassals, and seem to desire nothing more than Her Majesty's

*Cited in The Trinidad Historical Society, Publication No. 138, p. 2.
**Cited in Harvard Classics, de luxe edition, Vol. 33, p. 328.

protection and the return of the English nation.  It hath
another ground and assurance of riches and glory than the
voyage of the West Indies; an easier way to invade the best
parts thereof than by the common course....

But I hope it shall appear that there is a way found to
answer every man's longing; a better Indies for Her Majesty
than the King of Spain hath any....

But, if we now consider of the actions both of Charles
the Fifth, who had the maidenhead of Peru and the abundant treasures of Atabalipa, together with the affairs of the
Spanish king now living, what territories he hath purchased,
what he hath added to the acts of his predecessors, how many
kingdoms he hath endangered, how many armies, garrisons,
and navies he hath, and doth  maintain, the great  losses
which he hath repaired, as in eighty-eight above an hundred
sail of great ships with their artillery, and that no year is
less unfortunate, but that many vessels, treasures, and
people are devoured, and yet notwithstanding he beginneth
again like a storm to threaten shipwreck to us all; we shall
find that these abilities rise not from the trades of sacks and
Seville oranges, nor from aught else that, either Spain, Portugal, or any of his other provinces produce; it is his Indian
gold that  endangereth and disturbeth  all the nations  of
Europe....

Where  there is store  of gold  it is in effect  need-
less to remember other commodities for trade.  But it hath
....great  quantities  of  brazil-wood....All  places  yield
abundance of cotton, of silk....  The soil besides is so excellent, and so full of rivers, as it will carry sugar, ginger, and
all those other commodities which the West Indies have....

To conclude, Guiana  is a country that hath yet  her
maidenhead never sacked, turned, nor wrought; the face of
the earth  hath not been torn, nor the virtue and salt of the
soil spent by manurance.  The graves have not been opened
for gold, the mines not broken with sledges, nor their images
pulled down out of their temples....

....after the first or second year I doubt not but to see
in London a Contractation House* of more receipt for
Guiana than there is now in Seville for the West Indies....

....whatsoever prince shall possess it, shall be greatest;
and if the king of Spain enjoy it, he will become unresistible.

---

No. 231—TO SUPPLANT SPAIN IN THE WEST INDIES
(Sir Benjamin Rudyerd, Speech in the House of Commons,
March 17, 1623) **

Now, let us a little consider the enemy we are to encounter, the  King of Spain.  They are not his great terri-

* The reference is to the Casa de  Contratacion, or House of Trade.
**Cited in Stock, op. cit., Vol. I, p. 62.

tories which make him so powerful, and so troublesome to
all Christendom. For it is very well known, that Spain itself is but, weak in men, and barren of natural commodities.
As for his other territories, they lie divided and asunder,
which is a weakness in its self; besides, they are held by
force, and maintained at an extraordinary charge. Insomuch, as although he be a great king, yet he is like that
great giant, who was said to have 100 hands, but he had 50
bellies to feed, so that ratably, he had no more hands than
another man.

No sir, they are his mines in the West Indies, which
minister fuel to feed his vast ambitious desire of universal
monarchy: it is the money he hath from thence, which
makes him able to levy, and pay soldiers in all places; and
to keep an army continually on foot, ready to invade and
endanger his neighbours.

So that we have no other way, but to endeavour to cut
him up at root, and seek to impeach, or to supplant him in
the West Indies.

---

## No. 232 — THE FIRST FRENCH WEST INDIAN COLONY

*(Commission given by Cardinal de Richelieu to the Sieurs
d'Enambuc and du Rossey, for the establishment of a Colony
in the West Indies, October 21, 1626)\**

Be it known that Sieurs d'Enambuc and du Rossey
....with the permission of the King and Admiral of France,
have for fifteen years spent vast sums on the crews and
armour of ships and vessels in search of fertile lands in a
good climate which may be taken possession of and settled
by Frenchmen. They have been so active that some time
ago they discovered the islands of St. Christopher and Bar-
bádos....and other neighbouring islands all situated at the
entrance to Peru....forming part of the West Indies, which
do not belong to any Christian King or Prince. They
landed and stayed for one year....The climate is mild and
temperate, and the soil fertile and productive, yielding
many useful commodities....They even learned from the
native Indian inhabitants of the islands that there are some
gold and silver mines, which would have been sufficient
reason for numbers of Frenchmen to settle the islands and
instruct the inhabitants in the Apostolic and Roman Catholic
religion, and to plant the Christian Faith there to the glory
of God and the honour of the King....Wishing to spread the
Catholic Faith and to establish as much trade and commerce
as possible, and considering that the inhabitants of the
\*Cited in Moreau de Saint-Mery, *Loix et Constitutions des Colonies Francoises
de l'Amerique sous le Vent*, Paris, n.d., Tome I, 1550—1703, pp. 20—21.

islands are not friendly people, we have given Sieurs
d'Enambuc and du Rossey exclusive rights to settle the
islands of St. Christopher and Barbados and the surrounding islands. They are to fortify the islands, and carry over
a number of priests who are to instruct the Indian inhabitants in the Apostolic and Roman Catholic religion, say
Mass and administer the Sacraments. They shall take the
necessary steps for cultivating the land, and working all
mines and metals, subject to payment of one-tenth of the
profits....for the space of twenty years. They are charged
to bring the islands under the King's authority and reduce
the inhabitants to obedience to Your Majesty. For this
purpose they shall get ready and put in a state of defence
as many vessels, ships and boats as may be necessary, and
equip them with the necessary men, cannon, supplies and
ammunition for the voyages....These vessels are to leave
from Havre-de-Grace and Port Saint-Louis in Brittany,
where they must declare the number of vessels....They
must obey and see that their crew obey the Navy ordinances
and return with the ships to Havre-de-Grace.

---

## No. 233—RELIGION AND THE RISE OF BRITISH IMPERIALISM IN THE WEST INDIES

*(John Pym, Speech in the House of Commons,
April 17, 1640)\**

The differences and discontents betwixt his Majesty and
the people at home have in all likelihood diverted his royal
thoughts and counsels from those great opportunities which
he might have, not only to weaken the House of Austria and
to restore the Palatinate, but to gain a higher pitch of power
and greatness than any of his ancestors; for it is not unknown how weak, how distracted, how discontented the
Spanish colonies are in the West Indies. There are now in
those parts, in New England, Virginia, and the Carib Islands,
and in the Bermudos, at least sixty thousand able persons
of this nation, many of them well armed, and their bodies
seasoned to that climate, which, with a very small charge,
might be set down in some advantageous parts of these
pleasant, rich, and fruitful countries, and easily make his
Majesty master of all that treasure, which not only foments
the war but is the great support of Popery in all parts of
Christendom.

*Cited in Stock, *op. cit.*, Vol. I, p. 96.

## No. 234—THE END OF THE PAPAL DONATION

*(A Treaty of Peace between Philip IV, King of Spain, and the United Provinces of the Low Countries. Made at Munster, January 30, 1648)\**

V.    The navigation and trade of the East and West Indies shall be maintained according to and in conformity with the charters given, or hereafter to be given therefor; for the security of which the present treaty and its ratification, to be procured from both sides, shall serve.    And there shall be comprised under the above-mentioned treaty all potentates, nations and peoples with whom the said Lord States, or those of the Company of the East and West Indies in their name, are, within the limits of their said charters, in friendship and alliance, and each party, to wit, the above-mentioned Lords, the King and States respectively shall remain  in possession of and  enjoy such lordships,  towns, castles, fortresses, commerce and lands in the East and West Indies as also in Brazil and on the coasts of Asia, Africa, and America respectively as the above-mentioned Lords,  the King and States   respectively hold  and possess,  herein especially included the localities and places which the Portuguese have taken from the Lords States since the   year 1641 and occupied; including also the localities and  places which they, the Lord States, shall hereafter, without infraction of the present  treaty, come to conquer and  possess. And the Directors of the Company, both of the East and West Indies, of the United Provinces, as also the agents, officers high and low, soldiers and sailors being in the actual service of one or the other of said companies or having been in their service, as also those who (being) out of their  respective services, still remain or may hereafter be employed either in this country or in the district of the said two companies, shall be and  remain free and unmolested in all  countries being under the dominion of the said Lord King of Europe, and shall be permitted to travel, trade and frequent, like all other inhabitants of the countries of the said Lord States....

VI.    And as to the West Indies, the subjects and inhabitants of the kingdoms, provinces and lands of the  said Lords the King and States respectively, shall forbear sailing to, and trading in any of the harbours, localities and places, forts, lodgments or castles, and all others possessed by the one or the other Party, viz: the subjects of the said Lord the King shall not sail to, or trade in those held by the said Lords the States, nor the subjects of the said Lords  the States sail to or trade in those held by the said  Lord the

\*Cited in *British Guiana Boundary, Arbitration with the United States of Venezuela. Appendix to the Counter Case on behalf of the Government of Her Britannic Majesty,* London, 1898, pp. 351—352.

King. And among the places held by the said Lords the States shall be comprehended the places in Brazil which the Portuguese have taken from the States and occupied since the year 1641; as also all other places which they possess at present, so long as they shall continue in the hands of the said Portuguese, anything contained in the preceding Article notwithstanding.

---

*No. 235 — ENGLAND'S CLAIM TO A SHARE OF ADAM'S WILL*

*(Thomas Gage, The English-American, A New Survey of the West Indies, London, 1648, "Dedication to Sir Thomas Fairfax, Knight")* *

.... I offer a New World, to be the subject of your future pains, valour, and piety, beseeching your acceptance of this plain but faithful relation of mine, wherein Your Excellency, and by you the English Nation, shall see what wealth and honour they have lost by one of their narrow-hearted princes, who, living in peace and abounding in riches did notwithstanding reject the offer of being first discoverer of America, and left it unto Ferdinand of Aragon, who at the same time was wholly taken up by the wars in gaining of the city and kingdom of Granada from the Moors; being so impoverished thereby that he was compelled to borrow with some difficulty a few crowns of a very mean man to set forth Columbus upon so glorious an expedition. And yet, if time were closely followed at the heels, we are not so far behind but we may yet take him by the fore-top. To which purpose our plantations of the Barbados, St. Christophers, Nevis and the rest of the Caribbean Islands, have not only advanced our journey the better part of the way, but so inured our people to the clime of the Indies as they are the more enabled thereby to undertake any enterprise upon the firm land with greater facility. Neither is the difficulty of the attempt so great as many may imagine; for I dare be bold to affirm it knowingly that with the same pains and charge which they have been at in planting one of those petty islands they might have conquered so many great cities and large territories on the main continent as might very well merit the title of a kingdom. Our neighbours, the Hollanders, may be our example in this case; who whilst we have been driving a private trade from port to port, of which we are likely now to be deprived, have conquered so much land in the East and West Indies that it may be said of them, as of the Spaniards, *That the sun never sets upon their dominions.* And to meet with that

*Op. Cit., pp. 2—4.

objection by the way, *That the Spaniard being entitled to those countries, it were both unlawful and against all conscience to dispossess him thereof,* I anwer that (the Pope's donation excepted) I know no title he hath but, force, which by the same title and by a greater force may be repelled. And to bring in the title of first discovery, to me it seems as little reason that the sailing of a Spanish ship upon the coast of India should entitle the King of Spain to that country, as the sailing of an Indian or English ship upon the coast of Spain should entitle either the Indians or English unto the dominion thereof. No question but the just right or title to those countries appertains to the natives themselves, who, if they shall willingly and freely invite the English to their protection, what title soever they have in them no doubt but they may legally transfer it or communicate it to others. And to say that the inhuman butchery which the Indians did formerly commit in sacrificing of so many reasonable creatures to their wicked idols was a sufficient warrant for the Spaniards to divest them of their country, the same argument may by much better reason be enforced against the Spaniards themselves, who have sacrificed so many millions of Indians to the idol of their barbarous cruelty, that many populous islands and large territories upon the main continent are thereby at this day utterly uninhabited, as Bartholomeo de las Casas, the Spanish Bishop of Guaxaca in New Spain, hath by his writings in print sufficiently testified. But to end all disputes of this nature: since that God hath given the earth to the sons of men to inhabit, and that there are many vast countries in those parts not yet inhabited, either by Spaniard or Indian, why should my countrymen the English be debarred from making use of that which God from all beginning no question did ordain for the benefit of mankind? ....

---

## No. 236—CROMWELL'S WESTERN DESIGN

*("Instructions unto General Robert Venables given by His Highness by advice of his Council upon his Expedition to the West Indies," December 1654)\**

3.    The design in general is to gain an interest in that part of the West Indies in the possession of the Spaniard, for the effecting whereof We shall not tie you up to a method by any particular instructions, but only communicate to you what hath been under our consideration. Two or three ways have been thought of to that purpose.

*Cited in C. H. Firth (ed.), *The Narrative of General Venables*, London, 1900, pp. 112—114.

1st. The first is to land upon some of the Islands, and particularly Hispaniola, and St. John's Island,* one or both; the first of them hath no considerable place in the south part thereof but the City of Santo Domingo, and that not being considerably fortified may probably be possessed without much difficulty, which being done, and fortified, that whole Island will be brought under obedience; the chief place of St. John's Island is Porto Ricco.* The gaining of these Islands, or either of them, will as we conceive amongst many others have these advantages.

1st. Many English will come thither from other parts, and so those places become magazines of men and provisions for carrying on the design upon the Mainland.

2. They will be sure retreats upon all occasions.

3. They lie much to the windward of the rest of the K. of Spain's dominions, and being in the hand of the Spaniard will enable him to supply any part that is distressed on the main, and being in our hands will be of the same use to us.

4. From thence you may possibly after your landing there send force for the taking of the Havana, which lies in the Island of Cuba, which is the back door of the West Indies, and will obstruct the passing of the Spaniard's Plate Fleet into Europe, and the taking the Havana is so considerable that we have thoughts of beginning the first attempt upon that Fort and the Island of Cuba, and do still judge it worthy of consideration.

2. Another way we have had consideration of is, for the present to wave the Islands, and to make the first attempt upon the mainland, in one or more places between the River Orinoque and Porto Bello, aiming therein chiefly at Cartagena, which we would make the seat of the intended design, securing some places by the way thereto that the Spaniard might not be to the windward of us upon the mainland wherein if you have success, you will in all probability

1st Be master of the Spaniards' Treasure which comes from Peru by the way of Panama in the South sea to Porto Bello or Nombre de Dios in the North sea.

2. You will have houses ready built, a country ready planted, and most of the people Indians, who will submit to you, there being but few Spaniards there as is informed.

3. You will be able to put the country round about under contribution for the maintenance of the army, and therewith by the spoil and other ways probably make a great present return of profit to the Commonwealth.

There is a third consideration and that is mixed relating both to the Islands, and also to the mainland, which

**Today the island is known as Puerto Rico and the capital as San Juan.

is to make the first attempt upon Santo Domingo, or Porto Rico, one or both, and having secured them to go immediately to Carthagena, leaving that which is to the Windward of it to a farther opportunity, after you have secured and settled that City with what doth relate thereto, if God please to give that place into your hands.

These are the things which have been in debate here, and having let you know them We leave it to you, and the Commissioners aforesaid to be weighed upon the place, that after due consideration had amongst yourselves, and with such others as you shall think fit to advise with who have a particular knowledge of those parts, to take such resolutions concerning the making of the attempts, and the managing and carrying on this whole Design, as to you and the said Commissioners, or any two of them, shall seem most effectual, either by the way aforesaid, or such others as shall be judged more reasonable, and for the better enabling you to execute such resolutions as shall be taken in the premises, you are hereby authorised and required to use your best endeavours, wherein Gen. Penn Commander in Chief of the Fleet is by Us required to join with and assist you with the Fleet and sea forces as often as there shall be occasion to land your men upon the territories, dominions, and places belonging unto, in the possession of or claimed by the Spaniards in America, and to surprise their forts, take or beat down their castles and places of strength, and to pursue, kill and destroy by all means whatsoever all those who shall oppose or resist you therein, and also to seize upon all ships and vessels which you find in any of their harbours, and also upon all such goods as you shall find upon the land. . . .

5. In case it shall please God to give you success, such places as you shall take and shall judge fit to be kept, you shall keep for the use of Us and this Commonwealth, and shall also cause such goods and prizes as shall be taken to be delivered into the hands of the said Commissioners, that so they may be brought to a just and true account for the public advantage.

No. 237 — THE WESTERN DESIGN: THE INTELLECTUAL JUSTIFICATION

(Oliver Cromwell, Protector of England, Commission of the Commissioners for the West Indian Expedition, December 9, 1654)*

Oliver, Lord Protector of the Common Wealth of England, Scotland, and Ireland, and the Dominions thereto belonging. To our right trusty and wellbeloved General Robert Venables and General William Penn, and to our Trusty and beloved

*Cited in Firth, op. cit., pp. 149—161.

Edward Winslowe Esqr., Daniel Searle Esqr. Governor of our Island of Barbados, Gregory Butler Esqr. Greeting, We having taken into our serious consideration the state and condition of the English Plantations and Colonies in the Western part of the World called America, and the opportunity and means which God hath betrusted us and this Common Wealth with, both for the securing the interest we already have in those countries, which now lie open and exposed to the will and power of the King of Spain (who claims the same by colour of a Donation of the Pope) at any time when he shall have leisure to look that way; and also for getting ground and gaining upon the dominions and territories of the said King there.

Whereunto We also hold our self obliged in justice to the people of these nations for the cruelties, wrongs, and injuries done and exercised upon them by the Spaniards in those parts. Having a respect likewise in this our undertaking to the miserable thraldom and bondage, both spiritual and civil, which the natives and others in the dominions of the said King in America are subjected to and lie under by means of the Popish and cruel Inquisition and otherwise, from which if it shall please God to make us instrumental in any measure to deliver them, and upon this occasion to make way for the bringing in the light of the Gospel and power of true religion and godliness into those parts, We shall esteem it the best and most glorious part of any success or acquisition it shall please God to bless us with. And We having upon these and other considerations raised and set forth land and sea forces to send into the parts aforesaid for the ends and purposes before expressed, and considering how necessary it is that persons of known prudence, wisdom, and fidelity, should be authorized and commissionated by us for the better ordering and managing so great affairs upon all occasions, as things may emerge and fall out for the best advantage of the State, and for the improvement of this whole design....

## No. 238 — THE BRITISH CONQUEST OF JAMAICA

*(Henry Whistler, "Journal of the West Indian Expedition, 1654-1655")* *

(*April*) *The 9th Day 1655.*—Monday: this day all the land commanders were called aboard of us to a Council: their General did declare unto them that Hispaniola was the place resolved upon.

*Cited in Firth, op. cit., pp. 109—110.

*The 10th Day 1655.* — Tuesday: this morning all our land officers were called aboard again: to whom Comm. Winslow did declare that in their Instructions from my Lord Protector there was one Article that no soldier should plunder any place that they should take, upon pain of death, and that all plunder or goods that shall be taken at any place shall be put into a public store for the carrying on of the Design, and for the soldiers' encouragement when they had taken this Island they should have six weeks pay a man: but if any shall keep either goods or plate or money in their hands above 3 days, and not bring it in the public storehouse for the use of my Lord Protector, they should be proceeded against as felons. This put all the Commanders into a great passion: and those that durst did fully declare unto the two Generals and the Commrs, that had not me Lord Protector promised them and their soldiers free plunder wheresoever they did go, they would not have come out of England, and further told them that they had promised their soldiers for to encourage them to come with them all which me lord Protector did promise them: and that was that they should have free plunder in all enemies' countries which they came in, and that now they could not with honesty now deprive them of it: it being always their due; and that in all the wars in England they had it: and this being a foreign war they thought not just to deprive the soldiers of it. The Commrs. made answer to them, that seeing my Lord Protector had put it their Instructions they could not disannul it: the Officers departed saying that they did desire them to take it into further consideration, and not to discourage the soldiers, for by that means they never might attain to what they intended: this did put a great distraction among us all both seamen and soldiers. Now both our Generals and General Venables were willing to do anything to encourage the soldiers, but Commr. Winslow would not condescend to anything more than to give them their six weeks pay when they had taken this place. Now when we should have been asking the Lord to give us this place: we instead of that were a sharing the skin before we had cached the fox.

*The 15th Day 1655.* — Sabbath day: this day our army marched 12 miles, but the drought for want of water and the heat of the country did much discourage them. This day in their march they met with many houses and plantations: but the inhabitants all fled into the City, except one or two Spaniards that were eaten out with the pox and could not go. This day they met with a monastery, but all the ballpated friars were gone, but they left all their Images behind them, some of our soldiers found plate here: and one amongst the rest took the Virgin Mary upon his head, and brought her among the army, she was most richly clad: but the soldiers did fall a flinging of oranges at her, and did suddenly deform her, she had Christ in her arms, both these Images were very rich. Our soldiers did get a great deal of sugar at the plantations: but the heat and want of water did cause many to faint and die by the way, but they took all the care they could, and got wild horses to carry the sick. . . .

*The 17th Day 1655.*—Tuesday. . . .about 2 o clock they took an Irish man that did live in the city, and demanding of him where there was any water, he told them that he would bring them where there was water, and they being much joyed to hear of it, for many did faint for want of water. Now all our army did follow this Irish man, and marching carelessly, they having a very strong presumption in them that their enemy durst not face them, but all they thought they had to do was to march into the City there to inhabit. But this presumption was suddenly turned into a great terror, for this Irish man instead of bringing them where water was, brought them open with one of their forts before they did see it: this fort did fire very fast upon our army. But General Venables coming up to the head of our army to view this fort, there did fly forth of the woods a party of the enemy, which did lay in ambush upon our forlorn, and did do a great deal spoil upon our forlorn; and General Venables being one of the foremost, and seeing the enemy fall on so desperately with their lances, he very nobly run behind a tree; and our sea regiment having this day the forlorn hope did fall on most gallantly, and put the enemy to fly for their lives, and coming where General Venables was got behind a tree he came forth to them. But was very much ashamed, but made many excuses: being so much possessed with terror that he could hardly speak. . . .

*The 18th Day 1655.*—Wednesday: this morning General Venables came aboard of us to his Lady, and left his Army to look to themselves. . . .Here are a sort of vagabonds that are saved from the gallows in Spain and the king doth send them here: these go by the name of cow killers, and indeed it is their trade, for they live by killing of cattle for the hides and tallow: these are those that doth do all the mischief, and here are Negroes and Mulattoes which are their slaves: to these they did proclaim freedom if they could fight, telling them that if they would not fight that we would take and eat them as fast as we take them, and this did greatly encourage them to fight. If it were not for these cowkillers and the Negroes the Spaniards were not able to hold up his hand against any enemy, for the Spaniards are so rotten with the pox and so lethargic that they cannot

go 2 miles, but they are ready to die. But to those Spaniards that durst venture to command these Negroes and
cow killers, to these the Pope doth give a Bull, which is a
pardon for all (sins) past and to come, and many that our
men did take had their pardon hanging about their necks;
these men will fight with great confidence, and do believe
that if they die all dies, for they are pardoned: and when
you fire at them they will fall down upon their right knee,
and when you have fired then they will come on most
desperate....

*The 19th Day 1655.*— Thursday:.... But General
Venables, being aboard of our ship, and having a good ship
under him and his wife to lie by his side, did not feel the
hardship of the soldiers that did lie on the sand until the
rain did wash it from under them, and having little or no
victuals, and nothing to drink but water. But the General
did not consider that, but resolved to stay 2 or 3 days more,
pretending to refresh them, but the lying here did do
the army more hurt than their marching, for the fresh
meat and the abundant of fruit that they did eat, and lying
in the rain did cause most of them to have the bloody flux,
and now their hearts were got out of their doublets into
their breeches....for they were in a very sad condition....
and those that had it but 1 or 2 days it made them so
weak....Now the soldiers did begin to murmur at the
General lying aboard with his lady, and keeping them
ashore in this sad condition....

*The 21st Day 1655.*—Saturday:....But as soon as they
made it known to General Venables he made them this
answer, that it was in vain to talk any further of it, for he
did resolve not to go any more: but if our General would
ship the army again, and carry them for Jamaica, they
would do all that they could to take it, but as for this place
they did resolve never to attempt more this bout. Our
General did use all the means possible he could to persuade
them to try once more....and many of the Commanders
did seem willing to go again with a party of men which
should be picked out of the army. But General Venables
would not yield to it. Now our General being much ashamed
of their baseness, but not so much as they were themselves, did tell them that were it not for the sake of some
that were with them, he would set sail and leave them:
seeing they were so base to desire to come off from this
gallant island, and to leave it with so much shame and disgrace not only to themselves but to the Nation: he would
once more take them aboard. But he told them they must
shift for victuals ashore until our ships had got in water
and were fitted, telling them that he had taken care to feed

them long enough already, and now they were in a country where all things were plenty, and if they would not fight for it they should starve for him, until the fleet was fitted. Now the enemy had so much frightened our men in the last skirmish that now they would rather starve than they would go out of their quarters but one mile, where they might have killed as much as they would, but they were so much afraid of the cow killers that they would not budge out, and so many did starve upon that account. Now with lying in the rain and eating bad diet most of the army fell into bloody fluxes, and many did die with that, but more for want of victuals. Now they did begin to eat their dogs, and if a poor trooper did tie his horse to a bush but while he went to ease his body, they would have killed him, and half roasted him by that time he had done, if he were not nimble. This was our condition, these rats of men would rather starve and die than go but one mile into the woods where there is thousands of brave cattle. Here are an abundance of great crabs which live in the woods, they always come out of their holes in the night to feed, and here are such an abundance that as they go they will hit the one legs against the other, which will make a rattling. This noise did give many an alarm to our army in the night, and when they came to examine what they are that gave this alarm they would make answer they did hear a noise like the rattling of bandoliers, some of them did leap into the sea for fear that it had been the cow killers, and this was nothing but the crabs, which were looking for their meat when our army did not dare but did lie and starve. Here are also a great fly that the Spaniard doth call a firefly, these do fly in the night, and do show like a coal of fire: these did give our army many alarm, for the sentries would think them to be the enemy with light matches, and fire at them. This would give an alarm to all the army, and many would run into the woods for fear it was the cow killers and the Negroes come upon them....

*May the 5th, 1655.*—The army being all shipped we made sail and bore away to leeward, intending for Jamaica, and keeping close aboard this Island, and lamenting every time we did look on this Island, that it should be said that we Englishmen should leave such an Island so basely as we did leave this: our General being almost choked for want of venting and telling the army of their baseness: but he thought it wisdom rather to be silent, and to give them all the encouragement he could, lest they should do the like where we were going....

## No. 239—THE BRITISH ARMY OF OCCUPATION

### (An Anonymous Letter from Jamaica, November 5, 1655)*

The 11 ships lately arrived to this place with &c. poor men I pity them at the heart, all their imaginary mountains of gold are turned into dross, and their reason and affections are ready to bid them sail home again already. For my own part greater disappointments I never met with, having had no provision allowed me in 10 weeks last past, or above 3 biscuits this 14 weeks, so that all I can rake and scrape in ready money goes to housekeeping, and the shifts I make are not to be written here. We have lost half our army from our first landing on Spaniola, when we were 8000, besides 1000 or more seamen in arms. Never did my eyes see such a sickly time, nor so many funerals, and graves all the town over that it is a very Golgotha. We have a savannah or plain near us where some of the soldiery are buried so shallow that the Spanish dogs, which lurk about the town, scrape them up and eat them. As for English dogs, they are most eaten by our soldiery; not one walks the streets that is not shot at, unless well befriended or respected. We have not only eaten all the cattle within near 12 miles of the place, but now also almost all the horses, asses, mules flesh near us, so that I shall hold little Eastcheap in more esteem than the whole Indies if this trade last, and I can give nor learn no reason that it should not here continue; so beside this we expect no pay here, nor hardly at home now, but perhaps some ragged land at the best, and that but by the by spoken of, for us general officers not a word mentioned. I could dwell long upon this subject, and could tell you that still half our army lies sick and helpless, nor had we victuals for them before this fleet, nor expect aught now save some bread, and brandy, and oatmeal, and if that with physic will not keep them alive, we have no other remedy but death for them. For my own part in 25 years have not I endured so much sickness as here with bloody flux, rheum, ague, fever, so that I desire earnestly to go for England in March next, if permitted, for I am fallen away 5 inches about....

Amongst the dead persons your brother....is one, who died of the dropsy, consumption, and other complicated diseases, the 22 of August 1655 last....

*Cited in Firth, op. cit., pp. 141—142.

# CHAPTER VIII

# The Early Organisation of the Non-Spanish Colonies

## (i) — MERCANTILISM

## No. 240 — THE VISION

*(Richard Hakluyt, A particular discourse concerning the great necessity and manifold commodities that are like to grow to this Realm of England by the Western discoveries lately attempted, 1584)\**

.... I may well and truly conclude with reason and authority, that all the commodities of all our old decayed and dangerous trades in all Europe, Africa, and Asia haunted by us, may in short space for little or nothing, and many for the very workmanship, in a manner be had in that part of America which lieth between 30 and 60 degrees of northerly latitude, if by our slackness we suffer not the French or others to prevent us....

.... But we, for all the statutes that hitherto can be devised, and the sharp execution of the same in punishing idle and lazy persons, for want of sufficient occasion of honest employments, cannot deliver our commonwealth from multitudes of loiterers and idle vagabonds. Truth it is, that through our long peace and seldom sickness (two singular blessings of Almighty God) we are grown more populous than ever heretofore; so that now there are of every art and science so many, that they can hardly live one by another, nay rather they are ready to eat up one another; yea many thousands of idle persons are within this realm, which, having no way to be set on work, be either mutinous and seek alteration in the state, or at least very burdensome to the commonwealth, and often fall to pilfering and thieving and other lewdness, whereby all the prisons of the land are daily pestered and stuffed full of them, where either they pitifully pine away or else at length are miserably hanged, even 20 at a clap out of some one jail. Whereas if this voyage were put in execution, these petty thieves might be condemned for certain years in the western parts, especially in Newfoundland, in sawing and felling of timber for masts of ships, and deal boards; in burning of the firs and pine trees to make pitch, tar, rosen, and soap ashes; in beating and working of hemp for cordage; and, in the more southern parts, in setting them to work in mines of

*Cited in *The Two Richard Hakluyt's,* Document 46, pp. 233—238, 316.

gold, silver, copper, lead, and iron; in dragging for pearls
and coral; in planting of sugar canes, as the Portingales
have done in Madeira; in maintenance and increasing of
silk worms for silk, and in dressing the same; in gathering
of cotton whereof there is plenty; in tilling of the soil there
for grain; in dressing of vines whereof there is great abundance for wine; olives, whereof the soil is capable, for oil;
trees for oranges, lemons, almonds, figs, and other fruits,
all which are found to grow there already; in sowing of
woad and madder for dyers, as the Portingales have done
in the Azores; in dressing of raw hides of divers kinds of
beasts; in making and gathering of salt. . . .which may serve
for the new land fishing; in killing the whale, seal, porpoise,
and whirlpool for train oil; in fishing, salting, and drying
of linge, cod, salmon, herring; in making and gathering of
honey, wax, turpentine; in hewing and shaping of stone, as
marble, crystal, freestone, which will be good ballast for
our ships homewards, and after serve for noble buildings;
in making of cask, oars, and all other manner of staves; in
building of forts, towns, churches; in powdering and barrell-
ing of fish, fowls, and flesh, which will be notable
provision for sea and land; in drying, sorting, and packing
of feathers, whereof may be had there marvellous great
quantity.

Besides this, such as by any kind of infirmity cannot
pass the seas thither, and now are chargeable to the realm
at home, by this voyage shall be made profitable members,
by employing them in England in making of a thousand
trifling things, which will be very good merchandise for
those countries where we shall have most ample vent
thereof.

And seeing the savages of the Grand Bay, and all along
the mighty river that runneth up to Canada and Hochelaga,
are greatly delighted with any cap or garment made of
coarse wollen cloth, their countries being cold and sharp in
the winter, it is manifest we shall find great utterance of
our clothes, especially of our coarsest and basest northern
doosens, and our Irish and Welsh friezes and rugs;
whereby all occupations belonging to clothing and
knitting shall be freshly set on work, as cappers, knitters,
clothiers, woolmen, carders, spinners, weavers, fullers,
shearmen, dyers, drapers, hatters, and such like, whereby
many decayed towns may be repaired.

In sum, this enterprise will minister matter for all
sorts and states of men to work upon; namely, all several
kinds of artificers, husbandmen, seamen, merchants, soldiers,
captains, physicians, lawyers, divines, cosmographers,
hydrographers, astronomers, historiographers; yea, old
folks, lame persons, women, and young children, by many

means which hereby shall still be ministered unto them, shall be kept from idleness, and be made able by their own honest and easy labour to find themselves, without surcharging others....

This being so, it cometh to pass, that whatsoever cloth we shall vent on the tract of that firm, or in the islands of the same, or in other lands, islands, and territories beyond, ....are to pass out of this realm full wrought by our natural subjects in all degrees of labour....

And on the other side we are to note, that all the commodities we shall bring thence, we shall not bring them wrought, as we bring now the commodities of France and Flanders, &c., but shall receive them all substances unwrought, to the employment of a wonderful multitude of the poor subjects of this realm in return. And so to conclude, what in the number of things to go out wrought, and to come in unwrought, there need not one poor creature to steal, to starve, or to beg as they do....

No foreign commodity that comes into England comes without payment of custom once, twice, or thrice, before it come into the realm, and so all foreign commodities become dearer to the subjects of this realm; and by this course to Norumbega foreign princes customs are avoided; and the foreign commodities cheaply purchased, they become cheap to the subjects of England, to the common benefit of the people, and to the saving of great treasure in the realm; whereas now the realm becometh poor by the purchasing of foreign commodities in so great a mass at so excessive prices....

---

## No. 241 — THE BALANCE OF TRADE

*(Edward Misselden, The Circle of Commerce, London 1623)\**

For as a pair of scales is an invention to show us the weight of things, whereby we may discern the heavy from the light....so is also this balance of trade an excellent and politic invention to show us the difference of weight in the commerce of one kingdom with another: that is, whether the native commodities exported, and all the foreign commodities imported do balance or over-balance one another in the scale of commerce....If the native commodities exported do weight down and exceed in value the foreign commodities imported, it is a rule that never fails that then the kingdom grows rich and prospers in estate and stock: because the overplus thereof must needs come in in treasure ....But if the foreign commodities imported do exceed in value the native commodities exported, it is a manifest sign that trade decayeth, and the stock of the kingdom wasteth apace; because the overplus must needs go out in treasure.

No. 242—THE COLONIES AND THE BALANCE OF TRADE

(Reasons for Raising a Fund for the Support of a Colony at Virginia, London, 1607)*

That Realm is most complete and wealthy which either hath sufficient to serve itself or can find the means to export of the natural commodities than (if) it hath occasion, necessarily to import, consequently it must ensue that by a public consent, a Colony transported into a good and plentiful climate able to furnish our wants, our monies and wares that now run into the hands of our adversaries or cold friends shall pass unto our friends and natural kinsmen and from them likewise we shall receive such things as shall be most available to our necessities, which intercourse of trade may rather be called a home bred traffic than a foreign exchange.

No. 243 — THE THEORY OF BULLION

(Sir Edwyn Sandys, Speech in the House of Commons, February 27, 1620/1) **

There are three principal causes of want of money in the kingdom. 1. Defect of importation of money. 2. Excess of exportation of money. 3. Consumption of money in the kingdom. Merchandize and money is all one in matter of importation and exportation, but in the matter of consumption money is the chief. The fountain of money is Spain. By traffic we have had heretofore out of Spain, every year, 100,000 1. per ann. besides the wines and other commodities we have had from thence in exchange of our merchandizes. It is lawful to bring money out of Spain for victuals although it be prohibited otherwise. The cause we bring not money out of Spain, is, for that we have our return in tobacco; which, if we would bring out of other places which are under the protection of our king, we should have more money from Spain. The Summer Islands and Virginia have plenty of tobacco, and it grows every year better than other; for that country tobacco was worth 2 years since but 4/- s. the pound, and it is now so much bettered, as it was sold this last year for 8/- s. That it will be a double profit to us to divert the bringing in of tobacco out of Spain, and to cause it to be brought out of Virginia and the Summer Islands; for thereby we shall enrich those countries under our dominions, and

*Cited in K. E. Knorr, British Colonial Theories, 1570—1850, Toronto, 1944, p. 129.
**Cited in Stock, op. cit., Vol. I, pp. 28—29.

also England shall be better stored with money, when we will not take our return for our merchandize in tobacco, but in coin or bullion, as we were wont to do.

## No. 244 — THE DRAIN OF BULLION

*(Petition of the House of Commons to James I, King of England, May 28, 1624)* *

It is generally known, that the West Indies are at this day almost the only fountain, and Spain as it were the cistern, from whence silver is derived into all parts of Christendom.

The cause of the great importation of silver from thence, into this realm, hath been for that Spain having so great need of many English commodities, and being not able to counterbalance them with their own, they have been forced to make the account even with money.

But since this need of tobacco hath grown into request, they have paid (as their proverb is) for all our commodities with their smoke, and the rain of their silver to usward hath been in a manner dried up, to the loss of a million and a half in money in this fifteen years last past.

For upon very full and exact examination it hath very plainly and undeniably appeared, that what by under sale of our native commodities, to make ready money for their tobacco, what by the money it self paid unto them for that weed, there hath been loss to this kingdom of one hundred thousand pounds every year, which else would have returned in money from thence. And a miserable kind of trade hath been driven with that nation, our native commodities being undersold, and the foreign overbought, and the treasure of money transformed into a smoky weed.

Your humble Commons therefore most instantly crave of your Majesty that the importation of tobacco may be prohibited from all other parts, save your Majesty's own dominions, according to the practice in like cases of all other nations, in favour of their native commodity, and of their natural people.

## No. 245 — COMMERCIAL NATIONALISM
*(Jean Eon, Le Commerce Honorable, Nantes, 1646)* **

As I cast my glance throughout the length and breadth of France to find out what is the condition of its commerce,

---

*Cited in Stock, *op. cit.*, Vol. I, p. 72.
**Cited in *S. L. Mims, Colbert's West India Policy*, Yale Historical Studies I, Yale University Press, New Haven, 1921, p. 1.

I am dumbfounded to see into what a low state it has sunk.
I am seized with a feeling of disgrace and of sorrow, when
I see the greater part of our merchants idle, our sailors without employment, our harbours without vessels, and our ships
wrecked and stranded upon the beach....Like Diogenes I
might carry a lantern at noontide in our cities and our ports
in search of a French merchant.

## No. 246 — PLANNED ECONOMY

*(J. B. Colbert, Minister of Marine, to Cardinal Jules
Mazarin, Minister of France 1653)* *

We must re-establish or create all industries, even
those of luxury; establish a protective system in the customs; organise the producers and traders in corporations;
ease the fiscal bonds which are harmful to the people;
restore to France the marine transport of her productions;
develop the colonies and attach them commercially to
France; suppress all the intermediaries between France and
India; develop the navy to protect the mercantile marine.

## No. 247 — COLONISATION, THE THEORY

*(Francis Bacon, "Of Plantations", 1625)* **

Plantations are amongst ancient, primitive, and heroi-
cal works. When the world was young, it begat more children; but now it is old it begets fewer: for I may justly
account new plantations to be the children of former kingdoms. I like a plantation in a pure soil; that is, where
people are not displanted to the end to plant in others. For
else it is rather an extirpation than a plantation. Planting
of countries is like planting of woods; for you must make
account to leese*** almost twenty years profit, and expect
your recompense in the end. For the principal thing that
hath been the destruction of most plantations, hath been
the base and hasty drawing of profit in the first years. It is
true, speedy profit is not to be neglected, as far as may
stand with the good of the plantation, but no further. It is
a shameful and unblessed thing to take the scum of people,
and wicked condemned men, to be the people with whom
you plant; and not only so, but it spoileth the plantation;
for they will ever live like rogues, and not fall to work,

*Cited in *Cambridge History of the British Empire*, Vol. I, p. 207.
**Cited in *Bacon's Essays*, Cambridge University Press edition, 1937,
pp. 101—104.
***Lose.

but be lazy, and do mischief, and spend victuals, and be quickly weary, and then certify* over to their country to the discredit of the plantation. The people wherewith you plant ought to be gardeners, ploughmen, labourers, smiths, carpenters, joiners, fishermen, fowlers, with some few apothecaries, surgeons, cooks, and bakers. In a country of plantation, first look about what kind of victual the country yields of itself to hand; as chestnuts, walnuts, pineapples, olives, dates, plums, cherries, wild honey, and the like; and make use of them. Then consider what victual or esculent things there are, which grow speedily, and within the year; as parsnips, carrots, turnips, onions, radish, artichokes of Jerusalem, maize and the like. For wheat, barley, and oats, they ask too much labour; but with peas and beans you may begin, both because they ask less labour, and because they serve for meat as well as for bread. And of rice likewise cometh a great increase, and it is a kind of meat. Above all there ought to be brought store of biscuit, oat-meal, flour, meal, and the like, in the beginning; till bread may be had. For beasts, or birds, take chiefly such as are least subject to diseases, and multiply fastest; as swine, goats, cocks, hens, turkeys, geese, house-doves, and the like. The victual in plantations ought to be expended almost as in a besieged town; that is, with certain allowance. And let the main part of the ground employed to gardens or corn, be to a common stock; and to be laid in, and stored up, and then delivered out in proportion; besides some spots of ground that any particular person will manure for his own private. Consider likewise what commodities the soil where the plantation is doth naturally yield, that they may some way help to defray the charge of the plantation (so it be not, as was said, to the untimely prejudice of the main business), as it hath fared with tobacco in Virginia. Wood commonly aboundeth but too much; and therefore timber is fit to be one. If there be iron ore, and streams whereupon to set the mills, iron is a brave commodity where wood aboundeth. Making of bay-salt, if the climate be proper for it, would be put in experience. Growing silk likewise, if any be, is a likely commodity. Pitch and tar, where store of firs and pines are, will not fail. So drugs and sweet woods, where they are, cannot but yield great profit. Soap-ashes likewise, and other things that may be thought of. But moil** not too much under ground; for the hope of mines is very uncertain, and useth to make the planters lazy in other things. For government, let it be in the hands of one, assisted with some counsel; and let them have commission to exercise

*Send word.  **Toill.

martial laws, with some limitation.  And above all, let men make that profit of being in the wilderness, as they  have God always, and his service, before their eyes.  Let  not the government of the plantation  depend upon too many counsellors and undertakers in the  country that planteth, but, upon a temperate number; and  let those be rather noblemen and gentlemen,  than merchants; for they  look ever  to the present  gain.  Let  there be freedom  from custom,* till the plantation  be of strength; and  not only freedom from custom, but  freedom to carry their commodities where they may make their best of them, except, there be some special cause of caution.  Cram not in people, by sending  too fast  company  after company;  but  rather hearken how they waste, and send supplies proportionably; but so as the number may live well in the plantation,  and not by surcharge be in penury.  It hath been a great endangering to the health of some plantations, that they have built along the sea and rivers, in marish and unwholesome grounds.  Therefore, though  you  begin  there, to  avoid carriage and other like discommodities, yet build still rather upwards from the streams than along.  It concerneth likewise the health of the plantation that they have good store of salt with them, that, they may use it in their  victuals, when it shall be necessary.  If you plant where savages, are, do not only entertain them with trifles and gingles, but use them justly and graciously, with sufficient guard nevertheless; and do not win their favour by helping them to invade their enemies, but for their defence it is not amiss; and send oft of them over to the country that plants, that they may see a better condition than their own, and commend it when they return.  When the plantation grows to strength, then it is time to plant with women as well as with men; that, the plantation may  spread into generations, and not be  ever pieced from without.  It, is the sinfullest thing in the world to forsake or destitute a plantation once in forwardness; for besides the dishonour, it is the guiltiness of blood of many commiserable persons.

---

*No. 248—LIVING SPACE*

(*Sir Francis Bacon to James  I, King of England, 1606*)**

An effect of peace in fruitful kingdoms, where the stock of people, receiving no consumption nor diminution by war, doth continually multiply and increase, must in the end be a surcharge or overflow of people, more than the territories can well maintain, which many times insinuating a general

*Duties on imports and exports.
**Cited in Merivale, *op. cit.*, p. 140.

necessity and want of means into all estates, doth turn external peace into internal troubles and seditions. Now, what an excellent diversion of this inconvenience is ministered, by God's providence, to your Majesty in this plantation of Ireland, wherein so many families may receive sustentation and fortune, and the discharge of them out of England and Scotland may prevent many seeds of future perturbation; so that it is as if a man were troubled for the avoidance of water from the places where he hath built his house, and afterwards should advise with himself to cast those floods, pools, or streams, for pleasure, provision, or use. So shall your Majesty on this work have a double commodity, in the avoidance of people here, and in making use of them there.

---

### No. 249—RELIEVING UNEMPLOYMENT IN THE METROPOLITAN COUNTRY

(Robert Johnson, Nova Britannia, London, 1609)*

Two things are especially required herein, people to make the plantation, and money. . . . For the first, we need no doubt, our land abounding with swarms of idle persons, which having no means of labour to relieve their misery, do likewise swarm in lewd and naughty practices, so that if we seek not some ways for their foreign employment, we must provide shortly more prisons and corrections for their bad conditions. . . . so that you see it no new thing, but most profitable for our State, to rid our multitudes of such as lie at home, pestering the land with pestilence, and penury, and infecting one another with vice and villainy, worse than the plague itself.

---

#### (ii)—THE MONOPOLISTIC COMPANIES AND PRIVATE FIEFS

### No. 250 — THE DUTCH WEST INDIA COMPANY

(Charter granted by their High Mightinesses the Lords the States-General of Holland to the West India Company, June 3, 1621)**

Be it known that we, having taken into consideration that the prosperity of this country and the welfare of its inhabitants principally consist in the navigation and com-

*Cited in Knorr, op. cit., p. 43.
**Cited in Further Documents relating to the Question of Boundary between British Guiana and Venezuela, C. 8106, London, 1896, pp. 53—54,

merce which from time immemorial has been carried on
with good fortune and great blessing from out of this same
country with all countries and kingdoms:

And being desirous that the aforesaid inhabitants not
only be maintained in their navigation, commerce and trade,
but also that their commerce should increase as much as
possible, especially in conformity with the Treaties, Alliances, Conventions, and Agreements formerly made concerning the commerce and navigation with other Princes,
Republics and nations, which Treaties we intend shall be
punctually kept and observed in all their parts:

And we, finding by experience that without the common help, aid and means of a General Company no profitable business can be carried on, protected and maintained
in the parts hereafter enumerated, on account of the great
risks from sea pirates, extortions, and other things of the
same kind, which are incurred upon such long and distant
journeys:

We, therefore, being moved by many different and
pregnant considerations, have, after mature deliberation of
the Council and for very pressing causes, decided that the
navigation, trade, and commerce in the West Indies, Africa,
and other countries hereafter enumerated, shall henceforth
not be carried on otherwise than with the common united
strength of the merchants and inhabitants of these lands,
and that to this end there shall be established a General
Company which, on account of our great love for the
common welfare, and in order to preserve the inhabitants
of these lands in full prosperity, we shall maintain and
strengthen with our assistance, favour and help, so far as
the present state and condition of this country will in any
way allow, and which we shall furnish with a proper
Charter, and endow with the privileges and exemptions here
after enumerated, to wit:

(I)

That, for a period of twenty-four years no native or
inhabitant of this country shall be permitted, except in the
name of this United Company,' either from the United
Netherlands or from any place outside them, to sail upon
or to trade with the coasts and lands of Africa, from the
Tropic of Cancer to the Cape of Good Hope, nor with the
countries of America and the West Indies, beginning from
the southern extremity of Newfoundland through the
Straits of Magellan, Le Maire, and other straits and channels
lying thereabouts, to the Strait of Anjan, neither on the
North nor on the South Sea, nor with any of the islands
situated either on the one side or the other, or between
them both; nor with the Australian and southern lands
extending and lying between the two meridians, reaching

in the east to the Cape of Good Hope, and in the west to
the east end of New Guinea, inclusive. And therefore
whoever shall venture, without the consent of this Company,
to sail upon or trade with any places within the limits
granted to the said Company, shall do so at the risk of
losing the ships and merchandize which shall be found upon
the aforesaid coasts and districts, which it shall be competent to immediately seize on behalf of the said Company,
and to hold as confiscated property at the disposal of the
same. And in case such ships or merchandize should be
sold or taken to other lands or ports, the underwriters and
shareholders may be sued for the value of the said ships
and merchandize; with this exception only, that those ships
which, before the date of this Charter, have sailed from these
or other lands to any of the aforesaid coasts, shall be permitted to continue their trade until they have disposed of
their cargoes, and until their return to this country, or
until the expiration of their Charter, if they have been
granted any before this date, but no longer.

Provided, however, that after the 1st July, 1621, the
day and time of the commencement of this Charter, no one
shall be permitted to send any ships or merchandize to the
districts comprised in this Charter, even if it were before
the day on which the Company was finally established; but
we shall duly provide against those who wittingly and
fraudulently seek to frustrate our good intentions for the
commonwealth; it being understood that the salt trade to
Ponte de Re shall be permitted to be continued upon the
conditions and instructions laid down, or to be laid down,
by us in that matter without being otherwise connected with
this Charter.

(II)

That henceforth the aforesaid Company shall be permitted to make in our name and authority, within the
limits set forth above, contracts, leagues, and alliances with
the Princes and natives of the lands therein comprised;
they may also build there some fortresses and strongholds,
appoint Governors, soldiers, and officers of justice, and do
everything necessary for the preservation of the places and
the maintenance of good order, police, and justice....

(III)

In the event of their choosing a Governor–General, and
drawing up instructions for him, the same will have to be
approved and the Commission granted by us. And further,
such Governor–General, as also other Vice–Governors, Commanders, and officers shall be bound to take an oath of
loyalty to us and to the Company....

*No. 251 — THE FOUNDATION OF THE FRENCH WEST INDIAN EMPIRE*

*(Act of Association of the Lords of the Company of the Islands of America, October 31, 1626)* *

We.... acknowledge and admit that we have formed and form by these presents a faithful association between ourselves to send an expedition, under the leadership of the Sieurs d' Enambuc and du Rossey, Captains in the navy, or such others as we see fit to choose and name, to settle and people the Islands of St. Christopher and Barbados, and others situated at the entrance to Peru, from the eleventh to the eighteenth degree of the Equator, which are not in the possession of Christian princes, both to instruct the inhabitants of the aforesaid islands in the Catholic, Apostolic and Roman religion, and to trade and traffic in the products and merchandise which may be obtained and procured from the aforesaid islands and neighbouring places, to bring them to France to Havre-de-grace, in preference to all other ports, for the time and space of twenty years, as is more especially stipulated in the commission and authority which will be given to the said d'Enambuc and du Rossey by My Lord Cardinal Richelieu, Grand-Master, Chief and Superintendent of French commerce.... towards the execution of which design, there will be established a fund in the sum of forty-five thousand livres which will be furnished and paid by us the undersigned.... which sum.... will be employed for the purchase of three ships.... and for victualling, arming and equipping them with men and provisions necessary for the voyage....

---

*No. 252—THE FRENCH WEST INDIA COMPANY*

*(Contract for the Re-establishment of the Company of the Islands of America, with the articles granted by His Majesty to the Shareholders, February 12, 1635)* **

Art I. .... The shareholders shall continue the colony established in the island of St. Christopher and shall do their best to establish other colonies in the other principal islands of America.... which are not occupied by any Christian prince. If there are any islands inhabited by any Christian princes, on which they can establish joint settlements with their occupiers, they shall do so.

Art. II. The shareholders shall do their best to convert

*Cited in Moreau de Saint-Mery, *op. cit.*, Tome I, pp. 18—19.
**Cited in Moreau de Saint-Mery, *op., cit.*, Tome I, pp. 30—32.

the savages at present inhabiting the island.... to the Apostolic and Roman Catholic religion. To that effect, the shareholders shall maintain at least two or three Ecclesiastics in each island to teach the Word of God and administer the Sacraments to the Catholics, and to instruct the savages. They shall build places for them where they may say Mass, and to this end shall also furnish them with ornaments, books and other things necessary.

Art. III. The shareholders shall transport to the island, within twenty years from the day Your Majesty ratifies these articles, at least four thousand persons of both sexes....

Art. IV. They shall not admit to the islands, colonies and settlements any person who is not a Frenchman and who does not profess the Apostolic and Roman Catholic religion. If any other person should happen to enter the colony, he shall be forced to leave as soon as the governor of the island learns of it....

Art. VI. And so as not to have to compensate them for the expenses they have already incurred and may hereafter incur, Your Majesty shall grant in perpetuity.... to the shareholders and those who may hereafter be associated with them, their heirs, successors and assigns, the complete ownership and overlordship of the islands, lands, rivers, ports, harbours, streams, ponds, island, as well as mines and ores....Your Majesty will reserve only the jurisdiction of the islands, and the allegiance and the tribute due to him....and the appointment of the Members of the Supreme Court, who will be nominated and submitted to him by the shareholders, when the need arises for its establishment....

Art. X. For the space of twenty years, no subject of Your Majesty but the shareholders may trade with the islands, ports, harbours and rivers, unless with their written consent....on pain of the confiscation of the vessels and merchandise....to the profit of the Company....which shall henceforth be called the Company of the Islands of America....

Art. XIII. Artisans who go to the Islands, stay there for a period of six consecutive years, and practise their trade there must be master craftsmen....

---

### No. 253—THE "CARLISLE ISLANDS"

*(Grant of Charles I, King of England, to James, Earl of Carlisle, July 2, 1627)\**

Grant to James, Earl of Carlisle, entitled "the first grant of" the following islands called "The Caribbees", viz.,

*Cited in *Calendar of State Papers, Colonial Series, 1574—1660*, pp. 85—86.

St. Christopher's, Grenada, St. Vincent, St. Lucia, Barbados, Mittalanea, Dominico, Marigalante, Deseada, Todosantes, Guadaloupe, Antigua, Montserrat, Radendo, Barbuda, Nevis, Statia... St. Bartholomew, St. Martin, Anguilla, Sembrera, Enegada, and other islands, before found out to his great cost, and brought to a large and copious colony of English, to be hereafter named "the Carlisle or the islands of Carlisle province", reserving a yearly rent of 100 1., and a white horse when the King, his heirs and successors, shall come into those parts.

---

## No. 254 — THE NATIONAL STATE ASSUMES CONTROL

### (Ordinance of the Two Houses of Parliament, November 2, 1643)*

Whereas many thousands of the natives and good subjects of this kingdom of England, through the oppression of the prelates and other ill-affected ministers and officers of state, have of late years, to their great grief and miserable hardship, been enforced to transplant themselves and their families into several islands, and other remote and desolate parts of the West Indies, and having there, through exceeding great labour and industry (with the blessing of God), obtained for themselves and their families some competent and convenient means of maintenance and subsistence, so that they are now in a reasonable well-settled and peaceable condition; but fearing lest the outrageous malice of papists and other ill-affected persons should reach unto them in their poor and low (but as yet peaceable) condition, and having been informed that there hath been lately procured from His Majesty several grants under the great seal, for erecting some new governors and commanders amongst the said planters, in their aforementioned plantations; whereupon the said planters, adventurers, and owners of land, in the said foreign plantations, have preferred their petition unto this present Parliament, that, for the better securing of them, and their present estates there, obtained through so much extreme labour and difficulty, they might have some such governors and government as should be approved of and confirmed by the authority of both Houses of Parliament; which petition of theirs the Lords and Commons having taken into consideration, and finding it of great importance both to the safety and preservation of the aforesaid natives and subjects of this kingdom, as well from all foreign invasions and oppressions as from their own intestine distractions and

*Cited in Stock, op. cit., Vol. I, pp. 147—148.

disturbances, as also much tending to the honour and advantage of His Majesty's dominions, have thought fit, and do hereby constitute and ordain, Robert Earl of Warwick, governor in chief and lord high admiral of all those islands, and other plantations inhabited, planted, or belonging to any His Majesty's the King of England's subjects, or which hereafter may be inhabited, planted, or belonging to them, within the bounds and upon the coasts of America: and, for the more effectual, speedier, and easier transaction of this so weighty and important a buiness, which concerns the well-being and preservation of so many of the distressed natives of this and other His Majesty's dominions, the Lords and Commons have thought fit, that Phillip Earl of Pembroke, Edward Earl of Manchester, William Viscount Say and Seale, Phillip Lord Wharton, John Lord Roberts, members of the House of Peers, Sir Gilbert Gerrard knight and baronet, Sir Arthur Heselrigg baronet, Sir Henry Vane junior, knight, Sir Benjamin Rudyer knight, John Pym, Oliver Cromwell, Dennis Bond, Miles Corbett, Cornelius Holland, Samuel Vassall, John Rolls, and William Spurstowe, esquires, members of the House of Commons, shall be commissioners, to join in aid and assistance with the said Earl of Warwick, chief governor and admiral of the said plantations; which chief governor, together with the said commissioners or any four of them, shall hereby have power and authority to provide for, order, and dispose, all things which they shall from time to time find most fit and advantageous to the well-governing, securing, strengthening, and preserving of the said plantations, and chiefly to the preservation and advancement of the true Protestant religion amongst the said planters and inhabitants, and the further enlargement and spreading of the Gospel of Christ amongst those that yet remaineth there in great and miserable blindness and ignorance: and, for the better advancement of this so great a work it is hereby further ordained by the said Lords and Commons, that the aforesaid governor and commissioners shall hereby have power and authority, upon all weighty and important occasions which may concern the good and safety of the aforesaid planters, owners of land, or inhabitants of the said islands and plantations, which shall then be within twenty miles of the place where the said commissioners shall then be; and shall have power and authority to send for, view, and make use of, all such records, books, and papers, which do or may concern any of the said plantations....

### (iii)—THE ECONOMIC ORGANISATION OF THE COLONIES

## No. 255—THE WEST INDIES ARE MORE BENEFICIAL TO ENGLAND THAN THE EAST INDIES

*(Minutes of the Lords of Trade and Plantations, 1628 (?) )\**

Considerations upon the question, whether trade with the East or West Indies would be most beneficial to England; answered in favour of the West Indies. Appeal to the King to give encouragement to a company to be formed for working the mines there of gold and silver.

## No. 256—THE DISTRESS OF THE EARLY PLANTERS IN ST. KITTS

*(Petition of the Planters and Adventurers to the Caribbee Islands to the Lords of the Privy Council, February 4, 1630/1)\*\**

That the distressed planters and their servants his Majesty's most dutiful & loving subjects now upon the said Islands are at present in very great distress & want of victuals; many of them not having eaten one morsel of bread at least one month before divers people of good credit (who lately arrived here in England) departed thence; but are constrained to feed on land crabs & other unwholesome provisions & fruits, which the said Islands this winter season afford.

For prevention whereof, some of your petitioners have already provided a small quantity of victuals to be sent to the said Islands; some part whereof is already on board, & more ready to be shipped, to save the lives of his Majesty's said subjects; but that the petitioners are hindered by the officers of his Majesty's customs in as they cannot proceed; although their ships lie here at great expense.

May it therefore please your good Lordships, in tender consideration hereof to give order to the several officers of his Majesty's Customs, and ports, to permit & suffer your petitioners to transport a reasonable proportion of victuals unto the said Caribbee Islands (upon sufficient caution given to deliver the same there only) for the present supply of the foresaid distressed inhabitants his Majesty's subjects there. That they may but subsist with livelihood until the provisions by them planted shall be gathered; which are

\* Cited in *Calendar of State Papers, Colonial Series, 1574.1660*, p. 95.

\*\* Cited in V. L. Oliver, *The History of the Island of Antigua, one of the Leeward Caribbees in the West Indies, from the first settlement in 1635 to the present time*, Vol. I, London, 1894, p. 13.

hoped to be such, & so plentiful, that they shall never here-after have occasion to entreat supply from this Kingdom or any other place. . . .

## No. 257 — THE OVERPRODUCTION OF TOBACCO IN THE BRITISH WEST INDIES

*(Charles I, King of England, to Governor of Virginia, August 4, 1636)\**

And we being given to understand that at St. Christophers, Nevis and Barbados, the inhabitants finding by experience how incommodious it was to plant so much tobacco, of their own accord, for some years have inter-mitted the planting thereof, and employed themselves in cotton wools, which prosper well and yield the planters good profit for their labours: which course hath brought the price of tobacco from 2d the pound to 8d or more, clear of all charges.

## No. 258 — THE OVERPRODUCTION OF TOBACCO IN THE FRENCH WEST INDIES

*(Ordinance of M. de Poincy, Governor General of the French West Indies, May 26, 1639)\*\**

All planters and householders of the Island of St. Christopher, whatever their rank and condition, are ordered and enjoined to uproot all the tobacco on the lands of their plantations, without reserving a single plant, at the end of October next, that is, November 10, English style, and are forbidden to replant or make tobacco in any sort or form, on any pretext whatsoever, for eighteen months thereafter, and not before, on pain of confiscation of the plantations where any tobacco is found during the aforesaid period, contrary to the tenor of the present prohibition, confiscation also of all servants, men and women, whether whites, Negroes or Indians, together with an arbitrary fine to be imposed on the offender, and a year's imprisonment.

*Cited in Williamson, *op. cit.*, pp. 137—138.

**Cited in Moreau de Saint-Mery, *op. cit.*, Tom. I. pp. 43-44.

### No. 259 — BRITISH ENCOURAGEMENT OF AGRICULTURAL DIVERSIFICATION

*(Charles I, King of England, to the Feoffees of James, Earl of Carlisle, April (?) 1637)* *

It has been noticed that the inhabitants of St. Christopher's, Barbadoes, and the other Caribbee Islands, have mostly planted tobacco to the neglect of cotton, wools, and other useful commodities which they had begun, and of corn and grain sufficient for the support of those plantations, which compels them to receive supplies from the Dutch and other strangers. Directs them to send to the several Governors of the Caribbee Islands a perfect transcript of this letter, with instructions concerning the growth of their tobacco and the prohibition of trade in those islands, with strangers.

### NO. 260 — THE BEGINNINGS OF SUGAR CULTIVATION IN MARTINIQUE

*(Register of the French West India Company, October 6, 1638)* * *

After having taken note of the proposal made by Sieur Trezel of Rouen for the cultivation of sugar-cane and for the establishment of mills for the manufacture of sugar in the island of Martinique, and after having heard the aforesaid Sieur Trezel regarding his plans therefor, it was ordered that Mess. Martin and Chanut draw up a contract with him with the following stipulations: 2400 arpents of land to be granted by the company for the establishment of necessary building and the plantation of sugar-cane; a monopoly of the cultivation of sugar-cane in the aforesaid island of Martinique for the remainder of the current year and for six years following; the monopoly to be protected by the imposition of the penalty of confiscation and fines on all those who attempt to violate it;....the said six years to be prolonged in case of war;....the privilege of establishing one or two plantations of sugar-cane in the island of Guadeloupe without, however, a monopoly of its production in that island;.... a premium of one-tenth of all sugar and other products to be paid directly to the company and one-fortieth to some person designated by the company; the sugar produced to be transported only to France and its sale to foreigners to be strictly forbidden; no cultivation of tobacco to be permitted; at the expiration of the aforesaid six years

* Cited in *Calendar of State Papers, Colonial Series,* 1574-1660, p. 251.
* * Cited in Mims, *op. cit.,* pp. 31-32, footnote.

only the tax of one–tenth to be imposed by the company and
the monopoly to cease and all the planters of the said island
of Martinique thereafter to enjoy the liberty to plant sugar-
cane at their pleasure.

## No. 261 — THE EARLY DIFFICULTIES OF SUGAR MANUFACTURE

*(M. de Poincy, Governor of the French West Indies, to
Directors of the French West India Company, November
15, 1640)\**

We haven't enough land to produce roucou and cotton.
They are products which occupy too much space. I admit
that the soil is suited to the production of both.... The
planters do not know or wish to know anything except how
to produce tobacco, unless someone first shows them the
way. What I say about the cultivation of roucou and cotton
is also true of sugar–cane. In regard to that there is another
difficulty. It is the lack of water which is absolutely necessary and of which we have no supply except that from a
small brook.... This lack could of course be supplied, so
far as power to turn the mills is concerned, by the employment of horses or of oxen, but it would still be necessary to
have a supply of water.

## NO. 262 — SUGAR TECHNOLOGY IN BARBADOS

*(Petition of William Pennoyer to the House of Lords,
October 14, 1647)\*\**

Humbly shewing that your petitioner and divers others
planters at Barbados who are erecting sugar works there,
which are likely to prove very useful and beneficial in the
advancement of navigation, trade and the customs of this
kingdom, and tend to the employment of many thousands of
people in these affairs, have advice from thence, that the
plantation stand in great need of drawing horses and oxen
for the mills, without which a very great quantity of sugar
is likely to perish and be lost, and for want of grinding: all
which would tend to the great loss of the said plantation and
navigation of this kingdom.

Your petitioner humbly prayeth that it will please your
Lordships to appoint your petitioner by ordinance of Parlia-

* Cited in Mims, *op. cit.*, p. 35.
** Cited in Stock, *op. cit.*, Vol. I, pp. 196-197.

ment directed to the commissioners of customs, to send forth 120 nags and 40 steers from any the ports of this kingdom, for the supply of the said plantation by bill of store as usually for New England.

## No. 263 — THE BEGINNINGS OF MAINLAND TRADE WITH THE CARIBBEAN

### (Winthrop's Journal, 1630—49)*

As our means of returns for English commodities was grown very short it pleased the Lord to open to us a trade with Barbados and other islands in the West Indies, which as it proved gainful, so the commodities we had in exchange there for our cattle and provisions; as sugar, cotton, tobacco, and indigo were a good help to discharge our engagements in England.

## No. 264 — THE GARDEN OF THE INDIES : JAMAICA

### (Henry Whistler, "Journal of the West Indian Expedition, 1654-1655")**

(May) The 16th Day 1655.—The land is as good as any is in the Indies, and very fruitful if it be planted, but these people are a very lazy people, for by their goodwills none will work, nor take the pains to plant cassava to make them bread. But necessity doth move them to it: they do very few of them take care to be rich, for they say that they cannot want, for meat they have an abundance, and the hides and tallow will buy them clothes, and that is all they take care for most of them: here are some small plantations sugar, but they spend it most in the island: here is some cotton, both silk and other sorts: but the chiefest commodities are these: Lignum vitae and fastic wood, and hides and tallow, and pork fat tied up and put in gares: and that is not worth a going so far for. The Island as it is naturally (is) the best in all the Indies: it hath a great deal of level ground, and many brave savannas full of cattle, and abundance of brave horses, but they are all wild: and many hogs: and wild fowl an abundance: a many parrots: and monkeys: and plenty of fish: here are abundance of alligators and many large snakes. This ground will bear anything that they can plant on it: the Spaniard doth say that it will bear all sorts of

* Cited in V. T. Harlow, *A History of Barbados, 1625-1685*, Oxford University Press, 1926, p. 272.

**Cited in Firth, *op. cit.*, pp. 168—169.

spices, and sugar and indigo, and cotton, and tobacco, and very good grapes: but the Duke of Meden that it did belong to would not suffer them to plant grapes to make wine, for then he did know they would not care for Spain. This Island is bravely watered with fresh rivers: and hath 3 brave harbours in the South Side, and one in the North side: But the midellmust in the South Side is one of the best in the world: in it may ride 500 sail of ships from 50 fathom water to 8: and you may careen by the shore with your guns in 5 fathom water; this harbour is land locked, and the trade wind doth blow into the harbour all day and the land breeze out at night: here are many small Islands and shoals that lie before the harbour's mouth, but they are plain to be seen. The worst inconvenience of this harbour is that it is 6 miles from the town, but our English doth say that they will remove and build near the water side, for they may build such a town as that is in a small time, for the houses are but one storey high because of the hurricane, for he doth many times come and give them a visit. This is all I can say of this Island, for at present it is poor, but it may be made one of the richest spots in the world; the Spaniard doth call it the Garden of the Indies, but this I will say, the gardeners have been very bad, for here is very little more than that which groweth naturally.

---

### (iv) THE PROBLEM OF LABOUR

*No. 265 — THE WHITE INDENTURED SERVANT*

*(Ordinance of the Two Houses of Parliament, January 23, 1646/7)\**

And for that there is great want of servants in the said plantations, as well for the raising of commodities apt to be produced there, as for defence of themselves from being made a prey to the natives or foreign enemies; be it further ordained, by the said Lords and Commons, that it shall be lawful for any person or persons, subjects of this kingdom, to entertain and transport from hence, into the said several plantations, such persons, being fit to serve or advance the trade there, as shall be willing to serve or be employed in the said several foreign plantations: provided, that the names of all such persons, so to be transported to serve in the said plantations, be first registered in the custom-house; and that neither force be used to take up any such servants, nor any apprentices enticed to desert their masters, nor any children under age admitted without express consent of

* Cited in Stock, *op. cit.*, Vol. 1, pp. 185-186.

their parents: and provided also, that certificate within one
year be returned, from the governor or other chief officer
of such plantation where such persons shall be put on shore,
of the arrival of the said persons there, that no fraud be
used to carry any such persons to any other place.

### No. 266 — GETTING RID OF UNDESIRABLES

*(H. Robinson, England's Safety In Trades Encrease,*
*London, 1641)\**

....and send them for some of the new Plantations, all de-
linquents for matters which deserve not hanging, might be
served so too without sparing one of them.... so should we
not only free the streets and country of such rascals and
vagrant people that swarm up and down at present; but prevent many others, some whereof are successively born and
bred so the rest brought to the same begging lazy life by
their ill example, and a great sum of money saved, which
uses yearly to be given to such vagabonds to no purpose but
to make them worse....

### No. 267 — THE TRANSPORTATION OF CONVICTS TO BARBADOS

*(Petition of Thomas Devenish, Keeper of Winchester House*
*Prison, to the House of Lords, March 20, 1645/6)\* \**

Sheweth, that there are several prisoners committed to
him by the justice of peace of Surrey, most of them being for
petty misdemeanours (who have lain in his custody a long
time), at his great charge, he having had no allowance at all
for them since the time of their commitment.

For the easement of your petitioner's future charge; and
forasmuch as Captain William Fortescue (a gentleman of
quality) offers to give good security to transport to Barbadoes as many of them as the justices of peace in the said
county shall think fit to permit, so that this kingdom shall be
troubled with them no more, most of them being able young
men and fit to do that country service, who (if they be detained in prison till the next quarter sessions) will be discharged in course, their crimes being but for petty things as
aforesaid, whereby the country on their release will be in
danger of greater mischief done by them.

* Cited in Knorr, *op. cit.,* p. 44.
**Cited in Stock, *op. cit.,* Vol. I, pp. 175-176.

He therefore most humbly beseecheth Your Lordships, as well for the easing of the charge in their keeping; as for the kingdom's good and safety in their removal from hence, who else might prove dangerous if any sudden accident, should happen (which God forbid), to be pleased to recommend it to any two justices of peace of the said county, to examine the premises, and, finding them to be true, to give order for their present releasement, upon security to be taken for their transportation to the Barbadoes Islands, for the services aforesaid.

---

### No. 268 — TO "BARBADOES" THE IRISH

*(Oliver Cromwell to William Lenthall, "Speaker of the Parliament of England", Dublin, September 17, 1649)\**

The next day the other two towers were summoned, in one of which was about six or seven score, but they refused to yield themselves; and we knowing that hunger must compel them, set only good guards to secure them from running away, until their stomachs were come down. From one of the said towers, notwithstanding their condition, they killed and wounded some of our men. When they submitted, their officers were knocked on the head, and every tenth man of the soldiers killed, and the rest shipped for the Barbadoes. The soldiers in the other town were all spared as to their lives only, and shipped likewise for the Barbadoes....

---

### No. 269 — LAND HUNGER IN BARBADOS

*(Proclamation of the Earl of Carlisle, November 22, 1647)\*\**

Whereas divers People have been transported from the Kingdom of England to my Island of Barbados in America, and have there remained a long time as servants, in great labour for the profits of other persons, upon whose account they were first consigned thither, expecting that their faithful services according to the covenants agreed upon at their first entrance there to make some advantage to themselves by settling of plantations for their own use; but....the land is now so taken up as there is not any to be had but at great rates, too high for the purchase of poor servants. In consideration hereof....I have thought fit to declare that each freeman who is unprovided of land, and shall therefore desire to go off from the Barbados, shall have a proportion of land allotted to him in my Islands of Nevis, Antigua, or any other island under my command....

\* Cited in Stock, *op. cit.*, Vol I, p. 211.
\*\* Cited in Harlow, *op. cit.*, pp. '307—308 footnote.

## No. 270 — BARBADOS, ENGLAND'S DUNGHILL

*(Henry Whistler, "Journal of the West Indian Expedition, 1654-1655)\**

*(January) The 9th Day 1654*—....The gentry here doth live far better than ours do in England: they have most of them 100 or 2 or 3 of slaves apes whom they command as they please: here they may say what they have is their own.... This Island is inhabited with all sorts: with English, French, Dutch, Scots, Irish, Spaniards they being Jews; with Indians and miserable Negroes born to perpetual slavery they and their seed: these Negroes they do allow as many wives as they will have, some will have 3 or 4, according as they find their body able: our English here doth think a Negro child the first day it is born to be worth 05ll, they cost them nothing the bringing up, they go always naked: some planters will have 30 more or less about 4 or 5 years old: they sell them from one to the other as we do sheep. This Island is the dunghill whereon England doth cast forth its rubbish: rogues and whores and such like people are those which are generally brought here. A rogue in England will hardly make a cheater here: a bawd brought over puts on a demure comportment, a whore if handsome makes a wife for some rich planter. But in plain the Island of itself is very delightful and pleasant: it is manured the best of any Island in the Indies, with many brave houses, and here is a brave harbour for ships to ride in. The Island is but small: but it maintains more souls than any piece of land of the bigness in the world. It is but a little more than 30 miles long and eleven miles broad, and it does freight above a hundred sail of ships a year with commodities of the growth of the Island. This Island may be much improved if they can bring their design of wind mills to perfection to grind their sugar, for the mills they now use destroy so many horses that it beggars the planters, a good horse for the mills being worth 50ll sterling money.

## No. 271 — ENCOURAGING THE SETTLEMENT OF JAMAICA

*(Proclamation of Oliver Cromwell, Protector of England, 1655)\* \**

Whereas, by the good providence of God, our fleet, in their late expedition into America, have possessed them-

\* Cited in Firth, *op. cit.,* pp. 145-147.
\*\* Cited in *Interesting Tracts relating to the Island of Jamaica,* pp. 1—2.

selves of a certain island called Jamaica, spacious in its extent, commodious in its harbours and rivers within itself, healthful by its situation, fertile in the nature of the soil, well stored with horses and other cattle, and generally fit to be planted and improved, to the advantage, honour, and interest, of this nation.

And whereas divers persons, merchants, and others, heretofore conversant in plantations, and the trade of the like nature, are desirous to undertake and proceed upon plantations and settlements upon that island.

We, therefore, for the better encouragement of all such persons, so inclined, have, by the advice of our council, taken care not only for the strengthening and securing of that island from all enemies, but for the constituting and settling of a civil government, by such good laws and customs as are and have been exercised in colonies and places of the like nature, have appointed surveyors and other public officers, for the more equal distribution of public right and justice in the said island.

And, for the further encouragement to the industry and good affection of such persons, we have provided and given orders to the commissioners of our customs, that every planter or adventurer to that island shall be exempt and free from paying any excise, or custom, for any manufactures, provisions, or any other goods or necessaries, which he or they shall transport to the said island of Jamaica, within the space of seven years to come from Michaelmas next.

And also that sufficient caution and security be given by the said commissioners, that such goods shall be delivered at Jamaica only. And we have also, out of our special consideration of the welfare and prosperity of that island, provided that no customs, or other tax, or impost, be laid or charged upon any commodity, which shall be the produce and native growth of that island, and shall be imported into any of the dominions belonging to this commonwealth: which favour and exemption shall continue for the space of ten years, to begin and be accounted from Michaelmas next. We have also given our special orders and directions, that no embargo or other hindrance, upon any pretence whatsoever, be laid upon any ships, seamen, or other passengers or adventurers, which shall appear to be engaged and bound for the said island.

And we do hereby further declare, for ourselves and successors, that whatsoever other favour, or immunity, or protection, shall or may conduce to the welfare, strength, and improvement of the said island, shall from time to time be continued and applied thereunto.

*No. 272 — NEGROES THE LIFE OF BARBADOS*

*(George Downing to John Winthrop, Jr., August 26, 1645)\**

If you go to Barbados, you shall see a flourishing Island, many able men. I believe they have brought this year no less than a thousand Negroes, and the more they buy, the better able they are to buy, for in a year and half they will earn (with God's blessing) as much as they cost. . . .

A man that will settle there must look to procure servants, which if you could get out of England, for 6, or 8, or 9 years time, only paying their passages. . . .it would do very well, for so thereby you shall be able to do something upon a plantation, and in short time be able, with good husbandry, to procure Negroes (the life of this place) out of the increase of your own plantation.

*No. 273—SCIENTIFIC DETACHMENT : WHY ARE NEGROES BLACK ?*

*(Sir Thomas Browne, Pseudodoxia Epidemica, or Enquiries into very many received Tenets and Commonly presumed Truths, London, 1646)\*\**

. . . .Thus although a man understood the general nature of colours, yet were it no easy problem to resolve, why grass is green? Why garlic, molyes, and porrets have white roots, deep green leaves, and black seeds?  Why several docks and sorts of rhubarb with yellow roots send forth purple flowers? Why also from lactary or milky plants which have a white and lacteous juice dispersed through every part, there arise flowers blue and yellow ? Moreover, beside the specifical and first digressions ordained from the Creation, which might be urged to salve the variety in every species; why shall the marvel of *Peru* produce its flowers of different colours, and that not once, or constantly, but every day, and variously? Why tulips of one colour produce some of another, and running through almost all, should still escape a blue? And lastly, why some men, yea and they a mighty and considerable part of mankind, should first acquire and still retain the gloss and tincture of blackness? Which whoever strictly enquires, shall find no less of darkness in the cause, than in the effect itself; there arising unto examination no such satisfactory and unquarrelable reasons, as may confirm the causes generally received; which are but two in number. The

---

\* Cited in Donnan, *op. cit.*, Vol I, pp .25—126.

\*\* Cited in *Works of Sir Thomas Browne*, **Vol. 3, pp. 232—248.**

heat and scorch of the Sun; or the curse of God on *Cham* and his Posterity....

Thus having evinced, at least made dubious, the sun is not the author of this blackness, how, and when this tincture first began is yet a riddle, and positively to determine, it surpasseth my presumption. Seeing therefore we cannot discover what did effect it, it may afford some piece of satisfaction to know what might procure it. It may be therefore considered, whether the inward use of certain waters or fountains of peculiar operations, might not at first produce the effect in question....

Secondly, it may be perpended whether it might not fall out the same way that *Jacob's* cattle became speckled, spotted and ring-straked, that is, by the power and efficacy of imagination; which produceth effects in the conception correspondent unto the fancy of the agents in generation; and sometimes assimilates the idea of the generator into a reality in the thing engendered. For, hereof there pass for current many indisputed examples; so in *Hippocrates* we read of one, that, from an intent view of a picture conceived a *Negro*; and in the History of *Heliodore* of a Moorish Queen, who upon aspection of the picture of *Andromeda*, conceived and brought forth a fair one. And thus perhaps might some say was the beginning of this complexion: induced first by imagination, which having once impregnated the seed, found afterward concurrent co-operation, which were continued by climes, whose constitution advantaged the first impression. Thus Plotinus conceiveth white peacocks first came in. Thus many opinion that from aspection of the snow, which lieth long in northern regions, and high mountains, hawks, kites, bears, and other creatures become white; and by this way *Austin* conceiveth the devil provided, they never wanted a white spotted ox in *Egypt;* for such an one they worshipped, and called *Apis.*

Thirdly, it is not indisputable whether it might not proceed from such a cause and the like foundation of tincture, as doth the black jaundice, which meeting with congenerous causes might settle durable inclinations, and advance their generations unto that hue, which were naturally before but a degree or two below it. And this transmission we shall the easier admit in colour, if we remember the like hath been effected in organical parts and figures; the symmetry whereof being casually or purposely perverted; their morbosities have vigorously descended to their posterities, and that in durable deformities....

Artificial *Negroes,* or *Gypsies* acquire their complexion by anointing their bodies with bacon and fat substances, and so exposing them to the sun. In *Guinea Moors* and others, it hath been observed that they frequently moisten their skins with fat and oily materials, to temper the irksome dryness thereof from the parching rays of the sun. Whether this practice at first had not some efficacy toward this complexion, may also be considered.

Lastly, if we still be urged to particularities, and such as declare how, and when the seed of *Adam* did first receive this tincture; we may say that men became black in the same manner that some foxes, squirrels, lions, first turned of this complexion, whereof there are a constant sort in divers countries; that some chaughs came to have red legs and bills, that crows became pied: all which mutations however they began, depend on durable foundations; and such as may continue forever. And if as yet we must farther define the cause and manner of this mutation, we must confess, in matters of antiquity, and such as are decided by history, if their originals and first beginnings escape a due relation, they fall into great obscurities, and such as future ages seldom reduce unto a resolution. . . .

And if any will yet insist, and urge the question farther still upon me, I shall be enforced unto divers of the like nature, wherein perhaps I shall receive no greater satisfaction. I shall demand how the camels of *Bactria* came to have two hunches on their backs, whereas the camels of *Arabia* in all relations have but one? How oxen in some countries began and continue gibbous or hunch-back'd? what way those many different shapes, colours, hairs, and natures of dogs came in? How they of some countries became depilous, and without any hair at all, whereas some sorts in excess abound therewith? How the Indian hare came to have a long tail, whereas that part in others attains no higher than a scut? How the hogs of *Illyria,* which Aristotle speaks of, became solipedes or whole-hoofed, whereas in other parts they are bisulcous, and described clovenhoofed by God himself? All which with many others must needs seem strange unto those that hold there were but two of the unclean sort in the ark; and are forced to reduce these varieties to unknown originals.

However therefore this complexion was first acquired, it is evidently maintained by generation, and by the tincture of the skin as a spermatical part traduced from father unto son; so that they which are strangers contract it not, and the natives which transmigrate, omit it not without commixture, and that after divers generation. And this affection (if the story were true) might wonderfully be confirmed, by what *Maginus* and others relate of the Emperor of *Aethiopia,* or *Preston John,* who derived from *Solomon* is not yet descended into the hue of his country, but remains a *Mulatto,* that is, of a Mongrel complexion unto this day. Now although we conceive this blackness to be seminal, yet we are not of *Herodotus* conceit, that their seed is black. An opinion long ago rejected by *Aristotle,* and since by sense and enquiry. His assertion against the historian was probable, that all seed was white; that is without great controversy in viviparous animals, and such as have testicles, or preparing vessels wherein it receives a manifest dealbation. And not, only in them, but (for ought I know) in fishes not abating the seed of plants; whereof at least in most though the skin and covering be black, yet is the seed and fructifying part not so; as may be observed in the seeds of *onions, Pyonie* and Basil. Most controvertible it seems in the spawn of frogs, and lobsters, whereof notwithstanding at the very first the spawn is white, contracting by degrees a blackness, answerable in the one unto the colour of the shell, in the other unto the porwigle or tadpole; that is that animal which first proceedeth from it. And thus may it also be in the generation and sperm of Negroes; that being first and in its naturals white, but upon separation of parts, accidents before invisible become apparent; there arising a shadow or dark efflorescence in the outside; whereby not only their legitimate and timely births, but their abortions are also dusky, before they have felt, the scorch and fervour of the sun.

A second opinion there is, that this complexion was first a curse of God derived unto them from *Cham,* upon whom it, was inflicted for discovering the nakedness of Noah. Which notwithstanding is sooner affirmed than proved, and carrieth with it sundry improbabilities....

Lastly, in whatsoever its *theory* consisteth, or if in the general, we allow the common conceit of symmetry and of colour, yet to descend unto singularities, or determine in what symmetry or colour it consisted, were a slippery designation. For beauty is determined by opinion, and seems to have no essence that holds one notion with all; that seeming beauteous unto one, which hath no favour with another; and that unto every one, according as custom hath made it natural, or sympathy and conformity of minds shall make it seem agreeable. Thus flat noses seem comely unto the Moor, an aquiline or hawked one unto the *Persian,* a large and prominent nose unto the Roman; but none of all these are acceptable in our opinion. Thus some think it most ornamental to wear their bracelets on their wrists, others say it is better to have them about their ankles; some think it most comely to wear their rings and jewels in the ear, others will have them about their privities; a third will not think they are complete except they hang them in their lips, cheeks, or noses....Thus we that are of contrary complexions accuse the blackness of the Moors as ugly:

But the spouse in the Canticles excuseth this conceit, in that description of hers, I am black, but comely. And howsoever *Cerberus* and the furies of hell be described by the poets under this complexion, yet in the beauty of our Saviour blackness is commended, when it is said, his locks are bushy and black as a raven. So that to infer this as a curse, or to reason it as a deformity, is no way reasonable; the two foundations of beauty, symmetry and complexion, receiving such various apprehensions, that no deviation will be expounded so high as a curse or undeniable deformity, without a manifest and confessed degree of monstrosity.

Lastly, it is a very injurious method unto philosophy, and a perpetual promotion of ignorance, in points of obscurity; nor open unto easy considerations, to fall upon a present refuge unto miracles; or recur unto immediate contrivance, from the insearchable hands of God. Thus in the conceit of the evil odour of the Jews, Christians without a further research into the verity of the thing, or inquiry into the cause, draw up a judgement upon them from the passion of their Saviour. Thus in the wondrous effects of the clime of Ireland, and the freedom from all venomous creatures, the credulity of a common conceit imputes this immunity unto the benediction of *S. Patrick*, as *Beda* and *Gyraldus* have left recorded. Thus the ass having a peculiar mark of a cross made by a black list down his back, and another athwart, or at right angles down his shoulders, common opinion ascribes this figure unto a peculiar signation; since that beast had the honour to bear our Saviour on his back. Certainly this is a course more desperate than antipathies, sympathies, or occult qualities; wherein by a final and satisfactive discernment of faith, we lay the last and particular effects upon the first and general cause of all things; whereas in the other, we do but palliate our determinations, until our advanced endeavours do totally reject, or partially salve their evasions.

---

## (v)—THE STRUGGLE FOR THE CARIBBEAN

### (a)—METROPOLITAN RIVALRY

*No. 274—THE ANGLO-FRENCH PARTITION OF ST. KITTS*

*("Articles made between the gentlemen Governors Captain Warner & Captain Denumbuke, & Cap. Du Roissey, for the maintaining of their Commissions received from the King of England & the King of France", 1627)* \*

Seeing that the English & the French have together conquered the Island of St. Christopher in the West Indies & that their Kings have given them Commissions for the

\* Cited in Oliver, *op. cit.*, Vol. I, p. 10.

same place; they shall remain Governors of this Island, each of them in their several plantation, according to their agreement.

All the Englishmen that are upon the said Island shall live under the authority & command of the King & his Lieutenant Governors made by him.

No shipping that shall come to the said Island shall sell their merchandize without leave of the said Governors Cap. Warner, & Cap. Denumbuke, and Cap. Du Roissey. If it be an English ship, the Governor of the English shall set a price upon his merchandize. And if it be a French ship the French Governors shall do so likewise. But if here come any Flemish ship the Governors shall conclude together, & set a price upon his merchandize.

The Governors shall not entertain any men or slaves of either party, in their habitations, before they have given warning one to the other.

If any Indians shall be seen upon the said Island he that first discovereth them shall send word of it presently to the other nation.

If any Spaniards shall at any time invade the said Island, he that first discovereth them shall presently send word to the Governor or Governors of the other nation & they shall send forces immediately to aid them against the Spaniards, that they may not be suffered to land there.

If there be any quarrelling or fighting between any of the English and the French, they shall be judged by the Governors; & after judgment passed upon them they shall be sent each of them to their own plantations to be punished.

If there shall be any wars between England & France the Governors shall give warning thereof one to the other.

And although there be wars between England & France yet the English shall not make war against the French, nor the French against the English upon the said Island, unless they have special order for it from their King.

---

## No. 275 — DUTCH HOSTILITY TO SPAIN

### (Order and Regulations of the States-General, May 14, 1632 and July 15, 1633)*

First, none of the said vessels shall be permitted on any account whatever to sail to the coasts of Africa, nor to New Netherlands or any other place where the Company may trade; but shall be permitted to sail to the coasts of Brazil; item, in the West Indies, to wit, the River Oronocque westwards along the coast of Carthagena, Portobello, Honduras, Campeche, the Gulf of Mexico, and the coast of

* Cited in *Further Documents relating to the Question of Boundary between British Guiana and Venezuela*, p. 55.

Florida, together with all the islands lying within the boundaries, in order to injure and offer hostility to the King of Spain, his subjects and adherents, both on land and water.

---

## No. 276 — DUTCH FREE TRADE

*(Register of the Resolutions of their High Mightinesses the Lords the States-General of the United Netherlands, August 10, 1648)* *

The States-General of the United Netherlands having read and deliberated upon the Order and Regulation made, subject to our approval, by the General Chartered West India Company in the Council of Nineteen for each and all of the inhabitants of the United Provinces who shall henceforth desire to sail to certain districts within the limits of the Charter of the aforesaid Company hereinafter set forth, to fetch salt, timber, tobacco, cotton, and other wares or merchandize obtainable there; have, after due deliberation, approved and ratified the said Order and Regulation, as their High Mightinesses now approve and ratify them by these presents and in such manner as now hereinafter follows:—

Firstly, we hereby declare that we annul and quash all former Orders and Regulations according to which all ships in the respective provinces, either armed or unarmed, have been permitted to sail for private trade in timber, salt, tobacco, cotton, or other wares and products there obtainable to a certain area within the Charter of the West India Company, at whatever period, in what manner the said Regulations might have been issued, promulgated or drawn up; and we now decree, order, and ordain anew that the vessels of the aforesaid inhabitants shall henceforth be permitted to sail in the West Indies, to wit, from the River Oronocque westwards along the coasts of Paria, Cumana, Venezuela, Carthagena, Portobello, Honduras, Campeche, the Gulf of Mexico, and the coasts of Florida, as well as between and around all the islands situated in those parts, including even Curacoa, Buenayre, and Aruba, without permission to go east along the Wild Coast,** much less to the Amazon or the Maransan, or further north than Cape Florida, and equally without permission to come on any account whatever, or in any manner to the Virginias, New Netherlands, Nova Francia, and other places situated thereabouts, or to sail to or along the coasts of Africa, Brazil,

---

* Cited in *Further Documents relating to the Question of Boundary between British Guiana and Venezuela*, p. 57.

**The Wild Coast was the original name of the coast between the Orinoco and the Essequibo.

or anywhere else where the Company has trade, under the penalty that whoever shall be found to do or to have done contrary to this shall confiscate both ship and cargo, which also it shall be allowable to seize and to hold as confiscated property at the disposal of the Company without any action at law, and in case such ships or cargoes shall have been sold or have been put into other countries or ports, the captains, owners, or underwriters shall be used for the value of the said ships and cargoes according to Article I of the Charter....

And inasmuch as the inhabitants of these United Provinces and lands, as well as foreign vessels, shall be permitted to sail and trade, so shall all foreign ships bringing timber, salt, tobacco, and any other wares, products, or merchandize into this country from the West Indies, or the territories granted by Charter to the Company, whether it be for their own account, as freight, or on commission, be compelled to declare and deposit them in the warehouses of the Company in the manner hereinbefore expressed, and shall subsequently also to pay the above Company convoy dues, and such recognition money as the inhabitants and vessels of these countries have to pay, whether such foreign vessels come straight from the West Indies, and from within the limits of the Charter to this country, or whether they have, for any reason whatever, discharged their cargo in other countries or kingdoms, and exchanged their original cargoes in any of the ports at which they have touched for other goods and paid the duties of the country; anyone alleging this to be the case shall be held to produce sufficient proofs on entering his goods, so that the State and the Company may not be frustrated in their intentions in this matter.

---

## No. 277—ANGLO-DUTCH COLONIAL RIVALRY

*(Letters from Amsterdam, December 16 and 17, 1652)\**

Our people, though the vain reports of wholly destroying Blake's fleet prove lies, yet are they so puffed up with Tromp's sovereignty that an accommodation with England is spitted at without wholly satisfying for all ships taken and some harbours to boot; but our Lords at the Hague have sat close and resolved on the new placard which is augmented and absolutely to set up a West India Company, for taking of the Caribs' Islands, which is so forward that officers are appointed and divers have underwrote great

* Cited in S. R. Gardiner and C. T. Atkinson (eds.), *Letters and Papers relating to the First Dutch War, 1652-1654*, Publications of the Navy Records Society, Vol. XXX, London, 1906, Vol. III, pp. 179, 181-182.

sums near to the value of twenty tons of gold; such a height
hath this little skirmish brought them unto, though the
Garland, who is brought into Goree, witnesseth what they
paid for her, her small worth being considered; and that
Tromp's own ship and Evertsen's being so miserably
torn. . . .

They are so elevated here with the late unexpected
success that they spurn the thought of any accommodation,
unless it be upon their own terms. Great swelling words
abound, so that the scene is altered and nothing thought of
but domineering over England, which they say shall satisfy
them for the ships it hath taken, and secure them by yielding up some harbours. So much hath a slender advantage
for a season exalted these Low Countries and lower
souls. . . .

The new placard is now determined and much enlarged.
Besides, imagining nothing too hard for them, an absolute
resolution is taken to erect a West India Company for the
taking of the Caribbee Islands, which is so far promoted
already that officers are elected, and divers subscriptions of
great sums made; so besotted are they with the success of
this little skirmish, as if England were never likely to see
a ship again at sea. . .

---

### (b) COLONIAL SELF-GOVERNMENT

### No. 278—BARBADIAN DEMOCRACY

*(Henry Huncks to Earl of Carlisle, July 11, 1639)* *

A day I was appointed they would give me audience
that was, to speak: but I should read no Commission, but
they would take time to think of it. I presented them the
King's letter, which they did all extremely slight, bidding
lay it on the table. I desired them to take it. They would
not, but bid their Clerk to take it and lock it up; they would
read it at more leisure. Then I demanded the Government
according to my Commission. Captain Hawley told me he
knew not whether you had power or not, but my Commission they would have. (They) commanded me to yield it up.
I refusing, they told me they would seize my person. Some
said the right belonged to the ffeoffees, which when I gave
that letter, locked it up. And Capt. Hawley told me the
propriety to belong to the Lord of Warwick, and not to you
for aught he knew. I desired to know how he held that
then assuming power. He commanded the Marshall &
Sergeant to come into the room, and seize my Commission;
my Commission they had: I was forced to wait their leisure;
at last they after 4 days stay they had read the King's letter

(they said) He was misinformed, they would answer the King. But they would not obey nor acknowledge nor receive any Governor but Capt. Hawley, and bid me take that for an answer. A resolution was taken amongst them all of Parliament he should be chosen Governor, and was proclaimed, and with the greatest scorn towards you that I have seen. I was threatened to be pistolled if I demanded the Government. He means to bind you by the laws they now make. I cannot write one quarter of their designs, for I hear there is a ship going home. I therefore send this for present. He hath brought a master of ship to carry him for Florida; he pretends he hath a Commission from the King for what he doth. My Commission I got, but the Letters they have.

---

### No. 279 — BARBADOS' "DECLARATION OF INDEPENDENCE"

*(A Declaration of Lord Willoughby and the Legislature of the Island of Barbados against the British Parliament, 1651)**

A Declaration of my Lord Willoughby, Lieutenant-General, and Governor of Barbados, and other Caribbee Islands; as also the Council of the Island belonging to it; serving in answer to a certain Act formerly put forth by the Parliament of England, the 3rd October 1650.

A Declaration, published by Order of my Lord Lieutenant-General, the 18th of February 1651, the Lords of the Council, and of the Assembly, being occasioned at the sight of certain printed Papers, entitled, An Act forbidding Commerce and Traffic with the Barbados, Virginia, Bermudas, and Antigua.

The Lord Lieutenant-General, together with the Lords of this Council and Assembly, having carefully read over the said printed Papers, and finding them to oppose the freedom, safety, and well-being of this island, have thought themselves bound to communicate the same to all the inhabitants of this island; as also their observation and resolution concerning it, and to proceed therein after the best manner, wherefore they have ordered the same to be read publicly.

Concerning the abovesaid Act, by which the least capacity may comprehend how much the inhabitants of this island would be brought into contempt and slavery, if the same be not timely prevented :

* Cited in R. H. Schomburgh, *The History of Barbados; comprising a geographical and statistical description of the Island; a sketch of the historical events since the Settlement; and an account of its geology and natural productions,* London, 1848, pp. 706-708.

First — They allege that this island was first settled and inhabited at the charges, and by the especial order of the people of England, and therefore ought to be subject to the same nation. It is certain, that we all of us know very well, that we, the present inhabitants of this island, were and still be that people of England, who with great danger to our persons, and with great charge and trouble, have settled this island in its condition, and inhabited the same, and shall we therefore be subject to the will and command of those that stay at home? Shall we be bound to the Government and Lordship of a Parliament in which we have no Representatives, or persons chosen by us, for there to propound and consent to what might be needful to us, as also to oppose and dispute all what should tend to our disadvantage and harm? In truth, this would be a slavery far exceeding all that the English nation hath yet suffered. And we doubt not but the courage which hath brought us thus far out of our own country, to seek our beings and livelihoods in this wild country, will maintain us in our freedoms; without which our lives will be uncomfortable to us.

Secondly — It is alleged that the inhabitants of this island have, by cunning and force, usurped a power and Government.

If we, the inhabitants of this island, had been heard what we could have said for ourselves, this allegation had never been printed; but those who are destined to be slaves may not enjoy those privileges; otherwise we might have said and testified with a truth, that the Government now used amongst us, is the same that hath always been ratified, and doth every way agree with the first settlement and Government in these places; and was given us by the same power and authority that New England hold theirs; against whom the Act makes no objection.

And the Government here in subjection is the nearest model of conformity to that under which our predecessors of the English nation have lived and flourished for above a thousand years. Therefore we conclude, that the rule of reason and discourse is most strangely mistaken, if the continuation and submission to a right well-settled Government be judged to be an usurping of a new power, and to the contrary, the usurpation of a new Government be held a continuation of the old.

Thirdly — By the abovesaid Act all outlandish nations are forbidden to hold any correspondence or traffic with the inhabitants of this island; although all the ancient inhabitants know very well, how greatly they have been obliged to those of the Low Countries for their subsistence, and how difficult it would have been for us, without their assistance, ever to have inhabited these places, or to have brought them into order; and we are yet daily sensible, what necessary comfort they bring to us daily, and that they do sell their commodities a great deal cheaper than our own nation will do; but this comfort must be taken from us by those whose will must be a law to us: but we declare, that we will never be so unthankful to the Netherlanders for their former help and assistance, as to deny or forbid them, or any other nation, the freedom of our harbours, and the protection of our laws, by which they may continue, if they please, all freedom of commerce and traffic with us.

Fourthly — For to perfect and accomplish our intended slavery, and to make our necks pliable for to undergo the yoke, they got and forbid to our own countrymen, to hold any correspondence, commerce, or traffic with us, nor to suffer any to come at us, but such who have obtained particular licences from some persons, who are expressly ordered for that purpose, by whose means it might be brought about, that no other goods or merchandizes shall be brought hither, than such as the licensed persons shall please and think fit to give way to; and that they are to sell the same at such a price, as they shall please to impose on them; and suffer no other ships to come hither but their own: as likewise that no inhabitants of this island may send home upon their own account any island goods of this place, but shall be as slaves to the Company, who shall have the abovesaid licences, and submit to them the whole advantage of our labour and industry.

Wherefore, having rightly considered, we declare, that as we would not be wanting to use all honest means for the obtaining of a continuance of commerce, trade, and good correspondence with our country, so we will not alienate ourselves from those old heroic virtues of true Englishmen, to prostitute our freedom and privileges, to which we are born, to the will and opinion of any one; neither do we think our number so contemptible, nor our resolution so weak, to be forced or persuaded to so ignoble a submission, and we cannot think, that there are any amongst us, who are so simple, and so unworthily minded, that they would not rather choose a noble death, than forsake their old liberties and privileges.

---

## No. 280 — BARBADOS DEMANDS REPRESENTATION IN PARLIAMENT

*(Colonel Thomas Modyford to John Bradshaw, Barbados, February 16, 1652)* *

....The inhabitants of Barbadoes are now fully satisfied that they have fought for their bondage, and laid down their

* Cited in *Calendar of State Papers, Colonial Series, 1574-1660*, p. 373.

arms for their liberties; since the composure they have new
spirits in them. Entrusted with a share of the government,
he offers his advice how to preserve what has been gained,
and to enlarge the English dominions in the West Indies. The
people of Barbadoes would delight to have the same form of
government as England, and he desires, although it "may
seem immodest", that two representatives should be chosen
by the island to sit and vote in the English Parliament.

---

### No. 281 — THE INDEPENDENCE MOVEMENT IN BARBADOS

*(John Bayes to the Council of State in England, Barbados,
June 30, 1652)\**

.... They call themselves the representatives of the
island, but believe, if suffered, they will in time become the
sole power. State of feeling among the inhabitants; many, if
they could have preserved their families and estates from
ruin, "would never have complied with you, for their hearts
are not with you". Some persons had a design to make this
place a free state, and not run any fortune with England,
either in peace or war; "this I know to be a truth". Those
men now in the chiefest places of trust under the Government allow the Governor to be but a single person. Speaks
in high terms of Governor (Searle), "a man faithful to his
trust", but contends that he must have "power in his
management", an absolute power to choose his Council; for
when any dispute arises at the council table, he is over-
voted....

---

### No. 282 — THE BARBADOS FREE STATE

*(Daniel Searle, Governor of Barbados, to the Council of
State in England, September 19, 1653)\*\**

Restless spirits, unsatisfied with the Constitution of
England, would model "this little limb of the Commonwealth into a free state".

---

\* Cited in *Calendar of State Papers, Colonial Series, 1574-1660,* p. 384.
\*\* Cited in *Calendar of State Papers, Colonial Series, 1574-1660,* p. 408.

# INDEX

## COLLECT THESE OTHER SIGNIFICANT TITLES BY DR. ERIC WILLIAMS

***HISTORY OF THE PEOPLE OF TRINIDAD & TOBAGO***: A revealing portrait of the island nation, it's people and their rich heritage.
**$14.95**
• • • • • • • • • • • • • • • • • • • • • • • • • • • • • • • • • • • • • • • • • • •

***BRITISH HISTORIANS & THE WEST INDIES***: British Historians and their relationship and attitude to the Caribbean region and it's people, and the role they played in shaping the present day socio-economic and political landscape.
**$11.95**
• • • • • • • • • • • • • • • • • • • • • • • • • • • • • • • • • • • • • • • • • • •

***THE NEGRO IN THE CARIBBEAN***: Attitudes of former slave owners to the emerging movements of abolition and independence in the Caribbean.
**$ 9.95**
• • • • • • • • • • • • • • • • • • • • • • • • • • • • • • • • • • • • • • • • • • •

***INWARD HUNGER: THE EDUCATION OF A PRIME MINISTER***: Written with tremendous insight into his motivation, his achievements. and his rise to be the first Prime Minister of Trinidad & Tobago
**$ 14.95**
• • • • • • • • • • • • • • • • • • • • • • • • • • • • • • • • • • • • • • • • • • •

***COLUMBUS TO CASTRO***: A history of the Caribbean region from Columbus' voyage to the modern day vestige of Cuba.
**$ 16.00**
• • • • • • • • • • • • • • • • • • • • • • • • • • • • • • • • • • • • • • • • • • •

***DOCUMENTS OF WEST INDIAN HISTORY***: A look at the significant historical documents and writings of slavery in the West Indies.
**$ 12.95**
• • • • • • • • • • • • • • • • • • • • • • • • • • • • • • • • • • • • • • • • • • •

***CAPITALISM & SLAVERY***: Capitalism and it's undeniable contribution to the perpetration of slavery. The British and the Jewish question in slavery,
**$ 9.95**
• • • • • • • • • • • • • • • • • • • • • • • • • • • • • • • • • • • • • • • • • • •

***EDUCATION OF THE NEGRO IN THE BRITISH WEST INDIES***. Revelation of the contempt for the region and the education of it's peoples.
**$ 9.95**

Mail Order Form to **A&B BOOKS 149 LAWRENCE STREET, NEW YORK 11201**
TEL: (718) 596-3389 · FAX (718) 596-0968
Name:_____
Address_____
City_____ST_____Zip_____
Card Type_____
Card Number_____Exp____/____

*We accept VISA MASTERCARD AMERICAN EXPRESS & DISCOVER*

# SELECTED TITLES
## *Available from A&B BOOKS Publishers*

| | |
|---|---|
| BLACKMEN SAY GOODBYE TO MISERY | 10.00 |
| EDUCATION OF THE NEGRO | 9.95 |
| HEAL THYSELF | 9.95 |
| HEAL THYSELF COOKBOOK | 9.95 |
| VACCINES ARE DANGEROUS | 9.95 |
| COLUMBUS & THE AFRICAN HOLOCAUST | 10.00 |
| COLUMBUS CONSPIRACY | 11.95 |
| DAWN VOYAGE | 11.95 |
| AIDS THE END OF CIVILIZATION | 9.95 |
| GOSPEL OF BARNABAS | 8.95 |
| AFRICAN DISCOVERY OF AMERICA | 10.00 |
| GERALD MASSEY'S LECTURES | 9.95 |
| HISTORICAL JESUS & THE MYTHICAL CHRIST | 9.95 |
| FIRST COUNCIL OF NICE | 9.95 |
| ARAB INVASION OF EGYPT | 14.95 |
| ANACALYPSIS (SET) | 40.00 |
| ANACALYPSIS VOL. 1 | 25.00 |
| ANACALYPSIS VOL. 11 | 20.00 |
| HARLEM VOICES | 11.95 |
| HARLEM USA | 11.95 |
| LOST BOOKS OF THE BIBLE | 9.95 |
| OLUDUMARE: GOD IN YORUBA BELIEF | 12.95 |
| RAPE OF PARADISE | 14.95 |
| GLOBAL AFRICAN PRESENCE | 14.95 |
| SECRET SOCIETIES | 9.95 |
| FREEMASONRY:CHARACTER, CLAIMS & PRACTICAL WORKINGS OF | 9.95 |
| FREEMASONRY & THE VATICAN | 9.95 |
| FREEMASONRY INTERPRETED | 12.95 |
| FREEMASONRY EXPOSITION | 9.95 |
| FREEMASONRY & JUDAISM | 9.95 |
| HISTORY OF THEPEOPLE OF TRINIDAD & TOBAGO | 14.95 |
| THE NEGRO IN THE CARIBBEAN | 9.95 |
| EDUCATION IN THE BRITISH WEST INDIES | 9.95 |
| BRITISH HISTORIANS & THE WEST INDIES | 9.95 |
| DOCUMENTS OF WEST INDIAN HISTORY | 12.95 |
| BOOK OF THE BEGINNINGS VOL. I | 20.00 |
| BOOK OF THE BEGINNINGS VOL. II | 25.00 |
| BOOK OF THE BEGINNINGS VOL. II (SET) | 40.00 |

## *SEND FOR OUR COMPLETE CATALOG NOW*

Mail Order Form to **A&B BOOKS·149 LAWRENCE STREET· NEW YORK 11201**
TEL: (718) 596-3389 · FAX  (718) 596 -0968
Name:_____
Address_____
City_____ST_____Zip_____
Card Type_____
Card Number_____Exp_____/_____

*We accept VISA  MASTERCARD  AMERICAN EXPRESS & DISCOVER*